W9-AOM-644

BARRON'S

PTCE®

Pharmacy Technician Certification Exam

SECOND EDITION

Sacha Koborsi-Tadros, PharmD

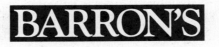
BARRON'S

PTCE® is a registered trademark of the Pharmacy Technician Certification Board, which neither sponsors nor endorses this product.

ABOUT THE AUTHOR

Sacha Koborsi-Tadros received her Doctor of Pharmacy degree from The Chicago College of Pharmacy at Midwestern University in Downers Grove, Illinois. She is an educator as well as a pharmacy consultant and professional speaker. She is an instructor in both the Allied Health department and the Social and Human Services department at Columbus State Community College in Columbus, OH. As an educator, Dr. Koborsi-Tadros has instructed dental hygiene students in pharmacology and has participated in professional board review courses. She also instructs pharmacology courses, specializing in substance abuse prevention and treatment. Most recently, she has helped develop and instruct pharmacy technician courses to prepare students for certification. As a consultant, Dr. Koborsi-Tadros has a vital role in promoting pharmacy technicians by serving as a consultant to other colleges in the area. As a professional speaker, she has presented on various topics including herbals, substances of abuse, and pharmacy technician training. She has also received recognition by the PTCB to serve as an advocate educator.

ACKNOWLEDGMENTS

For Nelson, Philip, Michael, Ava, and Matthew.

Note

While the content of this text was written based on all of the most current information available regarding the pharmacy technician profession and the PTCE exam, readers are still advised to consult with their employers and the Pharmacy Technician Certification Board website (*http://ptcb.org/*) for the latest pharmacy technician standards and guidelines that are applicable to their state.

The presence of knowledge domains in this publication has been determined subjectively by the author. While the author has made every attempt to categorize information by a singular knowledge domain, there may be times when the concepts relate to multiple domains.

This publication is designed to provide accurate information in regard to the subject matter covered as of its publication date, with the understanding that knowledge and best practice constantly evolve. The publisher is not engaged in rendering medical, legal, accounting, or other professional service. If medical or legal advice or other expert assistance is required, the services of a competent professional should be sought. This publication is not intended for use in clinical practice or the delivery of medical care. To the fullest extent of the law, neither the Publisher nor the Editors assume any liability for any injury and/or damage to persons or property arising out of or related to any use of the material contained in this book.

For the purposes of this publication, all trademark symbols have been deleted.

© Copyright 2019, 2016 by Kaplan, Inc., d/b/a Barron's Educational Series

All rights reserved.

No part of this publication may be reproduced or distributed in any form or by any means without the written permission of the copyright owner.

Published by Kaplan, Inc., d/b/a Barron's Educational Series
750 Third Avenue
New York, NY 10017
www.barronseduc.com

ISBN: 978-1-4380-1181-3

10 9 8 7 6 5 4 3 2 1

Kaplan, Inc., d/b/a Barron's Educational Series print books are available at special quantity discounts to use for sales promotions, employee premiums, or educational purposes. For more information or to purchase books, please call the Simon & Schuster special sales department at 866-506-1949.

Contents

APPENDIXES

Introduction

Pharmacy technicians play a major role in pharmacy practice. Ensuring patient safety and enhancing patient care are only a few of the many valuable contributions made by pharmacy technicians. Pharmacists rely on technicians to help provide patients with the best care possible. Pharmacy technicians who possess a comprehensive understanding of pharmacy practice are well sought after and are a valuable asset in pharmacy practice.

Certification is the process of granting recognition to an individual who has met predetermined qualifications. The CPhT designation is given to an individual with the knowledge, skills, and abilities necessary to function as a pharmacy technician. An individual proves that he/she has the necessary skills by passing either one of two national examinations: the Pharmacy Technician Certification Exam (PTCE®) or the Exam for the Certification of Pharmacy Technicians (ExCPT). The PTCE is provided by the Pharmacy Technician Certification Board; the ExCPT is offered by the National Healthcareer Association. This study guide will provide you with a comprehensive review of all the concepts tested on the Pharmacy Technician Certification Exam.

The Pharmacy Technician Certification Board, also known as the PTCB®, is a nongovernmental agency that administers the PTCE. In 2016, the Pharmacy Technician Certification Board conducted a job analysis survey to look at the current roles of pharmacy technicians. These results showed a strong need for an update to the exam blueprint. The updated PTCE will go into effect on January 1, 2020. The updated PTCE exam blueprint will assess knowledge comprehension in 4 knowledge domains, covering 26 knowledge areas; this is a significant change from the previous 9 knowledge domains covered in the past. No changes have been made to the format or length of the test. The PTCE is a 90-question, multiple-choice examination. Within a 2-hour time frame, 1 hour and 50 minutes are spent taking the test. The remaining 10 minutes are used for a tutorial and for a post-exam survey. This review book has been structured to review the content based on these domains. Each chapter focuses on one domain area and contains 10 practice questions and answers.

Included with this book is a full-length pretest, two full-length practice tests, and one full-length online exam. The pretest is designed to assess your strengths and weaknesses before beginning your review. The practice tests appear at the end of the book and test what you've learned. The full-length online exam completes your PTCE preparation. These examinations provide an in-depth review of all knowledge domains and are structured to mimic the certification examination. The practice tests assess your knowledge based on all domain areas, and the percentage of each content area is based on the actual PTCE exam structure. For every

---

PTCE® and PTCB® are registered trademarks of the Pharmacy Technician Certification Board.

question, a detailed answer explanation is included that outlines why one choice is correct and why the alternate choices are incorrect.

Use this book to supplement your current pharmacy-related knowledge as you prepare for your certification exam. Determine what you know. Make a list of topics that you need to review further as you continue to prepare for your test. Take the practice tests to simulate the conditions you will encounter on test day and to practice what you've learned. Congratulations on your journey to embark on a career in pharmacy. Best of luck on your examination!

> ## NOTE
>
> Go to *http://bit.ly/Barrons-PTCE* to access the full-length online PTCE exam. This practice test can be accessed on most mobile devices, including tablets and smartphones.
>
> *Be sure to have your copy of *PTCE: Pharmacy Technician Certification Exam, Second Edition* on hand to complete the registration process.

Overview of the Pharmacy Technician Certification Exam

2

PHARMACY TECHNICIAN CERTIFICATION BOARD

The Pharmacy Technician Certification Board (PTCB) is responsible for ensuring that pharmacy technicians meet predetermined standards that convey competency in the field of pharmacy. These standards include having knowledge and skills pertaining to pharmacy practice. In order to become a certified pharmacy technician, interested candidates need to apply for certification through the PTCB website, *http://ptcb.org/*. In order to qualify for certification, candidates must meet the following criteria:

- Have a high school diploma or an equivalent educational diploma (i.e., a GED or a foreign diploma)
- Provide full disclosure of all criminal actions and all State Board of Pharmacy registration or licensure actions
- Be in compliance with all applicable PTCB certification policies
- Receive a passing score on the Pharmacy Technician Certification Exam (PTCE)

The pharmacy technician must also attest to one of the following:

1. Completion of a PTCB-recognized pharmacy technician education/training program

OR

2. Equivalent work experience as a pharmacy technician (for a minimum of 500 hours)

NOTE

Candidates should also check with their State Board of Pharmacy for additional certification requirements.

Education Verification

PTCE applicants who are within 60 days of acquiring their high school diploma or equivalent educational diploma are eligible to apply for the PTCE. However, PTCB certified pharmacy technician (CPhT) certification will not be granted until proof of high school, or equivalent education, completion is provided to the PTCB. Acceptable documentation includes a copy of your high school diploma, a copy of your high school transcript with your graduation date, an official letter from a school official indicating your school and graduation date, your GED diploma, and/or your foreign diploma.

PHARMACY TECHNICIAN CERTIFICATION EXAM

The Pharmacy Technician Certification Exam (PTCE) is a computer-based, 90-question, multiple-choice examination given over a 2-hour time frame. Of that time, 1 hour and 50 minutes are allotted for the actual test. The remaining 10 minutes are for a tutorial and a post-exam survey. Eighty out of 90 questions are scored questions, and 10 questions are unscored. Test takers will not be able to differentiate between the scored and unscored questions because the unscored questions are randomly distributed throughout the exam.

TIP

Since you won't know which questions are scored and which are unscored, do your best on every question!

Scoring

For the PTCE exam, a passing score is determined by subject matter experts (SME) using a modified-Angoff method. For this method, a panel of field experts examine each test question and then predict the percentage of qualified pharmacy technicians who would be able to answer each question correctly. The estimates are averaged to produce a passing score, which is then reported, along with the candidate's results (a visual of each knowledge domain and how well the candidate did within each domain), as a scaled score. Candidates receive scores that range from 1,000 to 1,600. A passing score is 1,400.

Test Content

As per the Pharmacy Technician Certification Board, test questions are determined based on four knowledge domains. Table 2-1 lists these domains. Additional information, including subcategories, can be found in the "Knowledge Domain" boxes at the beginning of each review chapter.

Table 2-1. PTCE Knowledge Domains and Test Content

Knowledge Domain	Percentage of PTCE Content
1.0—Medications	40.00%
2.0—Federal Requirements	12.50%
3.0—Patient Safety and Quality Assurance	26.25%
4.0—Order Entry and Processing	21.25%

Scheduling Your Exam

Applications for certification are accepted continually, year-round by the PTCB. Candidates apply online through the PTCB website. First-time candidates must register for a new account, while returning candidates can log into their PTCB account to submit a new application.

The PTCE is administered at Pearson VUE testing centers. Pearson VUE testing centers are available nationwide. They offer computer-based testing (CBT) for a multitude of professions, including certification for pharmacy technicians.

Potential CPhT candidates can sign up for a testing slot by following these directions:

1. Go to *http://ptcb.org/*.
2. Click on "Apply for Certification," and then click on "Apply Online."
3. Create an account or log in to an existing account.
4. Pay the $129 fee.
5. Receive authorization to schedule and take the PTCE. Candidates are sent an authorization to schedule the PTCE via e-mail from the PTCB. The authorization period for test candidates is 90 days.
6. Go to *http://pearsonvue.com/ptcb/* or call 866-902-0593 to schedule an appointment.
7. Choose a date, time, and location that works for you to take your exam.

Applicants with a disability or a medical condition that requires an adjustment to standard testing conditions may apply for special accommodations. A "Special Testing Accommodations Form" is available for download on the PTCB website, and it must be submitted within 30 days of submitting your certification application.

Test-Taking Skills and Strategies Plus Steps for Recertification

3

BEFORE THE TEST

Using this book is an excellent way to review core concepts. However, the PTCB offers other options to help you prepare for the examination.

1. One option is to visit *http://ptcb.org/* and take a practice test provided by the PTCB:

   - PTCB official practice tests are aligned with recent changes to the testing blueprint. The format is similar in functionality and mirrors the look of the official examination. The practice test allows candidates to become familiar with the test and the testing environment. Once purchased, the test must be completed within 90 days.
   - The PTCB offers two versions of the practice test, and each contain unique questions that are aligned to current standards. Both also mimic the official PTCE formatting and specifications. A fee of $29 is required to take one exam, or there is an option to take both versions for $49.
   - A count of correct items will be provided once the exam is submitted. A 24-hour post-exam review period is also available to candidates within the 90-day window. There is an option to review all questions and solutions or just specific solutions.

   TIP
   The practice test may be stopped at any time by closing your browser. This will stop the clock. You may resume the test at any time during the 90-day window.

2. Another option allows candidates to become familiar with the testing atmosphere via a testing tutorial:

   - Visit *http://www.pearsonvue.com/athena/athena.asp* to download a simulated practice exam and participate in a testing tutorial.
   - The computerized testing tutorial allows users to navigate through the testing process. Users will have access to a sample, nonspecific, content-based exam where they can get a feel for the test-taking process.
   - The tutorial explains how to answer questions, change answers, and review questions.

3. A third option is to download the official "PTCB Calculations Questions app," which is available on both iOS and Android devices, as well as online on your computer.

   - The app contains 126 questions and detailed explanations to help you test your understanding of the calculations you will encounter in pharmacy practice. The questions in the app were selected from previous live PTCE tests and are no longer used on the actual PTCE. Each question is assigned a category based on the question's level of difficulty, and each question is labeled as easy, medium, or hard, based on the actual performance of past test-takers.
   - A fee of $14.99 will give users unlimited access to the questions with the ability to personalize their practice and track their progress.

TIP

After reviewing the exam material and scheduling your test date, be sure to get adequate sleep the night before the examination!

Remember these general rules:

- Review the PTCB blueprint to provide yourself with a basis about what you are expected to know.
- Review concepts that you need to understand better.
- Make a study timeline over several weeks or months. Stick to it!
- Test your knowledge by practicing how to answer test questions.
- Be confident in your abilities!

EXAM DAY

Candidates should arrive 30 minutes prior to the scheduled exam time in order to check in. Pearson VUE testing centers require you to bring positive proof of identification that matches your name as it appears in your PTCB account. Identification must be valid, unexpired, and government-issued. Examples of proper identification can be found on the PTCB website and include:

- A passport
- A government-issued driver's license
- A government-issued driving learner's permit
- An official ID issued by a government agency to non-drivers
- A military ID
- A permanent resident card
- A U.S. Department of Homeland Security-issued employment authorization card

The test center may provide lockers for the storage of personal items; be aware that this varies by location. Items brought to the test center are not allowed in the secure testing area. Examples of personal items include purses, wallets, and cell phones. You may not study in, or bring visitors into, the test center.

TIP

The following comfort items are provided by the testing center and may be requested by the candidate: ear plugs, noise-canceling headphones, and tissues.

After the testing assistant has checked you in and verified your authorization to take the exam, you will be escorted to the testing area. You will be given materials to take notes on or make calculations on as needed and as allowed by the PTCB. A calculator is available to candidates on the computer screen, but a physical calculator may also be requested. You must return all materials to the testing assistant upon completion of your exam. You will then be logged in to the testing computer to begin your exam. Candidates are monitored during the examination and may be recorded.

The PTCE examination has a maximum time allotment of 110 minutes (1 hour and 50 minutes). If you choose to take a break, you must alert the testing assistant by raising your hand. The time will not stop during the unscheduled break, so be aware that time will continue to run down if you do require a break.

AFTER THE EXAM

After completing the exam, you will receive an unofficial score on your computer screen. The test center will also provide you with an unofficial printed copy of the test results. You will have access to your official score report online approximately 1 to 3 weeks after your exam. Scores are not given via e-mail, phone, or U.S. mail.

Active PTCB-certified pharmacy technicians may request a certificate and a wallet-sized card (printed on fine paper) for a cost of $15 with a turnaround time of 3–4 weeks. Test-takers will also have access to an official downloadable certificate by logging in to their account. After successfully passing the PTCE, candidates are eligible to use the certified pharmacy technician (CPhT) designation immediately following their name.

You may also request for a test to be hand scored by downloading a "Hand Score Request Form" and submitting a $50 fee to the PTCB. These requests must be completed within 30 days of taking the exam. Results are provided in approximately 4 to 6 weeks.

Candidates are allowed 4 attempts to take the PTCE. They must wait 60 days before applying for the second and third attempts and 6 months before applying for the fourth attempt.

RECERTIFICATION

The CPhT credential will remain active for a period of two years. In order to maintain certification, every CPhT certificant must complete a minimum of 20 hours of continuing education (CE), sometimes referred to as continuing pharmacy education (CPE), during each 2-year recertification cycle. Continuing education is an educational activity that is designed to or intended to support the continuing education development of pharmacy technicians in order to maintain or enhance competency. The recertification cycle begins on the day that the certification or recertification is awarded to the certificant. The CE hours do not carry over to the next recertification cycle.

CPhT certificants must meet the following requirements to maintain their certification:

- They must complete a minimum of 20 hours of pharmacy technician CE during a 2-year recertification period.
- They must create an e-profile ID through the National Association of Boards of Pharmacy (NABP) via *https://nabp.pharmacy/* and include their PTCE certification number. The CPE Monitor is used to track CPE credits through a centralized system. Eventually, any CE that you enter into the CPE Monitor will automatically be recorded in your PTCB account.

Of the 20 CE hours that recertification candidates must complete, one hour must be on pharmacy law (pharmacy technician-specific subject matter) and one hour must be on patient safety (pharmacy technician-specific subject matter). A maximum of 10 hours may be earned by completing a relevant college course with a grade of "C" or better.

Examples of continuing education providers include:

- Accreditation Council for Pharmacy Education (*https://www.acpe-accredit.org/*)
- American Association of Pharmacy Technicians™ (*www.pharmacytechnician.com/*)
- American Pharmacists Association® (*www.pharmacist.com/*)
- American Society of Health-System Pharmacists (*www.ashp.org/*)
- Drug Store News (*www.drugstorenews.com/*)

- Drug Topics® (*http://drugtopics.modernmedicine.com/*)
- FreeCE (*www.freece.com/*)
- National Community Pharmacists Association (*https://www.ncpalearn.org/*)
- National Pharmacy Technician Association (*http://www.pharmacytechnician.org/*)
- PharmacyTechCE (*http://www.pharmacytechce.org/*)
- Pharmacy Technician's Letter™ (*http://pharmacytech.therapeuticresearch.com/*)
- Pharmacy Times® (*http://www.pharmacytimes.com/*)
- Power-Pak C.E.® (*http://www.powerpak.com/*)
- RxSchool® (*http://www.rxschool.com/*)
- U.S. Pharmacist® (*http://www.uspharmacist.com/*)
- State pharmacy associations

Recertification may be completed through your PTCB account via an online application and payment of a $40 recertification fee. Applications for recertification can be made 60 days prior to the certification expiration date but must be submitted at least 30 days prior to the certification expiration date.

REINSTATEMENT

In the event that a PTCB certificant fails to recertify by his or her certification expiration date, he or she will no longer be considered PTCB certified. In that case, the pharmacy technician may apply for reinstatement of his or her certification within one year of the original expiration date. A reinstatement fee of $80 will also be charged. Of the 20 CE hours that reinstatement candidates must complete, two hours must be on pharmacy law (pharmacy technician-specific subject matter) and one hour must be on patient safety (pharmacy technician-specific subject matter).

ANSWER SHEET
Pretest

1. Ⓐ Ⓑ Ⓒ Ⓓ	31. Ⓐ Ⓑ Ⓒ Ⓓ	61. Ⓐ Ⓑ Ⓒ Ⓓ
2. Ⓐ Ⓑ Ⓒ Ⓓ	32. Ⓐ Ⓑ Ⓒ Ⓓ	62. Ⓐ Ⓑ Ⓒ Ⓓ
3. Ⓐ Ⓑ Ⓒ Ⓓ	33. Ⓐ Ⓑ Ⓒ Ⓓ	63. Ⓐ Ⓑ Ⓒ Ⓓ
4. Ⓐ Ⓑ Ⓒ Ⓓ	34. Ⓐ Ⓑ Ⓒ Ⓓ	64. Ⓐ Ⓑ Ⓒ Ⓓ
5. Ⓐ Ⓑ Ⓒ Ⓓ	35. Ⓐ Ⓑ Ⓒ Ⓓ	65. Ⓐ Ⓑ Ⓒ Ⓓ
6. Ⓐ Ⓑ Ⓒ Ⓓ	36. Ⓐ Ⓑ Ⓒ Ⓓ	66. Ⓐ Ⓑ Ⓒ Ⓓ
7. Ⓐ Ⓑ Ⓒ Ⓓ	37. Ⓐ Ⓑ Ⓒ Ⓓ	67. Ⓐ Ⓑ Ⓒ Ⓓ
8. Ⓐ Ⓑ Ⓒ Ⓓ	38. Ⓐ Ⓑ Ⓒ Ⓓ	68. Ⓐ Ⓑ Ⓒ Ⓓ
9. Ⓐ Ⓑ Ⓒ Ⓓ	39. Ⓐ Ⓑ Ⓒ Ⓓ	69. Ⓐ Ⓑ Ⓒ Ⓓ
10. Ⓐ Ⓑ Ⓒ Ⓓ	40. Ⓐ Ⓑ Ⓒ Ⓓ	70. Ⓐ Ⓑ Ⓒ Ⓓ
11. Ⓐ Ⓑ Ⓒ Ⓓ	41. Ⓐ Ⓑ Ⓒ Ⓓ	71. Ⓐ Ⓑ Ⓒ Ⓓ
12. Ⓐ Ⓑ Ⓒ Ⓓ	42. Ⓐ Ⓑ Ⓒ Ⓓ	72. Ⓐ Ⓑ Ⓒ Ⓓ
13. Ⓐ Ⓑ Ⓒ Ⓓ	43. Ⓐ Ⓑ Ⓒ Ⓓ	73. Ⓐ Ⓑ Ⓒ Ⓓ
14. Ⓐ Ⓑ Ⓒ Ⓓ	44. Ⓐ Ⓑ Ⓒ Ⓓ	74. Ⓐ Ⓑ Ⓒ Ⓓ
15. Ⓐ Ⓑ Ⓒ Ⓓ	45. Ⓐ Ⓑ Ⓒ Ⓓ	75. Ⓐ Ⓑ Ⓒ Ⓓ
16. Ⓐ Ⓑ Ⓒ Ⓓ	46. Ⓐ Ⓑ Ⓒ Ⓓ	76. Ⓐ Ⓑ Ⓒ Ⓓ
17. Ⓐ Ⓑ Ⓒ Ⓓ	47. Ⓐ Ⓑ Ⓒ Ⓓ	77. Ⓐ Ⓑ Ⓒ Ⓓ
18. Ⓐ Ⓑ Ⓒ Ⓓ	48. Ⓐ Ⓑ Ⓒ Ⓓ	78. Ⓐ Ⓑ Ⓒ Ⓓ
19. Ⓐ Ⓑ Ⓒ Ⓓ	49. Ⓐ Ⓑ Ⓒ Ⓓ	79. Ⓐ Ⓑ Ⓒ Ⓓ
20. Ⓐ Ⓑ Ⓒ Ⓓ	50. Ⓐ Ⓑ Ⓒ Ⓓ	80. Ⓐ Ⓑ Ⓒ Ⓓ
21. Ⓐ Ⓑ Ⓒ Ⓓ	51. Ⓐ Ⓑ Ⓒ Ⓓ	81. Ⓐ Ⓑ Ⓒ Ⓓ
22. Ⓐ Ⓑ Ⓒ Ⓓ	52. Ⓐ Ⓑ Ⓒ Ⓓ	82. Ⓐ Ⓑ Ⓒ Ⓓ
23. Ⓐ Ⓑ Ⓒ Ⓓ	53. Ⓐ Ⓑ Ⓒ Ⓓ	83. Ⓐ Ⓑ Ⓒ Ⓓ
24. Ⓐ Ⓑ Ⓒ Ⓓ	54. Ⓐ Ⓑ Ⓒ Ⓓ	84. Ⓐ Ⓑ Ⓒ Ⓓ
25. Ⓐ Ⓑ Ⓒ Ⓓ	55. Ⓐ Ⓑ Ⓒ Ⓓ	85. Ⓐ Ⓑ Ⓒ Ⓓ
26. Ⓐ Ⓑ Ⓒ Ⓓ	56. Ⓐ Ⓑ Ⓒ Ⓓ	86. Ⓐ Ⓑ Ⓒ Ⓓ
27. Ⓐ Ⓑ Ⓒ Ⓓ	57. Ⓐ Ⓑ Ⓒ Ⓓ	87. Ⓐ Ⓑ Ⓒ Ⓓ
28. Ⓐ Ⓑ Ⓒ Ⓓ	58. Ⓐ Ⓑ Ⓒ Ⓓ	88. Ⓐ Ⓑ Ⓒ Ⓓ
29. Ⓐ Ⓑ Ⓒ Ⓓ	59. Ⓐ Ⓑ Ⓒ Ⓓ	89. Ⓐ Ⓑ Ⓒ Ⓓ
30. Ⓐ Ⓑ Ⓒ Ⓓ	60. Ⓐ Ⓑ Ⓒ Ⓓ	90. Ⓐ Ⓑ Ⓒ Ⓓ

Pretest

4

Directions: You will have 1 hour and 50 minutes to complete the following 90 questions. For each question, select the choice that best answers the question, and mark that answer letter on your answer sheet. Remember, this test should be used to help you determine areas that require additional review. Each question represents a particular area of the PTCE blueprint, which can help you pinpoint areas of mastery or concepts that require additional studying. The official PTCE exam uses a scaled score to determine your grade. Only 80 out of 90 questions on the PTCE are scored, and unscored questions are not identified. You should be able to answer about 72 of the questions on this test correctly, averaging an overall percentage of 80% or more on your attempt at this test.

1. For which of the following conditions would a patient receive an inhaler?

   (A) asthma
   (B) diabetes
   (C) hypertension
   (D) gout

2. A patient presents a prescription for Lasix 40 mg, which has been authorized for generic substitution. Which of the following medications may be substituted for Lasix 40 mg?

   (A) metoprolol
   (B) furosemide
   (C) alprazolam
   (D) diltiazem

3. Which of the following medications is available in a unit-of-use container?

   (A) metronidazole
   (B) azithromycin
   (C) oxycodone
   (D) gemfibrozil

4. What does the first set of numbers represent in the following National Drug Code (NDC) number?

   00456-012-03

   (A) package size
   (B) manufacturer
   (C) product
   (D) medication indication

5. What is a common side effect of diphenhydramine?

   (A) drowsiness
   (B) urticaria
   (C) angioedema
   (D) hyperkalemia

6. The following prescription has been received by your pharmacy:

Prednisone 5 mg #QS
Sig: 20 mg BID × 2D
15 mg BID × 2D
10 mg BID × 2D
5 mg BID × 2D
5 mg QD × 2D

What is the quantity needed to fill this prescription?

(A) 32 tablets
(B) 36 tablets
(C) 42 tablets
(D) 48 tablets

7. Which of the following auxiliary labels should be included on the label for Augmentin oral suspension?

(A) "Shake Well Before Using"
(B) "For The Nose"
(C) "For External Use Only"
(D) "Chew Tablets Before Swallowing"

8. A physician orders drug "x" 500 mg BID × 30D. The pharmacy has drug "x" 250 mg in stock. How many 250 mg tablets of drug "x" are needed to fill this order?

(A) 30 tablets
(B) 60 tablets
(C) 90 tablets
(D) 120 tablets

9. Which of the following medications may NOT have any refills on the same prescription?

(A) Actos
(B) Lasix
(C) Xanax
(D) Oxycontin

10. How many grams of glucose would you need to make 500 mL of a 10% glucose solution?

(A) 20 g
(B) 50 g
(C) 75 g
(D) 100 g

11. A 10 mL bottle of U-100 insulin is dispensed to a patient. A patient's prescription calls for 25 units of U-100 insulin to be injected subcutaneously daily. For how many days should this bottle last?

(A) 28 days
(B) 30 days
(C) 35 days
(D) 40 days

12. In the term "albuterol HFA," what does "HFA" stand for?

(A) high-frequency asthma
(B) hyper fast airway
(C) hydrofluoroalkane
(D) high-functioning autism

13. Acyclovir belongs to what drug classification?

(A) antibiotic
(B) antiviral
(C) antiemetic
(D) antihypertensive

14. What does the prefix "hyper-" mean?

(A) above
(B) below
(C) half
(D) fast

15. The process of dissolving powder drugs with diluents, such as water or normal saline, is known as _____.

(A) reconstitution
(B) levigation
(C) spatulation
(D) geometric dilution

16. Which schedule of controlled substances has the highest abuse potential and also an accepted medical use in the United States?

    (A) Schedule I
    (B) Schedule II
    (C) Schedule III
    (D) Schedule IV

17. A physician orders amiodarone (Cordarone) 300 mg in 100 mL of D5W to be infused over 30 minutes. Determine the IV flow rate in mL/hour.

    (A) 200 mL/hour
    (B) 100 mL/hour
    (C) 75 mL/hour
    (D) 50 mL/hour

18. Which of the following statements about drug classifications is true?

    (A) Paroxetine is an antidepressant.
    (B) Clopidogrel is an antibiotic.
    (C) Digoxin is an antiplatelet.
    (D) Furosemide is an antidiabetic.

19. The iPLEDGE program is designed to mitigate the risks that are associated with taking _____.

    (A) oxycodone
    (B) isotretinoin
    (C) quetiapine
    (D) amantadine

20. How many times can a Class III or a Class IV prescription be transferred by pharmacies that do not share the same online database?

    (A) once
    (B) twice
    (C) three times
    (D) never

21. Which of the following would be used to identify a medication in a recall situation?

    (A) lot number and NDC
    (B) drug name and NDC
    (C) drug strength and lot number
    (D) manufacturer and lot number

22. Which of the following dosage forms contains the highest concentration of alcohol?

    (A) solution
    (B) capsule
    (C) suspension
    (D) elixir

23. Which of the following vaccines is stored in a freezer?

    (A) HPV
    (B) hepatitis B
    (C) influenza
    (D) HZV

24. Biennial inventory is inventory of all controlled substances on hand that should be conducted _____.

    (A) every year
    (B) twice a year
    (C) every two years
    (D) every ten years

25. A prescription is filled with an incorrect strength of a medication due to the prescriber's illegible handwriting. How should this error be classified?

    (A) wrong dosage form error
    (B) prescribing error
    (C) unauthorized drug error
    (D) omission error

26. Which of the following best represents bioavailability?

   (A) the drug dosage form
   (B) the route of administration
   (C) the amount of the drug that enters circulation
   (D) the elimination half-life

27. In the absence of stability information, what is the appropriate beyond-use date for an oral suspension?

   (A) no later than 6 months
   (B) no later than 14 days
   (C) no later than 30 days
   (D) one year

28. What is the therapeutic classification of clopidogrel?

   (A) inhibitor of platelet aggregation
   (B) antidiabetic
   (C) antihyperlipidemic
   (D) antihypertensive

29. A patient requests a refill for Diazepam 10 mg. After reviewing the patient's profile, the pharmacy technician discovers that the prescription has been refilled 5 times. The pharmacy technician should _____.

   (A) refill the prescription
   (B) notify a pharmacist because the prescription cannot be refilled
   (C) ask the patient to provide a valid DEA 222 order form
   (D) refuse to fill the prescription since the strength of the requested medication is commercially unavailable

30. Which regulatory agency may issue a drug recall?

   (A) DEA
   (B) FDA
   (C) CDC
   (D) USP

31. How is pharmaceutical hazardous waste handled?

   (A) Personnel should consult the medication's SDS and handle the waste accordingly.
   (B) Personnel can throw hazardous waste into a regular trash bag.
   (C) Personnel should leave the hazardous waste in the compounding area until someone can pick up the hazardous waste and dispose of it.
   (D) Personnel should place the hazardous waste into a sharps container.

32. What is the brand name for duloxetine?

   (A) Lexapro
   (B) Cymbalta
   (C) Abilify
   (D) Zoloft

33. The Roman numeral CXIV is equal to _____.

   (A) 34
   (B) 54
   (C) 104
   (D) 114

34. PHI is regulated and protected under HIPAA. What does PHI stand for?

   (A) patient health information
   (B) protected health information
   (C) people health information
   (D) personal health information

35. Federal law requires prescriptions to be maintained in the pharmacy for how many years?

   (A) 1 year
   (B) 2 years
   (C) 3 years
   (D) 4 years

36. Which of the following drugs is classified as an antifungal agent?

    (A) itraconazole (Sporanox)
    (B) oseltamivir (Tamiflu)
    (C) clarithromycin (Biaxin)
    (D) doxycycline (Vibramycin)

37. You have on hand 250 mL of concentrated dextrose injection 40%. What is the resulting percentage of dextrose if you mix the dextrose with 150 mL of water for injection?

    (A) 10%
    (B) 20%
    (C) 25%
    (D) 30%

38. Which of the following nasal sprays is available over-the-counter (OTC)?

    (A) Nasonex
    (B) Omnaris
    (C) Nasacort
    (D) Veramyst

39. Which government agency oversees safety in the workplace?

    (A) ASHP
    (B) FDA
    (C) DEA
    (D) OSHA

40. What does "DAW" mean when it is present on a written prescription?

    (A) Refills are limited to 5 times within a 6-month period.
    (B) The medication should be taken with food.
    (C) The brand name medication is to be dispensed as written, with no generic substitution.
    (D) The medication is a controlled substance.

41. Nitroglycerin is available as a sublingual tablet, which means that _____.

    (A) the tablet should be dissolved under the tongue
    (B) the tablet should be swallowed whole, not chewed
    (C) the tablet is a sustained, released (long-acting) form
    (D) the tablet may be crushed and mixed with applesauce for patients with swallowing problems

42. A prescriber who is authorized to write prescriptions for the partial opioid agonist Subutex, which is used for the treatment of opioid addiction, must have a DEA number that starts with which of the following letters?

    (A) B
    (B) L
    (C) M
    (D) X

43. Which of the following medications uses the USAN suffix "-tidine?"

    (A) H_1 receptor antagonist
    (B) H_2 receptor antagonist
    (C) proton-pump inhibitor
    (D) beta-1 antagonist

44. If 200 mL of NS is infused, how many mg of sodium chloride will the patient receive?

    (A) 1,400 mg
    (B) 1,800 mg
    (C) 2,100 mg
    (D) 2,250 mg

45. A prescription calls for 15 mg/kg of vancomycin to be given every 6 hours. How many mg of vancomycin will a patient who weighs 198 pounds receive per day?

    (A) 1,350 mg
    (B) 2,700 mg
    (C) 4,050 mg
    (D) 5,400 mg

46. Which of the following OTC medications must be recorded, either electronically or written in a book, before being sold?

   (A) acetaminophen
   (B) cetirizine
   (C) pseudoephedrine
   (D) clotrimazole

47. How many milliliters of 95% (v/v) alcohol and 30% (v/v) alcohol should be mixed to prepare 1,000 mL of a 50% (v/v) solution?

   (A) 502 mL, 498 mL
   (B) 308 mL, 692 mL
   (C) 246 mL, 754 mL
   (D) 130 mL, 870 mL

48. Which disease state is characterized by polyuria, polydipsia, and polyphagia?

   (A) hypertension
   (B) gout
   (C) diabetes
   (D) arthritis

49. How many 30 mg tablets of codeine sulfate should be used in preparing the following prescription?

   Rx: Codeine sulfate 15 mg/tsp
   Robitussin at 120 mL

   (A) 10 tablets
   (B) 11 tablets
   (C) 12 tablets
   (D) 13 tablets

50. A patient has called in a refill for a selective COX-2 inhibitor. Which of the following drugs should be filled?

   (A) ibuprofen
   (B) naproxen
   (C) celecoxib
   (D) omeprazole

51. Where should a pharmacy store a policy and procedure manual?

   (A) The manual should be in the pharmacy library so it can be checked out.
   (B) The manual should be in the pharmacy manager's office.
   (C) The manual should be in the work area so it is accessible to all personnel.
   (D) A policy and procedure manual is not needed in a pharmacy.

52. Which of the following medications should be counted on a separate designated tray?

   (A) chemotherapeutic agents
   (B) antidepressants
   (C) diuretics
   (D) nonsteroidal anti-inflammatory drugs

53. The type of drug recall in which the drug may cause serious harm to a patient is called a _____ recall.

   (A) Class I
   (B) Class II
   (C) Class III
   (D) Class IV

54. Which of the following look-alike/sound-alike drug pairs contains a medication with a narrow therapeutic index (NTI)?

   (A) cycloSPORINE and cycloSERINE
   (B) medroxyPROGESTERone and methylPREDNISolone
   (C) predniSONE and prednisoLONE
   (D) traZODone and traMADol

55. What is the most important piece of information to verify before filling a patient's prescription?

   (A) the patient's identity
   (B) the patient's insurance
   (C) the patient's address
   (D) the patient's method of payment

56. What word should be used when giving directions for a topical medication?

(A) take
(B) insert
(C) apply
(D) inhale

57. The abbreviation "a.c." means _____.

(A) before meals
(B) after meals
(C) before bedtime
(D) before midnight

58. Which of the following safety strategies is used to distinguish medications that have look-alike/sound-alike names?

(A) short man lettering
(B) tall man lettering
(C) colored lettering
(D) bar codes

59. What volume of a 25 mg/mL solution should be measured to deliver a dose of 40 mg?

(A) 1.25 mL
(B) 1.6 mL
(C) 2.0 mL
(D) 2.4 mL

60. How many ounces of medication are needed to last 10 days if the dose of medication is one and one half teaspoonfuls twice a day?

(A) 2 oz
(B) 3 oz
(C) 4 oz
(D) 5 oz

61. Which of the following statements best represents the correct handling of hazardous drugs?

(A) Hazardous drugs may be prepared in the non-sterile compounding area.
(B) Hazardous drugs should be handled with at least two pairs of gloves.
(C) Hazardous drug spills may be thrown away in a regular waste bin.
(D) Safety data sheets (SDS) are not required for hazardous drug spills in the pharmacy.

62. A patient misinterprets her medication label when taking her lovastatin 20 mg tablet. She takes two tablets, instead of one as prescribed, at bedtime. This is an example of an error that occurs at which step of the medication-use process?

(A) transcription
(B) prescribing
(C) administration
(D) dispensing

63. A root-cause analysis is a method of problem solving that is used to _____.

(A) monitor drug therapy
(B) assess the patient's response
(C) prevent vaccination injuries
(D) prevent future medication errors

64. Which of the following medications does NOT need to be packaged in child-resistant containers?

(A) metoprolol
(B) lovastatin
(C) nitroglycerin sublingual
(D) penicillin

65. Which of the following is an example of a pair of drugs with look-alike/sound-alike names?

(A) buspirone/bupropion
(B) metoprolol/metoclopramide
(C) penicillin/ampicillin
(D) omeprazole/ritonavir

66. A patient tells you that he missed his last dose of glyburide. What should you do?

    (A) Tell the patient to take the next dose ASAP.
    (B) Call the pharmacist over to counsel the patient.
    (C) Call the doctor.
    (D) Tell the patient to skip the dose.

67. Convert 15°C to degrees Fahrenheit.

    (A) 55°F
    (B) 57°F
    (C) 59°F
    (D) 61°F

68. What does the last set of numbers of an NDC number indicate?

    (A) manufacturer
    (B) drug
    (C) strength
    (D) package size

69. Which of the following natural substances is used to treat hot flashes?

    (A) saw palmetto
    (B) resveratrol
    (C) ginger
    (D) black cohosh

70. At what standard time would a patient receive a medication if the military time is 0700 hours?

    (A) 7:00 A.M.
    (B) 7:00 P.M.
    (C) 11:00 A.M.
    (D) 11:00 P.M.

71. How many grams of hydrocortisone are needed to prepare 180 g of 3% hydrocortisone cream?

    (A) 2.6 g
    (B) 3.2 g
    (C) 5.4 g
    (D) 7.1 g

72. Ativan is the brand name for which drug?

    (A) enalapril
    (B) lorazepam
    (C) lisinopril
    (D) meloxicam

73. What is the name of a device that can be used to help actuate breaths while using an inhaler?

    (A) spacer
    (B) nebulizer
    (C) catheter
    (D) safety cap

74. What should pharmacy counting trays and counters be disinfected with?

    (A) water
    (B) 90% isopropyl alcohol
    (C) 70% isopropyl alcohol
    (D) antibacterial soap

75. What is the maximum weighable amount for a Class III prescription balance?

    (A) 12 g
    (B) 80 g
    (C) 100 g
    (D) 120 g

76. Which of the following dosage forms would be appropriate for a patient who is experiencing nausea and vomiting?

    (A) suppository
    (B) tablet
    (C) suspension
    (D) elixir

77. Inderal is to hypertension as Tazorac is to _____.

    (A) GERD
    (B) BPH
    (C) acne
    (D) psoriasis

78. Which of the following pharmacokinetic processes involves the movement of drug molecules from the site of administration into the bloodstream?

(A) absorption
(B) distribution
(C) metabolism
(D) excretion

79. An intravenous medication is administered directly into the _____.

(A) muscle
(B) vein
(C) eye
(D) skin

80. Where is the volume of an aqueous liquid read on a graduated cylinder?

(A) top surface of the liquid
(B) bottom surface of the liquid
(C) bottom of the meniscus
(D) top of the meniscus

81. A prescription is written for "ProAir HFA #1, Sig: 1–2 puffs q 4–6h prn." If there are 200 doses in one inhaler, what is the days supply?

(A) 5 days
(B) 16 days
(C) 30 days
(D) 50 days

82. Which of the following DEA forms should be used to surrender out-of-date controlled medications?

(A) DEA Form 222
(B) DEA Form 106
(C) DEA Form 41
(D) DEA Form 224

83. How much menthol is needed to prepare a prescription that requires 6 oz of menthol 0.5%?

(A) 0.9 g
(B) 9 g
(C) 0.9 mg
(D) 9 mg

84. Which of the following medications should be taken with a glass of water while sitting in an upright position for a minimum of 30 minutes?

(A) alendronate
(B) simvastatin
(C) oxycodone
(D) amoxicillin

85. Which of the following dosage forms bypasses the stomach when ingested?

(A) enteric coated tablet
(B) powder
(C) capsule
(D) suspension

86. Which of the following preparations is a coarse dispersion of insoluble solid particles in a liquid base?

(A) emulsion
(B) suspension
(C) solution
(D) elixir

87. Humulin R contains 100 units/mL. How much is needed for a 12-unit dose?

(A) 12 mL
(B) 1.2 mL
(C) 0.12 mL
(D) 1 mL

88. Calculate how many tablets are needed to fill the following prescription.

paroxetine 10 mg, 2 tabs qam, dispense 90 days supply

(A) 90 tablets
(B) 120 tablets
(C) 160 tablets
(D) 180 tablets

89. Why are medications rotated on pharmacy shelves?

(A) to move medications that will expire first in front of medications that have a longer shelf life
(B) to prevent dust from accumulating on stock bottles
(C) to consolidate medications for more shelf space
(D) to move newer bottles to the front of the shelf

90. Which of the following is a high-alert medication, as reported by the ISMP?

(A) amoxicillin
(B) warfarin
(C) naproxen
(D) lovastatin

1.	**A**	31.	**A**	61.	**B**
2.	**B**	32.	**B**	62.	**C**
3.	**B**	33.	**D**	63.	**D**
4.	**B**	34.	**B**	64.	**C**
5.	**A**	35.	**B**	65.	**A**
6.	**C**	36.	**A**	66.	**B**
7.	**A**	37.	**C**	67.	**C**
8.	**D**	38.	**C**	68.	**D**
9.	**D**	39.	**D**	69.	**D**
10.	**B**	40.	**C**	70.	**A**
11.	**D**	41.	**A**	71.	**C**
12.	**C**	42.	**D**	72.	**B**
13.	**B**	43.	**B**	73.	**A**
14.	**A**	44.	**B**	74.	**C**
15.	**A**	45.	**D**	75.	**D**
16.	**B**	46.	**C**	76.	**A**
17.	**A**	47.	**B**	77.	**C**
18.	**A**	48.	**C**	78.	**A**
19.	**B**	49.	**C**	79.	**B**
20.	**A**	50.	**C**	80.	**C**
21.	**A**	51.	**C**	81.	**B**
22.	**D**	52.	**A**	82.	**C**
23.	**D**	53.	**A**	83.	**A**
24.	**C**	54.	**A**	84.	**A**
25.	**B**	55.	**A**	85.	**A**
26.	**C**	56.	**C**	86.	**B**
27.	**B**	57.	**A**	87.	**C**
28.	**A**	58.	**B**	88.	**D**
29.	**B**	59.	**B**	89.	**A**
30.	**B**	60.	**D**	90.	**B**

ANSWERS EXPLAINED

1. **(A)** Patients who have asthma experience trouble breathing and require the use of an inhaler to open their airways, allowing for the passage of oxygen to their lungs more freely. Patients with type 1 or type 2 diabetes have high blood glucose levels and require the use of insulin and/or an oral hypoglycemic to correct one of the following: insulin resistance, insulin deficiency, or increased hepatic glucose output. Hypertensive patients experience high blood pressure. Treatment includes aerobic exercise, salt intake reduction, lifestyle changes, weight reduction, and antihypertensives. Gout is a condition that results when the body lacks the ability to process uric acid, resulting in increased levels of uric acid in the body. (*Knowledge Domain 1.6*)

2. **(B)** Furosemide is the generic equivalent for Lasix. Metoprolol is the generic equivalent for Toprol XL. Alprazolam is the generic equivalent for Xanax. Diltiazem is the generic equivalent for Cardizem. (*Knowledge Domain 1.1*)

3. **(B)** Azithromycin is available in a unit-of-use box that contains six tablets of azithromycin intended to last five days. Metronidazole, oxycodone, and gemfibrozil are not available in unit-of-use packages. (*Knowledge Domain 4.3*)

4. **(B)** The manufacturer, or labeler, is indicated by the first set of numbers in the NDC. The package size is indicated by the last set of numbers in the NDC. The product is indicated by the second, or middle, set of numbers in the NDC. The medication indication is not represented by the NDC. (*Knowledge Domain 4.4*)

5. **(A)** Diphenhydramine is the generic name for Benadryl, an H_1 antagonist that is used for the treatment of allergies and is used as a sleep aid. A common side effect is drowsiness. (*Knowledge Domain 1.5*)

6. **(C)** 20 mg BID $\times$ 2D = (4 tablets $\times$ 2) $\times$ 2 = 16 tablets
    15 mg BID $\times$ 2D = (3 tablets $\times$ 2) $\times$ 2 = 12 tablets
    10 mg BID $\times$ 2D = (2 tablets $\times$ 2) $\times$ 2 = 8 tablets
    5 mg BID $\times$ 2D = (1 tablet $\times$ 2) $\times$ 2 = 4 tablets
    5 mg QD $\times$ 2D = (1 tablet $\times$ 1) $\times$ 2 = 2 tablets
    16 + 12 + 8 + 4 + 2 = 42 tablets (*Knowledge Domain 4.2*)

7. **(A)** The label "Shake Well Before Using" is commonly placed on suspensions because they contain undissolved particles in a liquid solvent. "For The Nose" and "For External Use Only" are not appropriate auxiliary labels for an oral medication. "Chew Tablets Before Swallowing" is not an appropriate auxiliary label for an oral suspension. (*Knowledge Domain 1.4*)

8. **(D)** The prescription is written for 500 mg BID $\times$ 30D. The pharmacy has 250 mg BID $\times$ 30D. You will need 2 of the 250 mg tablets to equal 1 of the 500 mg tablets; (2 $\times$ 2) $\times$ 30 = 120 tablets. (*Knowledge Domain 4.2*)

9. **(D)** Oxycontin is a Class II substance. No refills are allowed for this substance (as per federal law). Actos and Lasix are both non-controlled substances. These medications do not have limitations on the amount of refills unless expressly written on the prescription. Xanax is a Class IV substance. Per federal law, up to 5 refills in 6 months are allowed for this substance. (*Knowledge Domain 2.2*)

10. **(B)** Set up a proportion:

$$\frac{10\text{ g}}{100\text{ mL}} = \frac{x}{500\text{ mL}}$$

$$x = 50\text{ g } (\textit{Knowledge Domain 4.2})$$

11. **(D)** U-100 insulin means that there are 100 units of insulin in 1 mL.

STEP 1 To determine the number of units in the vial, set up a proportion and solve for x:

$$\frac{100\text{ units}}{1\text{ mL}} = \frac{x\text{ units}}{10\text{ mL}}$$

$$x = 1{,}000\text{ units}$$

STEP 2 Determine the number of days that the vial will last:

$$\frac{1\text{ day}}{25\text{ units}} = \frac{x\text{ days}}{1{,}000\text{ units}}$$

$$x = 40\text{ days}$$

The answer is 40 days. (*Knowledge Domain 4.2*)

12. **(C)** "HFA" stands for hydrofluoroalkane, a propellant that is used in MDIs to move the medication out of the inhaler. HFAs replaced older chlorofluorocarbons (CFCs) that were phased out in 2008. (*Knowledge Domain 1.4*)

13. **(B)** Acyclovir is classified as an antiviral. (*Knowledge Domain 1.6*)

14. **(A)** The prefix "hyper-" means "over," "above," or "beyond" and is used to imply an excess or exaggeration. The prefix "hypo-" means "below," as in the word hypotension. The prefix "semi-" means "half," as in the word semicircle. The prefix "tachy-" means "fast," as in the word tachycardia. (*Knowledge Domain 4.2*)

15. **(A)** Reconstitution is the process of mixing a powder with diluents prior to administration. Levigation is the process of grinding a powder by incorporating a liquid. Spatulation is the process of using a spatula to mix ingredients in a plastic bag, on ointment paper, or on another medium. Geometric dilution is the process used when mixing two or more ingredients of different quantities to achieve a homogeneous mixture. (*Knowledge Domain 4.1*)

16. **(B)** Schedule II medications have a high potential for abuse and an accepted medical use in the United States. Schedule I medications have a high potential for abuse but do not have a currently accepted medical use in the United States. Schedule III medications have a potential for abuse that is less than that of Schedule I and Schedule II medications. Schedule IV medications contain a potential for abuse that is less than that of Schedule III medications. (*Knowledge Domain 2.2*)

17. **(A)** The IV flow rate is determined using the following formula:

$$\frac{\text{volume (mL)}}{\text{time (min)}} \times \frac{60\text{ min}}{1\text{ hour}} = \text{IV flow rate}\left(\frac{\text{mL}}{\text{hr}}\right)$$

$$\frac{100\text{ mL}}{30\text{ min}} \times \frac{60\text{ min}}{1\text{ hour}} = \text{IV flow rate}\left(\frac{\text{mL}}{\text{hr}}\right)$$

$$\frac{200\text{ mL}}{1\text{ hr}} = \text{IV flow rate } (\textit{Knowledge Domain 4.2})$$

18. **(A)** Paroxetine is used to treat depression and anxiety. Clopidogrel is an antiplatelet drug that is used in the treatment of a myocardial infarction, an acute coronary syndrome, and peripheral vascular disease. Digoxin is a calcium channel blocker (CCB) that is used to treat heart arrhythmias. Furosemide is a thiazide diuretic that is used to treat hypertension. (*Knowledge Domain 1.1*)

19. **(B)** The iPLEDGE program is a computer-based, risk management, distribution program for medications that contain isotretinoin. Oxycodone, quetiapine, and amantadine do not contain isotretinoin and are not monitored by this program. (*Knowledge Domain 2.4*)

20. **(A)** Controlled substances may be transferred only once if different online databases are used. (*Knowledge Domain 2.2*)

21. **(A)** The medication lot number and the NDC are used to identify a medication. The lot number is a production number that is used to track a product. (*Knowledge Domain 2.5*)

22. **(D)** Elixirs are hydroalcoholic liquids with an alcohol content range of 5–40% (10–80 proof). Solutions, capsules, and suspensions do not contain alcohol. (*Knowledge Domain 1.4*)

23. **(D)** The CDC recommends that the Herpes Zoster Vaccine (HZV) be stored in a freezer. The VAR (Varicella) vaccine, the MMR (measles, mumps, and rubella) vaccine, and the MMRV (measles, mumps, rubella, and varicella) vaccine are also stored in a freezer. The HPV (human papilloma virus) vaccine, the hepatitis B vaccine, and the influenza vaccine should be stored in a refrigerator. (*Knowledge Domain 1.7*)

24. **(C)** "Biennial" is a term that means "every two years." "Biannual," on the other hand, refers to an event that occurs "twice a year." "Yearly" may be used to describe an event that occurs "every year," and "decade" is used to describe "ten years." (*Knowledge Domain 4.2*)

25. **(B)** Prescribing errors occur when a prescriber orders a medication for a patient and uses either illegible handwriting and/or inadequate or incorrect instructions for medication use. Wrong dosage form errors occur when an incorrect dosage form is selected and may be due to deficiencies in product safety design or deficiencies in health care system safety processes. An unauthorized drug error can occur when a medication is administered but has not been authorized by the prescriber. An omission error occurs when there is a failure to administer the prescribed dose. (*Knowledge Domain 3.5*)

26. **(C)** Bioavailability is the amount of the drug that reaches circulation. Parenteral formulations are more bioavailable than oral formulations. (*Knowledge Domain 1.4*)

27. **(B)** Suspensions, oral solutions that contain water, have a beyond-use date of no later than 14 days from the reconstitution date. (*Knowledge Domain 4.4*)

28. **(A)** Plavix (clopidogrel) inhibits the aggregation of platelets, which is thought to be the primary mechanism of blood clotting. (*Knowledge Domain 1.1*)

29. **(B)** Prescriptions of Schedule III, IV, and V drugs cannot be refilled more than 5 times. A patient must bring in a new prescription after the last refill is executed. Prescriptions older than 6 months require a new prescription in order to be filled. (*Knowledge Domain 2.2*)

30. **(B)** The FDA may issue a drug recall. (*Knowledge Domain 2.5*)

31. **(A)** The Occupational Safety and Health Administration (OSHA) requires that Safety Data Sheets (SDS) be maintained for all hazardous chemicals. Proper handling procedures may be found in each chemical's SDS. (*Knowledge Domain 2.1*)

32. **(B)** The brand name for duloxetine is Cymbalta. Lexapro is the brand name for escitalopram. Abilify is the brand name for aripiprazole. Zoloft is the brand name for sertraline. (*Knowledge Domain 1.1*)

33. **(D)** CXIV = 100 + 10 + 4 = 114 (*Knowledge Domain 4.2*)

34. **(B)** The acronym PHI stands for protected health information. (*Knowledge Domain 3.3*)

35. **(B)** Federal law mandates that prescriptions be maintained in the pharmacy for a period of 2 years. (*Knowledge Domain 2.3*)

36. **(A)** Itraconazole (Sporanox) is classified as an antifungal agent. Oseltamivir (Tamiflu) is classified as an antiviral agent. Clarithromycin (Biaxin) is classified as a macrolide antibiotic. Doxycycline (Vibramycin) is classified as a tetracycline antibiotic. (*Knowledge Domain 1.1*)

37. **(C)**

STEP 1 The final percentage strength can be found by using the following formula:

$$C1 \times V1 = C2 \times V2$$

C1 is the initial concentration, V1 is the initial volume, C2 is the final concentration, and V2 is the final volume.

STEP 2 To determine the final volume, add the initial volume (V1) to the added volume. Therefore, the final volume, V2, is:

$$250 \text{ mL} + 150 \text{ mL} = 400 \text{ mL}$$

STEP 3 Solve for the final concentration:

$$C1 \times V1 = C2 \times V2$$

$$(40) \times (250 \text{ mL}) = (x) \times (400 \text{ mL})$$

$$x = 25\%$$

The answer is 25%. (*Knowledge Domain 4.2*)

38. **(C)** Nasacort (triamcinolone) is an intranasal corticosteroid that is available over-the-counter. Nasonex (mometasone furoate), Omnaris (ciclesonide), and Veramyst (fluticasone furoate) are all synthetic intranasal corticosteroids that are available by prescription only. (*Knowledge Domain 1.1*)

39. **(D)** The OSHA oversees safety in the workplace. The ASHP is an organization that oversees the accreditation of pharmacy technician training programs. The FDA oversees the marketing and approval of drugs. The DEA implemented the Controlled Substances Act. (*Knowledge Domain 2.1*)

40. **(C)** "DAW" is an acronym for "dispense as written." It indicates that the brand name drug should be dispensed. (*Knowledge Domain 4.2*)

41. **(A)** The word sublingual means "under the tongue." Therefore, nitroglycerin should be placed under the tongue. (*Knowledge Domain 4.2*)

42. **(D)** A prescriber who is designated by the DEA to write prescriptions for Subutex will have a DEA number that begins with the letter "X." The letter "B" is used to designate a hospital or an institution. The letter "L" is used to designate a reverse distributor. The letter "M" is used to designate a mid-level practitioner. (*Knowledge Domain 2.2*)

43. **(B)** The USAN suffix "-tidine" is associated with H2 receptor antagonists that are indicated in the treatment of excessive acid reflux. Medications such as nizatidine (Axid) or famotidine are commonly prescribed H2 receptor antagonists. H1 receptor antagonists do not have a common USAN suffix. Proton-pump inhibitors (PPIs) end in "-eprazole." Beta-1 antagonists end in "-lol." (*Knowledge Domain 1.1*)

44. **(B)**

   STEP 1 Set up a proportion:

   $$\frac{0.9 \text{ g}}{100 \text{ mL}} = \frac{x \text{ g}}{200 \text{ mL}}$$

   $$x = 1.8 \text{ g}$$

   STEP 2 Convert g to mg:

   $$\frac{1 \text{ g}}{1{,}000 \text{ mg}} = \frac{1.8 \text{ g}}{x \text{ mg}}$$

   $$x = 1{,}800 \text{ g}$$

   The answer is 1,800 mg. (*Knowledge Domain 4.2*)

45. **(D)**

   STEP 1 First convert pounds to kilograms:

   $$\frac{2.2 \text{ lbs}}{1 \text{ kg}} = \frac{198 \text{ lbs}}{x \text{ kg}}$$

   $$x = 90 \text{ kg}$$

   STEP 2 Set up a proportion to solve for the number of mg in one dose:

   $$\frac{15 \text{ mg}}{1 \text{ kg}} = \frac{x \text{ mg}}{90 \text{ kg}}$$

   $$x = 1{,}350 \text{ mg}$$

   STEP 3 Determine the total amount to be given in one day:

   $$\frac{1{,}350 \text{ mg}}{1 \text{ dose}} = \frac{x \text{ mg}}{4 \text{ doses}}$$

   $$x = 5{,}400 \text{ mg}$$

   The answer is 5,400 mg. (*Knowledge Domain 4.2*)

46. **(C)** The Combat Methamphetamine Epidemic Act of 2005 places limitations on the amount of pseudoephedrine- and ephedrine-containing products that may be purchased. (*Knowledge Domain 2.4*)

47. **(B)**

STEP 1 Set up an alligation (like the one pictured below), placing 95 in the top left corner and 30 in the bottom left corner. The final preparation concentration is placed in the middle. The "H" next to the "95" means that this is the highest concentration of alcohol. The "L" next to the "30" means that this is the lowest concentration of alcohol. The "P" next to the "50" means that this is the concentration of the final preparation.

95 (H)		20 (P – L)
	50 (P)	
30 (L)		45 (H – P)

STEP 2 Determine the number of parts by subtracting as indicated above in the right column.

STEP 3 Add the number of parts in the right column together to determine the total number of parts.

$$20 + 45 = 65 \text{ total parts}$$

STEP 4 Set up a proportion to determine the quantity needed of each solution.

$$95\%: \frac{20}{65} = \frac{x \text{ mL}}{1{,}000 \text{ mL}}$$

$$x = 308 \text{ mL}$$

$$30\%: \frac{45}{65} = \frac{x \text{ mL}}{1{,}000 \text{ mL}}$$

$$x = 692 \text{ mL}$$

The answer is 308 mL, 692 mL. (*Knowledge Domain 4.2*)

48. **(C)** Polyuria (increased urine output), polydipsia (increased thirst), and polyphagia (excessive hunger) are all symptoms of diabetes. (*Knowledge Domain 4.2*)

49. **(C)**

STEP 1 Set up a proportion to solve for the volume of Robitussin needed for 30 mg of codeine sulfate.

$$\frac{15 \text{ mg}}{5 \text{ mL}} = \frac{30 \text{ mg}}{x \text{ mL}}$$

$$x = 10 \text{ mL}$$

STEP 2 Determine the amount of 30 mg tablets needed to produce 120 mL.

$$\frac{120 \text{ mL}}{10 \text{ mL}} = 12 \text{ tablets}$$

The answer is 12 tablets. (*Knowledge Domain 4.2*)

50. **(C)** Celecoxib is a selective COX-2 inhibitor. Ibuprofen and naproxen are both nonselective inhibitors of both COX-1 and COX-2. Omeprazole is a proton-pump inhibitor (PPI). (*Knowledge Domain 1.1*)

51. **(C)** Policy and procedure manuals should be kept in an accessible work area. (*Knowledge Domain 1.10*)

52. **(A)** Chemotherapeutic drugs are considered hazardous drugs and should be counted on a separate counting tray that is labeled and designated as such. (*Knowledge Domain 3.6*)

53. **(A)** A Class I recall involves violative products that are likely to cause serious adverse health consequences or death. A Class II recall involves violative products that may cause temporary health issues or the probability of serious adverse health consequences is remote. A Class III recall involves violative products that are not likely to cause adverse health consequences. There are no Class IV recalls. (*Knowledge Domain 2.5*)

54. **(A)** Cyclosporine is an NTI drug that is also categorized by the ISMP and the FDA as a look-alike/sound-alike drug name. (*Knowledge Domain 1.8*)

55. **(A)** The patient's identity is the most important piece of information to verify. Do this by confirming the patient's date of birth, address, and phone number. (*Knowledge Domain 4.1*)

56. **(C)** "Apply" is used for medications that will be applied topically. "Take" is used for medications that will be ingested orally. "Insert" is used for medications that will be inserted vaginally or rectally. "Inhale" is used for medications that will be breathed or inhaled through the mouth. (*Knowledge Domain 4.2*)

57. **(A)** The abbreviation "a.c." means "before meals" and indicates that the patient should take the medication before eating. (*Knowledge Domain 4.2*)

58. **(B)** Tall man lettering is a strategy used to distinguish the parts of similar words that are different. (*Knowledge Domain 3.1*)

59. **(B)**

$$\frac{25 \text{ mg}}{1 \text{ mL}} = \frac{40 \text{ mg}}{x \text{ mL}}$$
$$x = 1.6 \text{ mL}$$

The answer is 1.6 mL. (*Knowledge Domain 4.2*)

60. **(D)** Remember that one and one half teaspoonfuls = 7.5 mL.

$$7.5 \text{ mL} \times 2 = 15 \text{ mL a day}$$
$$15 \text{ mL} \times 10 = 150 \text{ mL}$$
$$\frac{30 \text{ mL}}{1 \text{ oz}} = \frac{150 \text{ mL}}{x \text{ oz}}$$
$$x = 5 \text{ oz}$$

The answer is 5 oz. (*Knowledge Domain 4.2*)

61. **(B)** Additional training is necessary to properly handle, prepare, and dispose of hazardous drugs. This includes the use of special gowns, two pairs of gloves, and spill kits, and the use of safety data sheets (SDS). Hazardous drugs are also prepared in designated areas using a special laminar flow hood. (*Knowledge Domain 2.1*)

62. **(C)** This is an example of a medication error that is made during administration. Errors made during transcription are usually typographical errors. Errors made during prescribing include dosing errors, drug-drug interactions, and undocumented allergies. Dispensing errors may include situations in which a medication (other than the one that is prescribed) is dispensed, situations in which the drug bar code identifier is different than the one listed on the medication label, or situations in which a drug is dispensed to the wrong patient. (*Knowledge Domain 3.5*)

63. **(D)** A root-cause analysis (RCA) is a method employed by pharmacies to identify the root cause of an error in order to prevent future errors from occurring. (*Knowledge Domain 3.4*)

64. **(C)** Nitroglycerin sublingual is a tablet used for angina. It should be readily accessible to the patient in case of anginal pain. (*Knowledge Domain 1.10*)

65. **(A)** Buspirone/bupropion is an example of a pair of drugs that have similar-sounding names. (*Knowledge Domain 3.1*)

66. **(B)** The pharmacy technician should never counsel the patient. Instead, he or she should call over the pharmacist to address the situation. (*Knowledge Domain 3.3*)

67. **(C)**

$$°F = \left(°C \times \frac{9}{5} \right) + 32$$

$$°F = \left(15 \times \frac{9}{5} \right) + 32$$

$$°F = 59$$

The answer is 59°F. (*Knowledge Domain 4.2*)

68. **(D)** The package size is indicated by the last set of numbers of the NDC. (*Knowledge Domain 4.4*)

69. **(D)** Black cohosh is commonly used to treat symptoms of menopause, including hot flashes. Saw palmetto is commonly used to treat benign prostatic hyperplasia (BPH). Resveratrol is used for its antioxidant properties. Ginger is used for nausea and motion sickness. (*Knowledge Domain 1.6*)

70. **(A)** 0700 means 7 hours after midnight, which is 7:00 A.M. (*Knowledge Domain 4.2*)

71. **(C)** Set up a proportion:

$$\frac{3 \text{ g}}{100 \text{ g}} = \frac{x \text{ g}}{180 \text{ g}}$$

$$x = 5.4 \text{ g}$$

The answer is 5.4 g. (*Knowledge Domain 4.1*)

72. **(B)** Lorazepam is the generic drug name for Ativan. Enalapril is the generic drug name for Vasotec. Lisinopril is the generic drug name for Prinivil. Meloxicam is the generic drug name for Mobic. (*Knowledge Domain 1.1*)

73. **(A)** A spacer is attached to an inhaler and is used to help the patient get the medicine to his or her lungs. A nebulizer is a device that converts liquid medications into a mist for delivery to the lungs. A catheter is a thin tube that may be inserted in the body to treat diseases or to perform surgical procedures. A safety cap is a protective covering. (*Knowledge Domain 4.3*)

74. **(C)** 70% isopropyl alcohol is used as a disinfectant to clean counting trays, counters, and laminar flow hoods. (*Knowledge Domain 3.6*)

75. **(D)** A Class III prescription balance has a maximum weighable amount of 120 g. (*Knowledge Domain 4.1*)

76. **(A)** A suppository is inserted rectally or vaginally and bypasses the stomach (where nausea occurs), making it ideal for patients who have nausea and/or vomiting. (*Knowledge Domain 1.4*)

77. **(C)** Inderal is the brand name for the drug propranolol, which is a beta blocker indicated for hypertension. Tazorac is the brand name for the drug tazarotene, which is used for acne. (*Knowledge Domain 1.1*)

78. **(A)** The pharmacokinetic process of absorption is the movement of drug molecules from the initial site of administration into the bloodstream. Distribution is the movement of drugs throughout the body and is determined by the flow of blood to the tissues. Metabolism is the process of transforming and breaking down the drug to a more hydrophilic form so that it can be excreted from the body. Excretion, the final process, involves the removal of the drug from the body. (*Knowledge Domain 1.4*)

79. **(B)** Intravenous refers to an injection made into a vein. Intramuscular means an injection made into a muscle. Intraocular is an injection made into the eye. Intradermal is an injection made into the skin. (*Knowledge Domain 4.2*)

80. **(C)** The meniscus is the curved surface at the top of a column of liquid. The most accurate place to read the volume is at the bottom of the meniscus. (*Knowledge Domain 4.1*)

81. **(B)** When reading a prescription for an inhaler, it must be assumed that the patient will take the maximum amount of the drug. In the Rx described in the question, "1–2 puffs q 4–6h prn" means that the patient can take up to 2 puffs 6 times a day for a total of 12 puffs a day: $\frac{200}{12}$ = 16.66. The days supply for this medication is 16 days. Do not round up because the medication would not last a full 17 days. A higher days supply could potentially leave the patient without an inhaler. (*Knowledge Domain 4.2*)

82. **(C)** DEA Form 41 is used for outdated or damaged controlled substances that are to be surrendered or destroyed. (*Knowledge Domain 2.3*)

83. **(A)** To solve this problem, you need to understand conversions.

STEP 1 It is best to first convert 6 oz to grams:

$$\frac{1 \text{ oz}}{30 \text{ g}} = \frac{6 \text{ oz}}{x \text{ g}}$$
$$x = 180 \text{ g}$$

STEP 2 Solve for the amount of menthol required by setting up another proportion:

$$\frac{0.5 \text{ g}}{100 \text{ g}} = \frac{x \text{ g}}{180 \text{ g}}$$
$$x = 0.9 \text{ g}$$

The answer is 0.9 g. (*Knowledge Domain 4.2*)

84. **(A)** Alendronate is a medication used for the treatment of osteoporosis. Due to adverse effects, including stomach ulceration, it is best to take this medication with a full glass of water and sit in an upright position for 30 minutes afterward. (*Knowledge Domain 1.4*)

85. **(A)** The outer coating of an enteric coated tablet prevents dissolution in the stomach. As a result, the tablet breaks down in the intestines. (*Knowledge Domain 1.4*)

86. **(B)** A suspension is a liquid preparation in which the insoluble and coarse drug particles are evenly dispensed through a liquid medium. An emulsion is a mixture of two or more liquids that are normally immiscible, such as an oil-in-water mixture or a water-in-oil mixture. In a solution, the drug particles are completely dissolved in the liquid medium. An elixir is a liquid formulation that contains alcohol. (*Knowledge Domain 4.1*)

87. **(C)**

$$\frac{100 \text{ units}}{1 \text{ mL}} = \frac{12 \text{ units}}{x \text{ mL}}$$
$$x = 0.12 \text{ mL}$$

The answer is 0.12 mL. (*Knowledge Domain 4.2*)

88. **(D)** 90 days × 2 tablets/day = 180 tablets (*Knowledge Domain 4.2*)

89. **(A)** Stock with the closest expiration date is moved to the front of the pharmacy shelf to ensure that it is used before it expires. (*Knowledge Domain 4.5*)

90. **(B)** Warfarin is an example of an anticoagulant medication on ISMP's List of High-Alert Medications in Community/Ambulatory Healthcare. (*Knowledge Domain 3.1*)

Medications

5

KNOWLEDGE DOMAIN 1.0

Medications   **40.00%**
→ Knowledge Area 1.1: Generic names, brand names, and classifications of medications
→ Knowledge Area 1.2: Therapeutic equivalence
→ Knowledge Area 1.3: Common and life-threatening drug interactions and contraindications (e.g., drug-disease, drug-drug, drug-dietary supplement, drug-laboratory, drug-nutrient)
→ Knowledge Area 1.4: Strengths/dose, dosage forms, routes of administration, special handling and administration instructions, and duration of drug therapy
→ Knowledge Area 1.5: Common and severe medication side effects, adverse effects, and allergies
→ Knowledge Area 1.6: Indications of medications and dietary supplements
→ Knowledge Area 1.7: Drug stability (e.g., oral suspensions, insulin, reconstitutables, injectables, vaccinations)
→ Knowledge Area 1.8: Narrow therapeutic index (NTI) medications
→ Knowledge Area 1.9: Physical and chemical incompatibilities related to non-sterile compounding and reconstitution
→ Knowledge Area 1.10: Proper storage of medications (e.g., temperature ranges, light sensitivity, restricted access)

LEARNING OBJECTIVES

☐ Define terms associated with pharmacology.
☐ Be familiar with common terms used to describe drug interactions.
☐ Explain the drug approval process, including the timeline, clinical trial testing, and the FDA's role.
☐ Understand the importance of stability and beyond-use dating.
☐ Recognize commonly used auxiliary labels for prescribed medications.
☐ Define therapeutic index and narrow therapeutic index, and identify medications with a narrow therapeutic index profile.
☐ Understand common storage requirements.
☐ Identify brand and generic drug names of medications in each pharmaceutical classification.
☐ Identify common dosage forms, routes of administration, and the duration of drug therapy for each pharmaceutical agent.
☐ Identify common available doses of each pharmaceutical agent.
☐ Identify common side effects and therapeutic contraindications of frequently prescribed agents.
☐ List common indications associated with each pharmaceutical agent.

NOTE

Make sure to test
your knowledge
of the top brand
name drugs
by reviewing
Appendix A and
Appendix B in
this book!

A 2018 Gallup survey of consumers rated pharmacists as the third most trusted profession in terms of honesty and ethical standards. As a pharmacy technician, it is important to uphold those same standards. This starts with having a basic understanding of medications and being able to identify them.

The pharmacy contains thousands of medications that serve a wide range of indications and age ranges to help treat, prevent, or cure diseases. Pharmacy technicians should be able to classify drugs by major therapeutic categories, and they should be able to identify main indications (the therapeutic use of a drug). It is also essential for technicians to identify common brand and generic drug names. Look for commonly used drug prefixes and suffixes, dubbed "stems" as noted by the United States Adopted Names (USAN) Council, throughout this chapter. A stem refers to a unique pharmacological or chemical relationship between drugs and can be used to help recall a medication or a classification.

IMPORTANT TERMS TO KNOW

TIP

Remember
the difference:
Pharmacokinetics
is what the body
does to the drug.
Pharmacodynamics
can be remembered
as what the drug
does to the body.

- **PHARMACOLOGY:** Derived from the Greek words "pharmakon," meaning *remedy*, and "logos," meaning *knowledge*, the word *pharmacology* loosely translates to "the knowledge of drugs."
- **PHARMACOKINETICS:** A branch of pharmacology that refers to the rate of drug absorption, distribution, metabolism, and excretion (ADME).
- **PHARMACODYNAMICS:** A branch of pharmacology that refers to the biological and physical effects of the drug on the body.
- **BRAND NAME:** A proprietary name protected by a patent. This is often referred to as the manufacturer's trademarked name. The first letter of a brand name is always capitalized.
- **GENERIC NAME:** A nonproprietary name approved by the United States Adopted Names (USAN) Council. The generic drug must have the same active ingredient, dosage strength, and formulation as the brand name drug, but it may have different inactive ingredients. The first letter of a generic name is not capitalized.
- **CHEMICAL NAME:** A name given to a drug during the initial clinical investigation, referring to its atomic or molecular structure.
- **DOSAGE FORM:** The physical manifestation of the drug or how the drug is supplied. Table 5-1 lists the usual dosage forms.

Table 5-1. Dosage Forms

Form	Definition	Example
Aerosol spray	A solution containing an active ingredient with a propellant that is meant to carry the drug to the site of action	benzocaine aerosol spray
Caplet	A tablet shaped like a capsule, containing a solid inside	erythromycin caplet
Capsule	A dosage form containing powder or liquid in a gelatin coating	Nexium capsule
Cream	An oil-in-water emulsion for external use	hydrocortisone cream
Elixir	A flavored, sweetened hydroalcoholic solution	phenobarbital elixir
Emulsion	A dosage form made by the dispersion of one liquid into another that is immiscible	estradiol emulsion

Form	Definition	Example
Extract	A potent dosage form containing a powder, ointment-like form, or a solid produced by the evaporation of the aqueous solvent	peppermint extract
Gel	A dosage formed from ultrafine particles in a liquid	lidocaine gel
Intradermal implant, pellet	A dosage form placed under the skin via minor surgery, allowing the drug to be released slowly	Implanon
Lotion	A liquid suspension that is used for topical administration, containing insoluble dispersed solids	calamine lotion
Lozenge, pastilles, troches	A dosage form made with flavored or sweetened ingredients; generally designed to be dissolved in the mouth for a local effect	over-the-counter (OTC) cough drops
Micropump	A system of 5,000 to 10,000 microparticles contained within a tablet or capsule; each microparticle is released in the stomach and is able to deliver a drug over an extended period of time	Coreg CR
Ointment	A water-in-oil semisolid preparation for external use	lanolin ointment
Solution	A homogeneous liquid dosage form containing one or more solutes dissolved in a solvent	lactulose solution
Spirit	An alcoholic or hydroalcoholic solution containing volatile aromatic compounds	peppermint spirit, aromatic ammonia spirit
Suppository	A solid formulation intended for rectal or vaginal administration	promethazine suppository
Suspension	A dispersion containing an insoluble solid in a liquid	amoxicillin suspension
Syrup	An aqueous solution containing sugar	lithium citrate syrup
Tablet	A molded or compressed dosage form containing active ingredient(s) along with inert binder (inactive ingredients)	levothyroxine tablet
Tincture	An alcoholic or hydroalcoholic solution	Belladonna tincture, iodine tincture
Transdermal patch	A percutaneous delivery system consisting of a permeable polymer membrane, backing, drug reservoir, adhesive layer, and protective strip	fentanyl patch, nicotine patch

- **DRUG CLASSIFICATION:** Drugs are grouped by their common actions and effects on the body (e.g., anti-infective, anxiolytic, analgesic).
- **THERAPEUTIC EQUIVALENCE:** This classification is given to drugs that meet certain criteria. The drugs must be proven to be safe and effective, and they must be deemed as pharmaceutically equivalent. This means that identical amounts of active drug are present. The dosage form and route must also be the same. Standards of strength, purity, and quality must be met. Bioequivalence must also be proven. According to the FDA, this is completed through testing to prove the drugs have similar rates of absorption under similar conditions and dosage parameters. Therapeutic equivalence can be checked by looking at the *Approved Drug Products with Therapeutic Equivalence Evaluations*, which is commonly referred to as the *Orange Book*. This publication is the U. S. Food and Drug Administration's (FDA) official listing for prescription, over-the-counter, biologic, military, discontinued, or otherwise never-marketed drugs.
- **SIDE EFFECTS:** Secondary effects of the drug other than the primary therapeutic effect it was originally intended for.
- **DRUG INTERACTIONS:** A desirable or an undesirable effect that can occur when the effect of one drug is altered by the action of another drug or substance. This phenomenon can produce undesirable effects, resulting in a lack of efficacy or even toxicity. Factors that contribute to an increased number of drug interactions include multiple prescribers, poor patient compliance, taking multiple drugs, advanced age, and comorbidity. There are several different types of drug interactions.

   Drug-drug interactions occur when a drug interacts with or interferes with another drug. This interaction may be additive, synergistic, potentiated, or antagonistic. An **additive** interaction results when two drugs given in combination have an effect equal to the sum of the individual effects. A **synergistic** interaction results when drugs given in combination produce an effect greater than the sum of the individual effects. A **potentiated** interaction occurs when one drug intensifies the activity of another drug. An **antagonistic** interaction occurs when drugs given in combination cause a decreased, or diminished, effect in one or more drugs.

   Drug-food interactions occur when a drug reacts with a food. An example of this is when drinking grapefruit juice causes an increase in the serum concentration of the antihyperlipidemic drug lovastatin (Mevacor).

   Drug-disease interactions may occur when a prescription or an over-the-counter medication interacts or interferes with an existing medical condition. For example, a drug-disease interaction occurs when an individual with hypertension takes pseudo-ephedrine.

   Drug-nutritional supplement interactions occur when a drug affects vitamin absorption or metabolism. For example, anticonvulsants, such as phenytoin, can cause vitamin D deficiency.

   Drug-laboratory interactions occur when a drug or a substance alters the concentrations of substances in the body. For example, potassium-sparing diuretics, such as triamterene, increase serum potassium levels. In addition, the H_2 blocker cimetidine can elevate serum creatinine levels.

   Drug-nutrient interactions occur when a drug affects the use of a nutrient in the body. The drug may affect the nutrient's absorption, the use of the nutrient by the body, or the excretion of the nutrient. For example, antihyperlipidemic agents, such as cholestyramine, can decrease the absorption of the fat-soluble vitamins (vitamins A, D, E, and K).

THE FDA DRUG APPROVAL PROCESS

The FDA's Center for Drug Evaluation and Research (CDER) oversees clinical trial investigations used to explore the safety and effectiveness of medications, safety devices, and medical strategies for humans. Figure 5-1 provides more information about the process of drug approval.

	Discovery/ Preclinical Testing		Phase 1	Phase 2	Phase 3		FDA	Phase 4
Years	6.5		1.5	2	3.5		1.5	
Test Population	Laboratory and animal studies	File IND at FDA	20 to 100 healthy volunteers	100 to 500 patient volunteers	1,000 to 5,000 patient volunteers	File NDA at FDA		
Purpose	Assess safety, biological activity, and formulations		Determine safety and dosage	Evaluate effectiveness, look for side effects	Confirm effectiveness, monitor adverse reactions from long-term use		Review process/ approval	Additional postmarketing testing required by FDA
Success Rate	5,000 compounds evaluated		5 enter trials				1 approved	

Figure 5-1. The FDA drug approval process

STEP 1 **Preclinical Testing**

The FDA requires all drugs to undergo preclinical testing in a laboratory before testing in humans can begin. During this process, the developer or sponsor will compile data on dosing and toxicity levels. Researchers will evaluate the findings to determine if the drug should move to clinical testing.

STEP 2 **The Investigational New Drug Process**

The drug developer submits an Investigational New Drug (IND) application to the FDA. This application includes manufacturing information, animal safety data and toxicity, clinical protocols, and information about the investigator. An IND review team will review the data for potential approval. The review team has 30 days to review the application and indicate if the drug is approved, if it is stopped, or if additional information is required before a decision can be made.

STEP 3 **Clinical Trials**

Three phases of clinical trial testing are required before a drug may be considered for approval on the market. Phase 3 testing is contingent on successful completion of phase 2, which depends on the success of phase 1. (See Figure 5-1). As clinical trials progress, researchers will gather data on safety, appropriate dosage, side effects, interactions, and efficacy. If the drug is approved, the sponsor will conduct postmarketing testing to further evaluate the drug's safety and long-term side effects.

STEP 4 **New Drug Application**

The final step is for a New Drug Application (NDA) to be submitted to the FDA to approve the drug for marketing and distribution. The FDA has 60 days to accept the application for review. On average, the CDER will review and act on applications within 10–12 months after receiving the NDA.

On average, a drug takes 12 years to go from laboratory testing to the pharmacy shelf. During its development, the drug sponsor requests a **patent** to protect the company's interest in having an exclusive right to the drug. The patent excludes other companies from marketing, developing, or using the drug while the patent is valid. The term of a patent is 20 years from the initial filing date submitted with the IND application. A patent extension may be granted and is determined on an individual basis.

STABILITY AND BEYOND-USE DATING

Stability refers to the ability of a substance to remain unchanged over time while maintaining its initial characteristics. Chemical compatibility concerns, as well as proper beyond-use date labeling, are both vital to stability.

Chemical compatibility refers to stability, specifically the ability for the substance to remain stable when mixed with other substances. Chemical incompatibilities include visible as well as invisible changes. A change in color or the formation of a precipitate, such as calcium phosphate, are examples of visible changes. The formation of gases or of volatile chemicals, in contrast, are examples of invisible changes.

The **beyond-use date** is defined by the *USP-NF*, General Chapter <795>, as "the date after which a compounded preparation shall not be used and is determined from the date when the preparation is compounded." Medications may include stability information in their package insert or labeling. In the absence of stability information, packaged, light-resistant, temperature-controlled non-sterile compounded medications may use the beyond-use dates listed in Table 5-2.

Table 5-2. Maximum Non-Sterile Beyond-Use Dates

Formulation	Beyond-Use Date (BUD) Maximum
Nonaqueous solutions (i.e., capsule without water)	BUD no later than 6 months or BUD equal to earliest expiration date of any active pharmaceutical ingredient (API)
Oral solutions containing water (i.e., oral suspension)	BUD no later than 14 days from reconstitution date (must be kept at the controlled temperature as indicated on the package label)
Topical solutions and semisolid formulations containing water (i.e., ointment)	BUD no later than 30 days

AUXILIARY LABELS

Auxiliary labels are brightly colored medication labels that are added to prescription bottles in an effort to provide ancillary information to the patient regarding safe administration, use, storage, and disposal of the medication. Common examples of auxiliary labels are "Take with food" and "Medication should be taken with plenty of water." Prescriptions for controlled substances are required to carry an additional auxiliary label: "Caution: Federal law prohibits the transfer of this drug to any person other than the patient for whom it was prescribed."

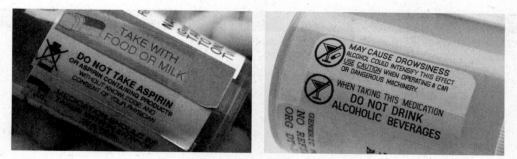

Figure 5-2. Auxiliary labels

Review Table 5-3, which outlines some of the most commonly used prescription auxiliary labels in pharmacy practice. For this exam and your career, learn to be comfortable identifying drugs that carry these labels.

Table 5-3. Examples of Prescription Auxiliary Labels

Prescription Auxiliary Labels	Medications
"Finish all of this medication unless otherwise directed by prescriber."	• antibiotics • antifungals • antivirals
"Take medication on an empty stomach 1 hour before or 2 hours after a meal unless otherwise directed by your doctor."	• ampicillin • azithromycin • bisphosphonates • captopril • Carafate • HIV medications (indinavir, efavirenz, didanosine) • levothyroxine (Synthroid) • methotrexate • penicillin • tetracycline • zarfirlukast (Accolate)
"Do not take dairy products, antacids, or iron preparations within one hour of this medication."	• selected antibiotics (tetracycline, doxycycline, ciprofloxacin, cefdinir, azithromycin, sucralfate)
"Medication should be taken with plenty of water."	• selected antibiotics (sulfonamides) • phenazopyridine • bisphosphonates • NSAIDs • potassium supplements • benzonatate • cyclophosphamide

Prescription Auxiliary Labels	Medications
"May cause discoloration of the urine or feces."	• cefdinir (Omnicef) • indomethacin (Indocin) • iron preparations • metronidazole (Flagyl) • nitrofurantoin (Furadantin) • phenazopyridine (Pyridium) • rifampin (Rifadin, Rimactane) • rifapentine (Priftin) • sulfasalazine (Azulfidine)
"Do not drink alcoholic beverages with this medication."	• metronidazole • sulfonylureas • NSAIDs • oral corticosteroids • phenytoin • disulfiram
"May cause drowsiness. Alcohol may intensify this effect. Use care when operating a car or dangerous machinery."	• opioid analgesics • tramadol • anticonvulsants • antidepressants • antipsychotics • antihistamines • benzodiazepines • hypnotics • skeletal muscle relaxants
"Swallow whole."	• sublingual tablets • film coated tablets • slow-release tablets • enteric-coated tablets • capsules
"For the ear only."	• otic preparations
"Rinse mouth thoroughly after each use."	• fluticasone (Flovent HFA) inhaler • fluticasone/salmeterol (Advair) inhaler • budesonide (Pulmicort) inhaler • budesonide/formoterol (Symbicort) inhaler • beclomethasone dipropionate (Qvar) inhaler • mometasone furoate (Asmanex HFA) inhaler • triamcinolone acetonide (Azmacort) inhaler

THERAPEUTIC INDEX

The **therapeutic index (TI)** is a ratio that compares a therapeutically effective dose to a toxic dose of a drug. It is a relative statement of safety. A dose-response curve is a visual representation of this relationship and is derived by dividing the toxic dose in an average population (TD50) by the effective dose in an average population (ED50).

$$TI = \frac{\text{toxic dose}}{\text{effective dose}} = \frac{TD50}{ED50}$$

A higher value therapeutic index is an indication of a more agreeable safety profile. For example, if Drug "X" had a TD50 of 100 and an ED50 of 10, its TI would be 10:

$$TI = \frac{TD50}{ED50} = \frac{100}{10} = 10$$

To put this into perspective, a drug with a TI of 10 would be considered safer than another drug with a TI of 5 or a TI of 2.

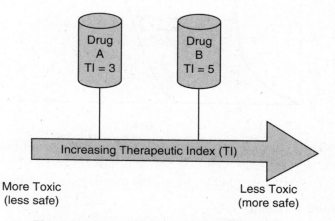

Figure 5-3. Increasing therapeutic index (TI)

Narrow therapeutic index (NTI) drugs are those drugs for which "small differences in dose or blood concentration may lead to serious therapeutic failures and/or adverse drug reactions that are life-threatening or result in persistent or significant disability or incapacity" as per the U.S. Food and Drug Administration, 2017. These drugs are subject to regular therapeutic drug monitoring to ensure that the patient's actual blood levels stay within therapeutic range.

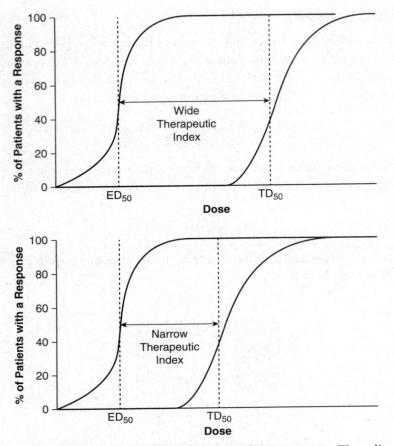

Figure 5-4. Dose response curve comparison: wide TI vs. narrow TI medications

The following is a list of drugs that are frequently monitored due to an NTI:

- carbamazepine (Tegretol)
- cyclosporine (Neoral, Sandimmune)
- digoxin (Lanoxin)
- ethosuximide (Zarontin)
- levothyroxine (Synthroid)
- lithium (Eskalith, Lithobid)
- phenytoin (Dilantin)
- theophylline (Theo-24 and Uniphyl)
- warfarin (Coumadin)

STORAGE REQUIREMENTS

The majority of prescription medications can be stored at room temperature: 15°C to 30°C or 59°F to 86°F. Some medications require refrigeration: 2°C to 8°C or 36°F to 46°F. A list of these medications can be found in Appendix C of this book. These drugs may also have special storage requirements after being dispensed to the patient. Drugs that must be frozen (–25°C to –10°C or –13°F to –14°F) are less common and are mainly vaccines. See Appendix D of this book for a list of vaccines, including those that must be frozen prior to use.

Medications that are stored outside of a recommended temperature range can incur a number of consequences, including a loss of physical integrity (e.g., suppositories melting), a reduced shelf life, or a partial or complete loss of effectiveness. Medications should be stored in their original packaging and placed in the appropriate storage area. Physical incompatibilities can occur between two or more substances, which can lead to a change in color, odor, taste, viscosity, or morphology. Chemical incompatibilities are the result of a reaction between two or more substances, leading to precipitation, effervescence, color change, decomposition, or an explosion.

Drugs can lose their potency due to exposure to light or moisture. This process can be slow, but some drugs are particularly sensitive to light and/or moisture and can lose their potency much more quickly. It is crucial that these drugs be stored in their original packaging to slow down the loss of potency. Medications should also be stored in their original packaging due to adherence issues or safety concerns.

Table 5-4. Medications That Should Be Stored in Their Original Containers

Medications That Are Sensitive to Light or Moisture	
Medication	**Sensitivity**
adalimumab inj. (Humira)	light
aliskiren (Tekturna)	moisture (Note that the original container has a desiccant.)
cyclosporine capsules, oral solution (Sandimmune, Neoral)	light (Note that this medication must be used within two months of opening the original container.)
dabigatran (Pradaxa)	moisture
dipyridamole and aspirin capsules (Aggrenox)	moisture
etanercept (Enbrel)	light
golimumab (Simponi)	light
nitroglycerin sublingual tablets (Nitrostat)	light and moisture
oxcarbazepine oral solution (Trileptal)	light (Note that this medication must be used within seven weeks of opening the original container.)
ritonavir capsules, oral solution, tablets (Norvir)	light and moisture
vaccines	light (Note that these medications should be stored in a refrigerator or in a freezer in their original packaging.)
zafirlukast (Accolate)	light and moisture
Medications with Adherence Issues	
Medication	**Adherence Issue**
oral contraceptives	These medications should be dispensed in their original packaging to alleviate confusion and to help with adherence.
Medications with Safety Concerns	
Medication	**Safety Concern**
finasteride (Proscar)	This medication is teratogenic. Dispense it in its original container to reduce exposure of the drug to individuals that may come in contact with it.

Medications with specific storage requirements may be flagged with shelf tags or stickers in the pharmacy to alert pharmacy staff. A "dispense after" auxiliary label should be placed on any prescription vial that requires special attention. Additional information on storage requirements can also be found in the "storage and handling" section of the medication package insert.

ANTI-ANXIETY, ANTIEPILEPTIC, ANTIDEPRESSANT, AND SEDATIVE AGENTS

You should familiarize yourself with the USAN stems for anti-anxiety, antiepileptic, antidepressant, and sedative agents, as outlined in Table 5-5.

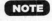

Antidepressants work by altering chemicals known as neurotransmitters in the brain. These agents may take 4–6 weeks to become effective.

Table 5-5. USAN Stems for Anti-anxiety, Antiepileptic, Antidepressant, and Sedative Agents

Stem	Description	Example
-azepam	Benzodiazepine anxiolytic	temazepam
-pidem	Zolpidem-type sedative/hypnotic	zolpidem
-plon	Nonbenzodiazepine anxiolytic	zaleplon

Table 5-6 lists vital information about common anti-anxiety, antiepileptic, antidepressant, and sedative agents, including common strengths/dosages, dosage forms, routes, and indications.

Table 5-6. Anti-anxiety, Antiepileptic, Antidepressant, and Sedative Agents

Generic Name	Brand Name	Common Strengths/Dosages	Dosage Forms	Route	Indication
alprazolam	Xanax	0.25 mg, 0.5 mg, 1 mg, 2 mg, 3 mg, 1 mg/mL	Tablet, liquid solution	PO	Treatment of anxiety (C-IV)
chlordiazepoxide	Librium	5 mg, 10 mg, 25 mg, 100 mg	Tablet, parenteral	IV, PO, IM	Treatment of anxiety (C-IV)
clonazepam	Klonopin	0.125 mg, 0.25 mg, 0.5 mg, 1 mg, 2 mg	Tablet	PO	Treatment of anxiety (C-IV)
clorazepate	Tranxene	3.75 mg, 7.5 mg, 15 mg	Tablet	PO	Treatment of anxiety (C-IV)
diazepam	Valium	2 mg, 5 mg, 10 mg, 5 mg/mL	Tablet, oral solution, parenteral	PO, IV, IM	Treatment of anxiety (C-IV)
lorazepam	Ativan	0.5 mg, 1 mg, 2 mg, 2 mg/mL	Tablet, oral concentration, parenteral	PO, IV	Treatment of anxiety (C-IV)
meprobamate	Equanil	200 mg, 400 mg	Tablet	PO	Treatment of anxiety (C-IV)
oxazepam	Serax	10 mg, 15 mg, 30 mg	Capsule	PO	Treatment of anxiety (C-IV)

Generic Name	Brand Name	Common Strengths/Dosages	Dosage Forms	Route	Indication
buspirone	Buspar	5 mg, 7.5 mg, 10 mg, 15 mg, 30 mg	Tablet	PO	Treatment of anxiety
carbamazepine	Tegretol	100 mg, 200 mg, 300 mg, 400 mg, 100 mg/5 mL	Tablet, capsule, oral suspension	PO	Treatment of epilepsy
divalproex sodium	Depakote	125 mg, 250 mg, 500 mg, 100 mg/mL	Tablet, capsule	PO	Treatment of epilepsy
ethosuximide	Zarontin	250 mg, 250 mg/mL	Capsule, oral suspension	PO	Treatment of epilepsy
gabapentin	Neurontin	100 mg, 300 mg, 400 mg, 600 mg, 800 mg, 250 mg/mL	Tablet, capsule, oral solution	PO	Treatment of epilepsy
lamotrigine	Lamictal	2 mg, 5 mg, 25 mg, 100 mg, 150 mg, 200 mg	Tablet	PO	Treatment of epilepsy
levetiracetam	Keppra	250 mg, 500 mg, 750 mg, 1,000 mg, 100 mg/mL	Tablet, oral solution	PO	Treatment of epilepsy
oxcarbazepine	Trileptal	150 mg, 300 mg, 600 mg, 300 mg/5 mL	Tablet, oral suspension	PO	Treatment of epilepsy
phenytoin	Dilantin	50 mg, 125 mg/5 mL	Tablet, capsule, oral solution, parenteral	PO, IV, IM	Treatment of epilepsy
pregabalin	Lyrica	50 mg, 75 mg, 100 mg, 150 mg, 200 mg, 225 mg, 20 mg/mL	Capsule, oral solution	PO	Treatment of epilepsy
tiagabine	Gabitril	2 mg, 4 mg, 12 mg, 16 mg	Tablet	PO	Treatment of epilepsy
topiramate	Topamax	15 mg, 25 mg, 50 mg, 100 mg, 200 mg	Tablet, capsule	PO	Treatment of epilepsy
valproic acid	Depakene	250 mg, 250 mg/5 mL	Capsule, oral solution	PO	Treatment of epilepsy
zonisamide	Zonegran	25 mg, 50 mg, 100 mg	Capsule	PO	Treatment of epilepsy
amitriptyline	Elavil	10 mg, 25 mg, 50 mg, 75 mg, 100 mg, 150 mg	Tablet	PO	Treatment of depression
bupropion	Wellbutrin	75 mg, 100 mg, 150 mg, 200 mg, 300 mg	Tablet	PO	Treatment of depression
citalopram	Celexa	10 mg, 20 mg, 40 mg, 10 mg/5 mL	Tablet, oral solution	PO	Treatment of depression
desipramine	Norpramin	25 mg, 50 mg, 75 mg, 100 mg, 150 mg	Tablet	PO	Treatment of depression
doxepin	Sinequan	10 mg, 25 mg, 50 mg, 75 mg, 100 mg, 150 mg, 10 mg/mL	Tablet, oral solution	PO	Treatment of depression
duloxetine	Cymbalta	20 mg, 30 mg, 60 mg	Capsule	PO	Treatment of depression
escitalopram	Lexapro	5 mg, 10 mg, 20 mg, 5 mg/5 mL	Tablet, oral solution	PO	Treatment of depression

Generic Name	Brand Name	Common Strengths/Dosages	Dosage Forms	Route	Indication
fluoxetine	Prozac	10 mg, 20 mg, 40 mg, 90 mg	Capsule	PO	Treatment of depression
fluvoxamine	Luvox	25 mg, 50 mg, 100 mg	Tablet	PO	Treatment of depression
imipramine	Tofranil	10 mg, 25 mg, 50 mg, 75 mg, 100 mg, 125 mg, 150 mg	Tablet, capsule	PO	Treatment of depression
isocarboxazid	Marplan	10 mg	Tablet	PO	Treatment of depression
maprotiline	Ludiomil	25 mg, 50 mg, 75 mg	Tablet	PO	Treatment of depression
mirtazapine	Remeron	15 mg, 30 mg, 45 mg	Tablet	PO	Treatment of depression
nefazodone	Serzone	50 mg, 100 mg, 150 mg, 200 mg, 250 mg	Tablet	PO	Treatment of depression
nortriptyline	Pamelor	10 mg, 25 mg, 50 mg, 75 mg	Tablet	PO	Treatment of depression
paroxetine	Paxil	10 mg, 12.5 mg, 20 mg, 25 mg, 30 mg, 37.5 mg, 40 mg	Tablet	PO	Treatment of depression
phenelzine	Nardil	15 mg	Tablet	PO	Treatment of depression
sertraline	Zoloft	25 mg, 50 mg, 100 mg, 20 mg/mL	Tablet, oral solution	PO	Treatment of depression
trazodone	Desyrel	50 mg, 100 mg, 150 mg, 300 mg	Tablet	PO	Treatment of depression
venlafaxine	Effexor	25 mg, 37.5 mg, 50 mg, 75 mg, 100 mg, 150 mg	Tablet, capsule	PO	Treatment of depression
eszopiclone	Lunesta	1 mg, 2 mg, 3 mg	Tablet	PO	Treatment of insomnia (C-IV)
temazepam	Restoril	7.5 mg, 15 mg, 22.5 mg, 30 mg	Capsule	PO	Treatment of insomnia (C-IV)
triazolam	Halcion	0.125 mg, 0.25 mg	Tablet	PO	Treatment of insomnia (C-IV)
zaleplon	Sonata	5 mg, 10 mg	Capsule	PO	Treatment of insomnia (C-IV)
zolpidem	Ambien	5 mg, 6.25 mg, 10 mg, 12.5 mg	Tablet	PO	Treatment of insomnia (C-IV)
ramelteon	Rozerem	8 mg	Tablet	PO	Treatment of insomnia

ANTI-INFECTIVE AGENTS

Refer to Table 5-7 for the USAN stems for anti-infective agents that you should know.

Table 5-7. USAN Stems for Anti-Infective Agents

Stem	Description	Example
-bactam	Beta-lactamase	sulbactam
cef-/ceph-	Cephalosporins	cefepime
-cillin	Penicillins	piperacillin
-conazole	Miconazole-type antifungal	itraconazole
-cycline	Tetracyclines	doxycycline
-ezolid	Oxazolidone antibiotics	linezolid
-mycin	Macrolides	azithromycin
-oxacin	Quinolones	levofloxacin
sulfa-	Sulfonamides	sulfamethoxazole with trimethoprim
-vir	Antivirals (general undefined)	acyclovir

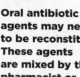

TIP

Oral antibiotic agents may need to be reconstituted. These agents are mixed by the pharmacist or technician upon dispensing due to their short shelf life. Oral syringes or dosing spoons should also be dispensed with pediatric oral medications.

Anti-infective agents, or antimicrobials, are agents that either kill microorganisms or slow the spread by inhibiting growth. These agents are classified as either **bactericidal** (kill the microorganisms) or **bacteriostatic** (inhibit the growth of the microorganisms). Antibiotics are agents produced by microorganisms and, at low concentrations, kill or inhibit the growth of bacteria.

Microorganisms most commonly include bacteria (antibacterial) and viruses (antiviral) but could also refer to fungi (antifungal) and protozoa (antiprotozoal). Selection of an agent depends on the following:

- Pathogen—determined via previous acquisition, antimicrobial testing, or from a disease state
- Drug—attributes to be considered include pharmacokinetics, pharmacodynamics, and toxicity
- Cost—low cost vs. high cost, insurance, and so on
- Administration—oral vs. I.V., hospital or home infusion, and so on
- Host—variables that must be considered include age, liver and/or kidney function, and immune status

Antibacterial agents are categorized by the spectrum of activity (Gram-positive and/or Gram-negative), bacterial effect (bactericidal or bacteriostatic), and mechanism of action.

Tables 5-8 to 5-15 provide information on the most commonly prescribed anti-infective drug classifications. Each table provides information on drug classifications, mechanisms of action, bacterial effects, spectrums of action, common indications and side effects, and the duration of therapy.

Table 5-8. Penicillins

Classification: penicillin
Mechanism of Action: inhibitor of cell wall synthesis
Bacterial Effect: bactericidal
Spectrum of Action: usually Gram-positive
Common Indications: prophylaxis, respiratory infections, otitis media, pneumonia, meningitis, syphilis
Common Side Effects: stomach upset, diarrhea, and allergic reactions (i.e., rash, hives, edema, and anaphylactic shock)
Typical Duration: 3-, 7-, or 10-day therapy

Generic Name	Brand Name	Common Strengths	Dosage Forms	Route
amoxicillin	Amoxil, Moxatag, Trimox	250 mg, 500 mg, 125 mg/5 mL, 200 mg/5 mL, 250 mg/5 mL, 400 mg/5 mL	Capsule, powder for suspension, chewable tablet, extended-release tablet, tablet	PO
amoxicillin and clavulanate	Augmentin	250 mg, 500 mg, 875 mg, 125 mg/5 mL, 200 mg/5 mL, 250 mg/5 mL, 400 mg/5 mL, 600 mg/5 mL	Tablet, powder for suspension, extended-release tablet	PO
ampicillin	Omnipen	125 mg, 250 mg, 125 mg/5 mL, 250 mg/5 mL	Capsule, oral suspension	PO
ampicillin and sulbactam	Unasyn	150 mg, 300 mg, 1.5 g, 3 g	Parenteral	IV, IM
dicloxacillin	Dynapen	250 mg, 500 mg	Capsule	PO
penicillin G	Bicillin-L-A	600,000 units/1 mL, 1.2 million units/2 mL, 2.4 million units/4 mL	Parenteral	IV, IM
penicillin V potassium	Penicillin VK, Pen-Vee K, Penicillin V, Veetids	250 mg, 500 mg, 125 mg/5 mL, 250 mg/5 mL	Tablet, liquid	PO
piperacillin and tazobactam	Zosyn	2.25 g, 3.375 g, 4.5 g	Parenteral	IV
ticarcillin and clavulanate	Timentin	3.1 g	Parenteral	IV

Table 5-9. Cephalosporins

Classification: cephalosporin
Mechanism of Action: inhibitor of cell wall synthesis
Bacterial Effect: bactericidal
Spectrum of Action: Gram-positive and some Gram-negative
Common Indications: prophylaxis, respiratory infections, pneumonia, dental procedures, genitourinary tract infections
Common Side Effects: upset stomach, diarrhea, and allergic reactions (i.e., rash, hives, edema, and anaphylactic shock)
Contraindications: hypersensitivity to penicillin, renal impairment
Special Considerations: 1–3% cross-sensitivity to penicillin
Typical Duration: 7–14 day therapy

Generic Name	Brand Name	Common Strengths	Dosage Forms	Route
cefaclor	Ceclor	250 mg, 500 mg, 125 mg/5 mL, 250 mg/5 mL, 375 mg/5 mL	Capsule, tablet, suspension	PO
cefadroxil	Duricef	250 mg, 500 mg, 250 mg/5 mL, 500 mg/5 mL, 1 g	Capsule, suspension, tablet	PO
cefazolin	Ancef	500 mg, 1 g	Parenteral	IV
cefdinir	Omnicef	300 mg, 125 mg/5 mL, 250 mg/5 mL	Capsule, suspension	PO
cefepime	Maxipime	500 mg, 1 g, 2 g	Parenteral	IV
cefixime	Suprax	400 mg, 100 mg/5 mL, 200 mg/5 mL, 500 mg/5 mL	Tablet, suspension	PO
cefprozil	Cefzil	250 mg, 500 mg, 125 mg/5 mL, 250 mg/5 mL	Tablet, suspension	PO
ceftazidime	Fortaz	1 g, 2 g, 6 g	Parenteral	IV
ceftriaxone	Rocephin	250 mg, 500 mg, 1 g, 2 g	Parenteral	IV
cefuroxime	Ceftin	250 mg, 500 mg, 125 mg/5 mL, 250 mg/5 mL	Tablet, suspension	PO
cephalexin	Keflex	250 mg, 500 mg, 750 g, 125 mg/5 mL, 250 mg/5 mL	Capsule, suspension	PO

Table 5-10. Macrolides

Classification: macrolide
Mechanism of Action: inhibitor of protein synthesis
Bacterial Effect: bacteriostatic
Spectrum of Action: mostly Gram-positive and some Gram-negative
Common Indications: respiratory infections, skin infections, pneumonia, chlamydia, sinusitis
Common Side Effects: upset stomach, diarrhea
Contraindications: QT prolongation, hepatic impairment, renal impairment
Special Considerations: intensifies the effect of warfarin, digoxin, and cyclosporine; take on an empty stomach; potential ototoxicity after IV administration of erythromycin
Typical Duration: 7–14 day therapy

Generic Name	Brand Name	Common Strengths	Dosage Forms	Route
azithromycin	Zithromax, Zmax	250 mg, 500 mg, 600 mg, 100 mg/5 mL, 200 mg/5 mL, 1 g	Tablet, suspension, parenteral, powder	IV, PO
clarithromycin	Biaxin	250 mg, 500 mg, 125 mg/5 mL, 250 mg/5 mL	Tablet, suspension	PO
erythromycin base	Ery-tab, PCE Dispertab	250 mg, 500 mg, 1 g	Tablet, capsule	PO

Table 5-11. Tetracyclines

Classification: tetracycline
Mechanism of Action: inhibitor of protein synthesis
Bacterial Effect: bacteriostatic
Spectrum of Action: Gram-positive and Gram-negative
Common Indications: acne, chronic bronchitis
Common Side Effects: upset stomach
Contraindications: children, pregnancy, renal impairment, hepatic impairment
Special Considerations: photosensitivity resulting in sunburn and rashes; may stain teeth; antacids and dairy products should be taken several hours before or after tetracycline therapy (will decrease the effectiveness of the antibiotic); ingesting expired tetracycline can result in kidney damage; expired tetracycline should be discarded appropriately
Typical Duration: Daily; up to 14 days

Generic Name	Brand Name	Common Strengths	Dosage Forms	Route
doxycycline	Vibramycin	50 mg, 75 mg, 100 mg, 25 mg/5 mL	Parenteral, tablet, capsule, suspension	IV, PO
minocycline	Minocin	50 mg, 75 mg, 100 mg	Parenteral, capsule	IV, PO
tetracycline	Sumycin	250 mg, 500 mg	Capsule	PO

Table 5-12. Quinolones

Classification: quinolone
Mechanism of Action: inhibit bacterial DNA synthesis
Bacterial Effect: bactericidal
Spectrum of Action: Gram-positive and Gram-negative
Common Indications: pneumonia, sinusitis, respiratory infections, urinary tract infections, chronic bronchitis
Common Side Effects: nausea, vomiting, joint swelling
Contraindications: myasthenia gravis, patients < 18 years and patients > 60 years
Special Considerations: black box warning: increased risk of tendinitis and tendon rupture; phototoxicity; antacids should be avoided or taken several hours before or after quinolone therapy (may interfere with absorprtion)
Typical Duration: 3–7 day therapy

Generic Name	Brand Name	Common Strengths	Dosage Forms	Route
ciprofloxacin	Cipro	250 mg, 500 mg, 250 mg/5 mL, 500 mg/5 mL	Tablet, parenteral	IV, PO
levofloxacin	Levaquin	250 mg, 500 mg, 750 mg, 250 mg/10 mL, 25 mg/mL, 0.5%	Tablet, parenteral, solution, ophthalmic drops	IV, PO, ophthalmic
moxifloxacin	Avelox, Vigamox	400 g, 0.5%	Tablet, ophthalmic drops	PO, ophthalmic
norfloxacin	Noroxin	400 mg	Tablet	PO
ofloxacin	Floxin	400 mg, 0.3%	Tablet, ophthalmic, otic	PO, ophthalmic, otic

Table 5-13. Ketolide

Classification: ketolide
Mechanism of Action: inhibit protein synthesis
Bacterial Effect: bacteriostatic
Spectrum of Action: Gram-positive, Gram-negative, atypicals
Common Indications: community-acquired pneumonia
Common Side Effects: blurred vision, upset stomach, diarrhea
Contraindications: QT prolongation, hepatic impairment, renal impairment
Special Considerations: life-threatening respiratory failure seen in patients with myasthenia gravis
Typical Duration: 7–10 days

Generic Name	Brand Name	Common Strengths	Dosage Forms	Route
telithromycin	Ketek	400 mg	Tablet	PO

Table 5-14. Aminoglycosides

Classification: aminoglycoside
Mechanism of Action: inhibit bacterial protein synthesis
Bacterial Effect: bactericidal
Spectrum of Action: broad Gram-negative activity
Common Indications: endocarditis, sepsis, immunocompromised patients
Common Side Effects: renal toxicity, neurotoxicity (vestibular and auditory toxicity)
Contraindications: neuromuscular blockage, neurotoxicity
Special Considerations: may prolong the activity of neuromuscular blockers
Typical Duration: dosed every 8–12 hours

Generic Name	Brand Name	Common Strengths	Dosage Forms	Route
amikacin	Amikin	500 mg/2 mL, 1,000 mg/4 mL	Parenteral	IV, IM
gentamicin	Gentak	0.1%, 0.3%, 40 mg/mL	Cream ointment, ophthalmic cream, ophthalmic drops, parenteral	Topical, IV
streptomycin*		1 g	Parenteral	IM
tobramycin	Tobrex	28 mg, 300 mg, 3 mg/mL, 300 mg/4 mL, 300 mg/5 mL, 0.3%	Solution, inhalation, capsule, ophthalmic solution, ophthalmic ointment	IV, ophthalmic, inhaler

*No brand name formulation is currently available.

Table 5-15. Carbapenems and Monobactams

Classification: carbapenem and monobactam
Mechanism of Action: inhibit bacterial cell wall synthesis
Bacterial Effect: bactericidal
Spectrum of Action: Gram-positive and Gram-negative
Common Indications: community-acquired pneumonia, complicated UTI, complicated skin infections, complicated intra-abdominal infections
Common Side Effects: upset stomach, diarrhea
Contraindications: history of seizures, CNS disorders
Special Considerations: sensitivity to beta-lactams or ertapenem
Typical Duration: 7–14 days

Generic Name	Brand Name	Common Strengths	Dosage Forms	Route
aztreonam	Azactam	1 g, 2 g	Parenteral	IV
ertapenem	Invanz	1 g	Parenteral	IV, IM
imipenem and cilastatin	Primaxin	250 mg, 500 mg, 1 g	Parenteral	IV
meropenem	Merrem	1 g	Parenteral	IV

Miscellaneous Anti-Infective Agents

These agents, as outlined in Table 5-16, are used to treat a variety of infections. Proper selection of an agent is determined by an initial accurate diagnosis, the duration of therapy, the need for cost-effective agents, and individual host characteristics, including state of mind. Appropriate selection can maximize the effect of treatment while minimizing side effects and unintended consequences, such as microbial resistance.

Table 5-16. Miscellaneous Anti-Infective Agents

Drug Class	Cyclic Lipopeptide
Mechanism of Action	inhibit DNA and RNA synthesis
Indication	skin infections, complicated gram-positive infections, endocarditis
Side Effects	insomnia, pharyngeal pain, elevated CPK, abdominal pain, hypertension
Example	daptomycin (Cubicin)
Common Strengths	500 mg
Dosage Forms	parenteral
Route	IV
Special Considerations	monitor creatine phosphokinase (CPK)
Drug Class	**Lincosamide**
Mechanism of Action	inhibits protein synthesis
Indication	acne, dental prophylaxis, anaerobic infections, bone infections
Side Effects	jaundice, pseudomembranous colitis, vomiting, diarrhea
Example	clindamycin (Cleocin)
Common Strengths	1%, 2%, 100 mg, 150 mg, 300 mg, 600 mg/4 mL, 900 mg/6 mL
Dosage Forms	gel, solution, suppository, capsule, parenteral, topical, rectal
Route	PO, IV
Special Considerations	reconstituted oral solution should not be refrigerated because it will thicken; IM injection may increase creatine phosphokinase (CPK), should not be used while breastfeeding
Drug Class	**Nitrofuran**
Mechanism of Action	inhibition of bacterial growth
Indication	uncomplicated UTI and UTI prophylaxis
Side Effects	nausea, vomiting, flatulence
Examples	nitrofurantoin (Macrobid, Macrodantin, Furadantin)
Common Strengths	25 mg, 50 mg, 100 mg
Dosage Forms	oral
Route	PO
Special Considerations	may cause urine to turn dark yellow to brown in color

Drug Class	Oxazolidinone
Mechanism of Action	inhibits the initiation of bacterial protein synthesis
Indication	treatment of multi-resistant bacteria, including streptococcus and MRSA
Side Effects	fungal infection, oral thrush, abdominal pain, alterations in taste
Example	linezolid (Zyvox)
Common Strengths	600 mg, 2 mg/mL, 100 mg/mL
Dosage Forms	parenteral, oral
Route	IV, PO
Special Considerations	linezolid is a known MAOI; may cause hypoglycemia

Drug Class	Streptogramin
Mechanism of Action	inhibition of protein synthesis
Indication	complicated skin and skin structure infections
Side Effects	nausea, vomiting, and in rare cases, C. diff-associated diarrhea
Examples	quinupristin and dalfopristin (Synercid)
Common Strengths	500 mg
Dosage Forms	parenteral
Route	IV
Special Considerations	does not contain any antibacterial preservatives; should not be diluted with normal saline; should not be mixed or added to other drugs because of incompatibility issues

Drug Class	Sulfonamide
Mechanism of Action	inhibits folate synthesis, resulting in a bacteriostatic effect
Indication	UTI, respiratory tract infection, pneumocystis pneumonia, toxoplasmosis, MRSA skin infections
Side Effects	nausea, vomiting, rash, diarrhea
Examples	sulfamethoxazole/trimethoprim (Bactrim, Bactrim DS, Septra)
Common Strengths	800 mg/160 mg, 400 mg/80 mg, 200 mg/40 mg
Dosage Forms	parenteral, oral
Route	IV, PO
Special Considerations	contraindicated in patients with sulfite sensitivity

Drug Class	Vancomycin
Mechanism of Action	interferes with bacterial cell wall formation
Indication	pseudomembranous colitis, endocarditis, MRSA
Side Effects	hypotension, itching, flushing, bitter taste, nausea, erythematous rash on face and upper body
Example	vancomycin HCl (Vancocin)
Common Strengths	125 mg, 250 mg, 1,000 mg, 5 g, 10 g
Dosage Forms	capsule, parenteral
Route	PO, IV
Special Considerations	a rate-dependent infusion reaction called Red Man Syndrome (characterized by flushing, erythema, and pruritus and usually affects the upper body, neck, and face) may occur and does not represent an allergic reaction, but rather an idiopathic rate-related infusion reaction

ANTIFUNGAL AGENTS

Antifungal agents, listed in Table 5-17, are used to treat fungal infections, such as athlete's foot and candidiasis (thrush). They can also be used to treat more complicated conditions such as aspergillosis and blastomycosis. Some antifungal drugs are found over-the-counter, while others require prescriptions. Long-term antifungal use requires monitoring of the liver functions and enzymes due to the potential for liver toxicity. Patients with CHF should not use itraconazole due to enzyme inhibition. Therapy may last a few weeks to several months depending on the type of fungal infection.

Table 5-17. Antifungal Agents

Generic Name	Brand Name	Common Strengths/Dosages	Dosage Forms	Route
amphotericin b	AmBisome, Amphocin, Fungizone	50 mg, 100 mg	Parenteral	IV
butenafine	Mentax	1%	Cream	Topical
caspofungin	Cancidas	50 mg, 70 mg	Parenteral	IV
ciclopirox	Loprox, Penlac	0.77%, 1%, 8%	Gel, cream, shampoo	Topical
clotrimazole	Lotrimin *OTC formulation available	10 mg, 1%	Troche, lozenge, cream	Topical, vaginal
fluconazole	Diflucan	50 mg, 100 mg, 150 mg, 200 mg, 10 mg/mL, 40 mg/mL	Tablet, liquid, parenteral	PO, IV
itraconazole	Sporanox	100 mg, 10 mg/mL	Capsule, liquid	PO
ketoconazole	Nizoral	200 mg, 400 mg, 1%, 2%	Tablet, cream, shampoo	PO, topical
miconazole	Monistat 1, Monistat 3, Monistat 7 *OTC formulation available	100 mg, 200 mg, 1,200 mg	Cream	Vaginal
nystatin	Mycostatin	100,000 U	Liquid, topical	PO, topical
terbinafine	Lamisil *OTC formulation available	250 mg, 500 mg	Cream	Topical
terconazole	Terazol	0.4%, 0.8%	Cream	Topical
voriconazole	Vfend	200 mg, 200 mg/5 mL	Tablet, parenteral, suspension	IV, oral

ANTIVIRAL AGENTS

Antiviral drugs, described in Table 5-18, are used to treat viral infections. These drugs prevent the growth of the offending pathogen by inhibiting replication (acyclovir, famciclovir, ganciclovir, valacyclovir), stopping the release of the virus from the cell (oseltamivir, zanamivir), preventing DNA synthesis (cidofovir), or preventing the virus from affecting the cell (palivizumab). Antivirals can be used to treat herpes simplex virus, respiratory syncytial virus (RSV), influenza, HIV, herpes zoster (shingles), and varicella zoster (chickenpox). The length of therapy varies. Patients may require medication daily, for a few weeks, or for months.

Table 5-18. Antiviral Agents

Generic Name	Brand Name	Common Strengths/Dosages	Dosage Forms	Route
acyclovir	Zovirax	200 mg, 400 mg, 800 mg, 5%, 200 mg/5 mL	Capsule, tablet, ointment, suspension	Oral, topical
amantadine	Symmetrel	100 mg, 50 mg/5 mL	Tablet, capsule, solution	Oral
cidofovir	Vistide	75 mg/mL	Parenteral	IV
famciclovir	Famvir	125 mg, 250 mg, 500 mg	Tablet	Oral
ganciclovir	Cytovene, Zirgan	500 mg, 0.15%	Parenteral, gel	IV, topical
oseltamivir	Tamiflu	30 mg, 45 mg, 75 mg, 6 mg/mL	Capsule, suspension	Oral
palivizumab	Synagis	100 mg/mL	Parenteral	IV
valacyclovir	Valtrex	500 mg, 1,000 mg	Tablet	Oral
zanamivir	Relenza	5 mg	Diskhaler	Inhalation

ANTIRETROVIRAL AGENTS

Antiretroviral agents, listed in Table 5-19, are used for the treatment of the human immunodeficiency virus (HIV) and are categorized based on their reaction with HIV replication. **Nucleoside (NRTIs)/nucleotide (NtRTI)** reverse transcriptase inhibitors stop HIV DNA synthesis by attaching to the HIV DNA chain. Side effects of NRTIs and NtRTIs may include anemia, hepatotoxicity, lactic acidosis, lipodystrophy (fat redistribution), and skin rash. **Non-nucleoside reverse transcriptase inhibitors (NNRTIs)** inhibit the conversion of HIV RNA to HIV DNA. These agents may have adverse effects, including hepatotoxicity, lipodystrophy, and skin rash. **Protease inhibitors (PIs)** exert their action by interfering with protease, an enzyme that breaks the HIV virus into small segments. Side effects of protease inhibitors include hepatotoxicity, hyperglycemia, hyperlipidemia, lipodystrophy, osteonecrosis (bone death), and skin rash. A **C-C motif chemoreceptor 5 (CCR5)** inhibitor interferes with the HIV virus's ability to bind to the outer surface of a cell. This class of drug may cause hepatotoxicity. **Integrase inhibitors** block the HIV enzyme integrase; the virus uses the enzyme to help transfer its genetic material into the DNA of infected cells. **Fusion inhibitors** prevent HIV from entering a cell by interfering with the virus's ability to fuse with the cell membrane.

Table 5-19. Antiretroviral Agents

Drug Class and Indication	Generic Name	Brand Name	Common Strengths/Dosages	Dosage Forms	Route
Nucleoside/nucleotide reverse transcriptase inhibitors (NRTI); human immunodeficiency virus (HIV)	abacavir	Ziagen	300 mg, 20 mg/mL	Tablet, oral solution	PO
	abacavir, lamivudine	Epzicom	600 mg/300 mg	Tablet	PO
	abacavir, zidovudine, lamivudine	Trizivir	300 mg/300 mg/ 150 mg	Tablet	PO
	didanosine	Videx, Videx EC	125 mg, 200 mg, 250 mg, 400 mg, 10 mg/mL	Capsule, powder for oral solution	PO
	emtricitabine	Emtriva	200 mg, 10 mg/mL	Capsule, oral solution	PO
	emtricitabine, tenofovir disoproxil	Truvada	100 mg/150 mg, 133 mg/200 mg, 167 mg/250 mg, 200 mg/300 mg	Tablet	PO
	lamivudine	Epivir, Epivir HBV	100 mg, 150 mg, 300 mg, 5 mg/mL, 10 mg/mL	Tablet, oral solution	PO
	lamivudine, tenofovir	Cimduo	300 mg/300 mg	Tablet	PO
	stavudine	Zerit	15 mg, 20 mg, 30 mg, 40 mg, 1 mg/mL	Capsule, oral solution	PO
	tenofovir, emtricitabine	Descovy	25 mg/200 mg	Tablet	PO
	tenofovir disoproxil	Viread	300 mg	Tablet	PO
	zidovudine	Retrovir	100 mg, 300 mg, 10 mg/mL	Tablet, capsule	PO
	zidovudine, lamivudine	Combivir	300 mg/150 mg	Tablet	PO
Non-nucleoside reverse transcriptase inhibitors (NNRTI); human immunodeficiency virus (HIV)	doravirine	Pifeltro	100 mg	Tablet	PO
	efavirenz	Sustiva	50 mg, 200 mg, 600 mg	Tablet, capsule	PO
	etravirine	Intelence	100 mg, 200 mg	Tablet	PO
	nevirapine	Viramune	200 mg, 400 mg, 50 mg/5 mL	Tablet, oral suspension	PO
	rilpivirine	Edurant	25 mg	Tablet	PO

Drug Class and Indication	Generic Name	Brand Name	Common Strengths/Dosages	Dosage Forms	Route
Protease inhibitor (PI); human immunodeficiency virus (HIV)	atazanavir	Reyataz	50 mg, 150 mg, 200 mg, 300 mg	Capsule, oral powder	PO
	atazanavir, cobicistat	Evotaz	300 mg/150 mg	Tablet	PO
	darunavir	Prezista	150 mg, 400 mg, 600 mg, 800 mg	Tablet	PO
	darunavir, cobicistat	Prezcobix	800 mg/150 mg	Tablet	PO
	fosamprenavir	Lexiva	700 mg, 50 mg/mL	Tablet, oral suspension	PO
	indinavir	Crixivan	200 mg, 400 mg	Capsule	PO
	lopinavir, ritonavir	Kaletra	100 mg/25 mg, 200 mg/50 mg, 400 mg/100 mg/5 mL	Tablet, oral solution	PO
	nelfinavir	Viracept	250 mg, 625 mg	Tablet	PO
	ritonavir	Norvir	100 mg, 80 mg/mL	Tablet, oral solution, oral powder	PO
	saquinavir	Invirase	200 mg, 500 mg	Tablet, capsule	PO
	tipranavir	Aptivus	250 mg, 100 mg/mL	Capsule, oral solution	PO
C-C motif chemoreceptor 5 (CCR5) inhibitor; human immunodeficiency virus (HIV)	maraviroc	Selzentry	150 mg, 300 mg	Tablet	PO
Integrase strand transfer inhibitor (INSTI); human immunodeficiency virus (HIV)	dolutegravir	Tivicay	50 mg	Tablet	PO
	raltegravir	Isentress	100 mg, 400 mg	Tablet, powder for oral solution	PO
Fusion inhibitor; human immunodeficiency virus (HIV)	enfuvirtide	Fuzeon	90 mg	Parenteral	PO

CARDIOVASCULAR AGENTS

Table 5-20 reviews commonly used USAN stems for cardiovascular agents.

Table 5-20. USAN Stems for Cardiovascular Agents

Stem	Description	Example
-arone	Antiarrhythmics	amiodarone
-azosin	Prazosin-type antihypertensive	terazosin
-dralazine	Hydrazinophthalazine-type antihypertensive	hydralazine
-lol	Beta blockers	metoprolol
-pril	ACE inhibitor–type hypertensive	lisinopril
-sartan	Angiotensin II receptor antagonist	losartan
-statin	HMG-CoA reductase inhibitor–type antihyperlipidemics	simvastatin
-teplase	Plasminogen activator	reteplase

NOTE

Sublingual nitroglycerin should be kept in the original container and at room temperature away from heat, light, and moisture. Pharmacy technicians may be required to label the medication container along with the prescription vial. Make sure to check with your pharmacist for state-specific requirements.

The **ACE (angiotensin-converting enzyme) inhibitors** prevent the conversion of angiotensin I to angiotensin II. This inhibition results in vasodilation and indirectly inhibits the increase of fluid from aldosterone. Medications in this class end in the suffix "-pril" and include lisinopril (Prinivil, Zestril). Common side effects include hyperkalemia (an increase in serum potassium), a dry hacking cough, rash, and hypotension.

Beta blockers, such as atenolol (Tenormin), block the stimulatory effects of epinephrine by exerting antagonist effects on beta-1 and beta-2 receptors. Medications such as atenolol (Tenormin) are used as antihypertensive agents to reduce the workload of the heart and to reduce blood pressure. Common side effects include drowsiness, weakness, and dry mouth. Caution should be observed in patients with diabetes because these agents have been found to mask symptoms of hypoglycemia.

Calcium channel blockers (CCB) block the entry of calcium into the heart muscle and vessel walls. The conduction of electrical signals depends on the movement of calcium into the cell. A blockage of calcium results in relaxation of the vessel wall, causing dilation of the arteries. The relaxed vessels allow blood to flow easier, thereby lowering blood pressure. Medications that reduce the strength and rate of the heart's contraction include diltiazem (Cardizem) and verapamil (Isoptin, Calan). These drugs are primarily used as antiarrhythmics. Amlodipine (Norvasc) is recommended for the treatment of heart failure due to its vasodilatory effects. CCB side effects include edema, rash, hypotension, and gingivitis. Patients should be advised to avoid concomitant consumption of grapefruit juice to avoid increased serum concentrations of the CCB.

Diuretic agents promote the excretion of salt and water from the kidneys, thus, resulting in an increase in urine production. These agents are generally used to treat hypertension and CHF (congestive heart failure). **Loop diuretics**, including furosemide (Lasix), prevent the reabsorption of chloride and sodium in the loop of Henle. Both thiazide and potassium-sparing diuretics exert effects on the distal convoluted tubules. **Thiazide diuretics**, such as hydrochlorothiazide (Microzide), prevent the reabsorption of sodium, whereas **potassium-sparing diuretics** prevent an excessive loss of sodium ions. Thiazide diuretics may cause photosensitivity, dizziness, blurred vision, and hypokalemia. Potassium-sparing diuretics may cause hyperkalemia, diarrhea, rash, edema, and—in some cases—gynecomastia (an enlargement of breasts in males).

Statins are a class of antihyperlipidemics that inhibit the enzyme HMG-CoA reductase, resulting in decreased cholesterol production. This class includes agents such as atorvastatin (Lipitor) and simvastatin (Zocor). These agents are commonly taken at night when the body produces endogenous cholesterol. Side effects may include muscle pain and weakness, hyperglycemia, rash, flushing, and liver damage.

Thrombolytic drugs are also called plasminogen activators or fibrinolytic drugs due to mechanisms used to dissolve blood clots. These agents activate plasminogen, forming a product called plasmin. This resulting compound is an enzyme that breaks cross-links between fibrin molecules, resulting in the compromised structural integrity of a blood clot.

Table 5-21. Cardiovascular Agents

Drug Class and Indication	Generic Name	Brand Name	Common Strengths/Dosages	Dosage Forms	Route
ACE inhibitor; antihypertensive	benazepril	Lotensin	5 mg, 10 mg, 20 mg, 40 mg	Tablet	PO
	captopril	Capoten	12.5 mg, 25 mg, 50 mg, 100 mg	Tablet	PO
	enalapril	Vasotec, Epaned	2.5 mg, 5 mg, 10 mg, 20 mg, 1 mg/mL	Tablet, oral solution	PO
	fosinopril	Monopril	10 mg, 20 mg, 40 mg	Tablet	PO
	lisinopril	Prinivil, Zestril	2.5 mg, 5 mg, 10 mg, 20 mg, 30 mg, 40 mg	Tablet	PO
	moexipril	Univasc	7.5 mg, 15 mg	Tablet	PO
	perindopril	Aceon	2 mg, 4 mg, 8 mg	Tablet	PO
	quinapril	Accupril	5 mg, 10 mg, 20 mg, 40 mg	Tablet	PO
	ramipril	Altace	1.25 mg, 2.5 mg, 5 mg, 10 mg	Capsule	PO
	trandolapril	Mavik	1 mg, 2 mg, 4 mg	Tablet	PO
Angiotensin II receptor blocker (ARB); antihypertensive	candesartan	Atacand	4 mg, 8 mg, 16 mg, 32 mg	Tablet	PO
	eprosartan	Teveten	400 mg, 600 mg	Tablet	PO
	irbesartan	Avapro	75 mg, 150 mg, 300 mg	Tablet	PO
	losartan	Cozaar	50 mg, 75 mg, 100 mg	Tablet	PO
	olmesartan	Benicar	5 mg, 20 mg, 40 mg	Tablet	PO
	telmisartan	Micardis	20 mg, 40 mg, 80 mg	Tablet	PO
	valsartan	Diovan	40 mg, 80 mg, 160 mg, 320 mg	Tablet	PO
Antiarrhythmic	amiodarone	Cordarone, Pacerone	100 mg, 200 mg, 400 mg, 50 mg/mL	Tablet, parenteral	PO, IV
	digoxin	Lanoxin	125 mcg, 250 mcg, 50 mcg/mL, 100 mcg/mL, 250 mcg/mL	Tablet, parenteral	PO, IV

Drug Class and Indication	Generic Name	Brand Name	Common Strengths/Dosages	Dosage Forms	Route
Beta blocker (BB); antihypertensive	acebutolol	Sectral	200 mg, 400 mg	Capsule	PO
	atenolol	Tenormin	25 mg, 50 mg, 100 mg	Tablet	PO
	bisoprolol fumarate	Monocor, Zebeta	5 mg, 10 mg	Tablet	PO
	carvedilol	Coreg	3.125 mg, 6.25 mg, 12.5 mg, 25 mg,	Tablet	PO
	labetalol	Trandate	100 mg, 200 mg, 300 mg, 5 mg/mL	Tablet, parenteral	PO, IV
	metoprolol succinate	Toprol XL	25 mg, 50 mg, 100 mg, 200 mg	Tablet	PO
	metoprolol tartrate	Lopressor	5 mg, 50 mg, 100 mg	Tablet, solution	PO, IV
	nadolol	Corgard	20 mg, 40 mg, 80 mg	Tablet	PO
	nebivolol	Bystolic	2.5 mg, 5 mg, 10 mg, 20 mg	Tablet	PO
Calcium channel blocker (CCB); antihypertensive, antianginal, antiarrhythmic	amlodipine	Norvasc	2.5 mg, 5 mg, 10 mg	Tablet	PO
	diltiazem	Cardizem, Cardizem SR, Cardizem LA	30 mg, 60 mg, 90 mg, 120 mg, 180 mg, 240 mg, 300 mg, 360 mg, 420 mg, 5 mg/mL	Tablet, capsule, parenteral	PO, IV
	felodipine	Plendil	2.5 mg, 5 mg, 10 mg	Tablet	PO
	nifedipine	Adalat CC, Procardia, Procardia XL	10 mg, 20 mg, 30 mg, 60 mg, 90 mg	Tablet, capsule	PO
	nisoldipine	Sular	8.5 mg, 17 mg, 20 mg, 25.5 mg, 30 mg, 34 mg, 40 mg	Tablet	PO
	propranolol	Inderal LA, Inderal XL	10 mg, 20 mg, 40 mg, 60 mg, 80 mg, 120 mg, 160 mg, 1 mg/mL	Tablet, capsule, parenteral	PO, IV
	sotalol	Betapace, Sotylize	80 mg, 120 mg, 160 mg, 240 mg, 5 mg/mL, 15 mg/mL	Tablet, oral solution, parenteral	PO, IV
	verapamil	Isoptin, Isoptin SR, Calan, Calan SR	40 mg, 80 mg, 100 mg, 120 mg, 180 mg, 200 mg, 240 mg, 300 mg, 360 mg, 2.5 mg/mL	Tablet, capsule, parenteral	PO, IV

Drug Class and Indication	Generic Name	Brand Name	Common Strengths/Dosages	Dosage Forms	Route
Diuretic; antihypertensives	bumetanide	Bumex	0.5 mg, 1 mg, 2 mg, 0.25 mg/mL	Tablet, parenteral	PO, IV, IM
	chlorthalidone	Hygroton	25 mg, 50 mg	Tablet	PO
	furosemide	Lasix	20 mg, 40 mg, 80 mg, 10 mg/mL, 40 mg/5 mL	Tablet, oral solution, parenteral	PO, IV, IM
	hydrochloro-thiazide	Hydrodiuril, Microzide	12.5 mg, 25 mg, 50 mg	Tablet, capsule	PO
	indapamide	Lozol	1.25 mg, 2.5 mg	Tablet	PO
	metolazone	Zaroxolyn	2.5 mg, 5 mg, 10 mg	Tablet	PO
	spironolactone	Aldactone	25 mg, 50 mg, 100 mg,	Tablet	PO
	torsemide	Demadex	5 mg, 10 mg, 20 mg, 100 mg	Tablet	PO
	triamterene	Dyrenium	50 mg, 100 mg	Capsule	PO
Alpha blocker; antihypertensives	doxazosin	Cardura	1 mg, 2 mg, 4 mg, 8 mg	Tablet	PO
	prazosin	Minipress	1 mg, 2 mg, 5 mg	Capsule	PO
	terazosin	Hytrin	1 mg, 2 mg, 5 mg, 10 mg	Capsule	PO
Miscellaneous; antihypertensives	aliskiren	Tekturna	150 mg, 300 mg	Tablet	PO
	clonidine	Catapres	0.1 mg/24 hr, 0.2 mg/24 hr, 0.3 mg/24 hr	Patch	Topical
	hydralazine	Apresoline	10 mg, 25 mg, 50 mg, 100 mg, 20 mg/mL	Tablet, parenteral	PO, IV, IM
HMG-CoA reductase inhibitors; antihyperlipidemics	atorvastatin	Lipitor	10 mg, 20 mg, 40 mg, 80 mg	Tablet	PO
	fluvastatin	Lescol, Lescol XL	20 mg, 40 mg, 80 mg	Tablet, capsule	PO
	lovastatin	Mevacor, Altoprev	10 mg, 20 mg, 40 mg, 60 mg	Tablet	PO
	pitavastatin	Livalo	1 mg, 2 mg, 4 mg	Tablet	PO
	pravastatin	Pravachol	10 mg, 20 mg, 40 mg, 80 mg	Tablet	PO
	rosuvastatin	Crestor	5 mg, 10 mg, 20 mg, 40 mg	Tablet	PO
	simvastatin	Zocor	5 mg, 10 mg, 20 mg, 40 mg, 80 mg	Tablet	PO

Drug Class and Indication	Generic Name	Brand Name	Common Strengths/Dosages	Dosage Forms	Route
Miscellaneous antihyperlipidemics	cholestyramine	Prevalite, Questran, Questran Light	5 mg, 9 mg	Powder	PO
	ezetimibe	Zetia	10 mg	Tablet	PO
	fenofibrate	TriCor, Lofibra	40 mg, 50 mg, 54 mg, 67 mg, 120 mg, 134 mg, 150 mg, 160 mg, 200 mg	Tablet, capsule	PO
	gemfibrozil	Lopid	600 mg	Tablet	PO
	niacin	NIASPAN	100 mg, 250 mg, 500 mg, 750 mg, 1,000 mg	Tablet, capsule	PO
	omega-3-carboxylic acids	Epanova	1,000 mg	Capsule	PO
Thrombolytic agents	alteplase	Activase, Cathflo Activase	1 mg, 100 mg	Parenteral	IV
	reteplase	Retavase	50 mg, 100 mg	Parenteral	IV
	streptokinase	Streptase	250,000 IU, 750,000 IU, 1,500,000 IU	Parenteral	IV
	tenecteplase	TNKase, TNK-tPA	50 mg	Parenteral	IV
	urokinase	Abbokinase	1.5 mg	Parenteral	IV
Miscellaneous agents used to prevent or reduce the risk of blood clot formation	heparin	Hep-Lock	10 U/mL, 100 U/mL, 1,000 IU, 5,000 IU, 10,000 IU, 20,000 IU	Parenteral	IV, SQ
	warfarin	Coumadin, Jantoven	1 mg, 2 mg, 2.5 mg, 3 mg, 4 mg, 5 mg, 6 mg, 7.5 mg, 10 mg	Tablet	PO
Miscellaneous agents used to prevent heart attacks and strokes or for the prevention or treatment of chest pain	acetylsalicylic acid	Bayer Aspirin *Available OTC	81 mg, 325 mg, 500 mg, 650 mg	Tablet, capsule, caplet, gelcap	PO
	clopidogrel	Plavix	75 mg	Tablet	PO
	dipyridamole	Persantine	25 mg, 50 mg, 75 mg, 5 mg/mL	Tablet	PO, IV
	prasugrel	Effient	5 mg, 10 mg	Tablet	PO
	ticlopidine	Ticlid	250 mg	Tablet	PO
Miscellaneous agents used to prevent angina	isosorbide dinitrate	Isordil	5 mg, 10 mg, 20 mg, 30 mg, 40 mg	Tablet	PO
	isosorbide mononitrate	Imdur	10 mg, 20 mg, 30 mg, 60 mg, 120 mg	Tablet	PO
	nitroglycerin	Nitro-Bid ointment, Nitro-Dur, Nitrolingual	0.1 mg/hr, 0.2 mg/hr, 0.4 mg/hr, 0.6 mg/hr, 0.3 mg, 0.4 mg, 0.6 mg	Ointment, patch, spray	Topical, sublingual

TIP

Determining a days supply for creams and ointments may require making estimates. Looking at the package size, application amount, frequency of administration, and application area can help you determine an accurate representation of the days supply.

DERMATOLOGICAL AGENTS

Dermatological agents may be identified by recognizing prefixes and suffixes used in USAN stem names. Table 5-22 lists commonly used stems for dermatological agents that are recognized by the USAN Council.

Table 5-22. USAN Stems for Dermatological Agents

Stem	Description	Example
-cort	Cortisone derivative	hydrocortisone
-olone	Steroids	triamcinolone
-onide	Steroids	fluocinonide
sulfa-	Antimicrobial (sulfonamide derivative)	silver sulfadiazine
-vir	Antiviral	acyclovir

Dermatological agents, such as those listed in Table 5-23, are used to treat a variety of skin conditions, including acne, burns, itching, infections, rashes, and psoriasis. Most agents can be applied topically to the site of the irritation or condition. Topical agents have fewer side effects because they are not absorbed systemically. The effect of the topical agent is contained to the application site. Potential side effects include irritation, dryness, and redness. The drug isotretinoin is an oral acne agent that is reserved for the treatment of cystic acne. It is also a **Risk Evaluation and Mitigation Strategies (REMS)** agent that has restricted prescribing due to the teratogenic effects of the drug. The patient, prescriber, and pharmacy must be registered through the iPLEDGE program, which requires the patient to follow monthly precautions and guidelines.

Table 5-23. Dermatological Agents

Generic Name	Brand Name	Common Strengths/ Dosages	Dosage Forms	Route	Indication
adapalene	Differin	0.1 %	Cream, solution, gel	Topical	Treatment of acne
benzoyl peroxide	Benoxyl, Benzac, Panoxyl	2.5–10%	Lotion, cream, gel	Topical	Treatment of acne
clindamycin	Cleocin	1%	Gel, lotion	Topical	Treatment of acne
clindamycin and benzoyl peroxide	BenzaClin, Duac	1%, 5%	Gel	Topical	Treatment of acne
erythromycin and benzoyl peroxide	Benzamycin	3%, 5%	Gel	Topical	Treatment of acne
isotretinoin	Claravis, Amnesteem, Absorica, Myorisan	10 mg, 20 mg, 30 mg, 40 mg	Capsule	PO	Treatment of acne
tazarotene	Tazorac	0.05%, 0.1%	Cream, gel	Topical	Treatment of acne
tretinoin	Retin-A	0.025%, 0.04%, 0.05%, 0.1%	Cream, gel	Topical	Treatment of acne

Generic Name	Brand Name	Common Strengths/ Dosages	Dosage Forms	Route	Indication
betamethasone dipropionate, clotrimazole	Lotrisone	0.05%, 1%	Cream, lotion	Topical	Treatment of minor skin redness, itching, and swelling
clobetasol propionate	Temovate	0.05%	Cream, ointment	Topical	Treatment of minor skin irritations, rashes, and itching
desoximetasone	Topicort	0.25%	Cream	Topical	Treatment of minor skin irritations, rashes, and itching
fluocinonide	Lidex	0.2%	Cream, ointment	Topical	Treatment of minor skin irritations, rashes, and itching
fluticasone propionate	Cutivate	0.005%, 0.05%	Cream, ointment	Topical	Treatment of minor skin irritations, rashes, and itching
hydrocortisone	Cortaid *Available OTC	0.5%, 1%, 2.5%	Cream	Topical	Treatment of minor skin irritations, rashes, and itching
mometasone furoate	Elocon	0.1%	Cream, ointment	Topical	Treatment of minor skin irritations, rashes, and itching
triamcinolone	Kenalog	0.025%, 0.1%, 0.5%	Cream, ointment	Topical	Treatment of minor skin irritations, rashes, and itching
bacitracin	Baciguent *Available OTC	500 iU/g	Ointment	Topical	Treatment or prevention of an infection of minor skin wounds
mupirocin	Bactroban	2%	Ointment	Topical	Treatment or prevention of an infection of minor skin wounds
neomycin, polymyxin, bacitracin	Neosporin *Available OTC	3.5 mg/5,000 U/ 400 U/1g	Ointment	Topical	Treatment or prevention of an infection of minor skin wounds
acyclovir	Zovirax	5%	Ointment	Topical	Treatment of cold sores
docosanol	Abreva *Available OTC	10%	Cream	Topical	Treatment of cold sores
pyrithione zinc	Head & Shoulders *Available OTC	1%	Shampoo	Topical	Treatment of dandruff
selenium disulfide	Selsun Blue	1%	Shampoo	Topical	Treatment of dandruff

Generic Name	Brand Name	Common Strengths/ Dosages	Dosage Forms	Route	Indication
ketoconazole	Nizoral *Available OTC	2%	Cream, shampoo	Topical	Treatment of fungal infections
terbinafine	Lamisil *Available OTC	1%	Cream	Topical	Treatment of fungal infections
acitretin	Soriatane	10 mg, 17.5 mg, 22.5 mg, 25 mg	Capsule	PO	Treatment of psoriasis
calcipotriene	Dovonex	0.005%	Cream, ointment	Topical	Treatment of psoriasis
pimecrolimus	Elidel	1%	Cream	Topical	Treatment of psoriasis
diphenhydramine	Benadryl *Available OTC	1% (OTC), 2%	Ointment	Topical	Used as an antihistamine for the treatment of rashes, itches, or skin irritations
imiquimod	Aldara	5%	Cream	Topical	Used to treat actinic keratosis
silver sulfadiazine	Silvadene	1%	Cream	Topical	Treatment of infections due to second- and third-degree burns

EARS, EYES, NOSE, AND THROAT AGENTS

Medications in this category treat a variety of conditions and are sometimes referred to as medications pertaining to the senses. Use Table 5-24 to help you recognize common stems used by the USAN Council.

Table 5-24. USAN Stems for Ears, Eyes, Nose, and Throat Agents

Stem	Description	Example
-astine	H$_1$ receptor	azelastine
-olol	Beta antagonists	betaxolol
-onide	Corticosteroid	budesonide

Ears, eyes, nose, and throat agents are used to treat a variety of disease states and symptoms (see Table 5-25). Varying formulations within routes are also available. Proper selection is based on the condition treated. Ophthalmic (eye) and otic (ear) formulations include drops and ointments. Medications for these routes may have anti-infective properties like ciprofloxacin (Ciloxan), may act as histamine blockers like oloptadine (Pataday, Patanol), or may be used to decrease ocular pressure like brimonidine (Alphagan P). Treatment may last a few days for conditions like redness or ear pain. In contrast, infections may require a 7–10 day course of therapy. Patients who have chronic conditions, including glaucoma, must con-

TIP

A pharmacy technician should pay attention to the package quantity input in the pharmacy computer when transcribing the script. Most pharmacy systems ask for the total package size (e.g., 1 g or 5 mL), not the number of units (e.g., 1 box or 1 bottle). Make sure to check with the pharmacist before proceeding.

tinue medications long term. Medications for the nose are used to treat allergy symptoms or nasal congestion. These medications may be taken long term, seasonally, or for a few days. Oxymetazoline (Afrin, Vicks Sinex) is an alpha-adrenergic agonist used to produce vasoconstriction in the nasal arteries, therefore, increasing airflow and reducing nasal congestion. These agents should not be used for more than three to five days because of the possibility of causing rebound congestion. Medications for the throat have anesthetic properties used as needed to treat pain in the oral mucosa and throat.

Table 5-25. Ears, Eyes, Nose, and Throat Agents

Generic Name	Brand Name	Common Strengths/ Dosages	Dosage Forms	Route	Indication
azelastine	Astelin, Astepro	0.1%, 0.15%	Nasal spray	Intranasal	Treatment of allergic rhinitis
beclomethasone	Beconase AQ	168 mcg	Nasal spray	Intranasal	Treatment of allergic rhinitis
budesonide	Rhinocort Aqua	32 mcg	Nasal spray	Intranasal	Treatment of allergic rhinitis
ciclesonide	Omnaris, Zetonna	37 mcg, 50 mcg	Nasal spray	Intranasal	Treatment of allergic rhinitis
mometasone	Nasonex	50 mcg	Nasal spray	Intranasal	Treatment of allergic rhinitis
triamcinolone	Nasacort *Available OTC	110 mcg	Nasal spray	Intranasal	Treatment of allergic rhinitis
fluticasone	Flonase *OTC formulation available	27.5 mcg, 50 mcg	Nasal spray	Intranasal	Treatment of nonallergic rhinitis
oxymetazoline	Afrin, Vicks Sinex *Available OTC	0.05%	Nasal spray	Intranasal	Treatment of nasal congestion
sodium chloride	Ayr, Ocean, Simply Saline *Available OTC	0.65%	Nasal spray	Intranasal	Treatment of nasal congestion
azelastine	Optivar	0.05%	Eye drop	Ophthalmic	Treatment of allergic conjunctivitis
ketorolac	Acular	0.4%, 0.5%	Eye drop	Ophthalmic	Treatment of allergic conjunctivitis
ketotifen fumarate	Alaway, Zaditor *Available OTC	0.025%	Eye drop	Ophthalmic	Treatment of allergic conjunctivitis
loteprednol	Alrex, Lotemax	0.2%, 0.5%	Eye drop	Ophthalmic	Treatment of allergic conjunctivitis
olopatadine	Pataday, Patanol, Pazeo	0.1%, 0.2%, 0.7%	Eye drop	Ophthalmic	Treatment of allergic conjunctivitis

Generic Name	Brand Name	Common Strengths/ Dosages	Dosage Forms	Route	Indication
lodoxamide	Alomide	0.1%	Eye drop	Ophthalmic	Treatment of conjunctivitis
naphazoline	Naphcon-A, Opcon-A, Visine-A	0.025%	Eye drop	Ophthalmic	Treatment of decongestion, ocular vasoconstrictor
betaxolol	Betoptic, Betoptic S	0.25%, 0.5%	Eye drop	Ophthalmic	Treatment of glaucoma
bimatoprost	Lumigan	0.03%	Eye drop	Ophthalmic	Treatment of glaucoma
brimonidine	Alphagan P	0.1%, 0.15%	Eye drop	Ophthalmic	Treatment of glaucoma
brinzolamide	Azopt	1%	Eye drop	Ophthalmic	Treatment of glaucoma
dorzolamide	Trusopt	2%	Eye drop	Ophthalmic	Treatment of glaucoma
erythromycin	Ilotycin Ophthalmic	0.5%	Ointment	Ophthalmic	Treatment of glaucoma
gatifloxacin	Zymar, Zymaxid	0.3%	Eye drop	Ophthalmic	Treatment of glaucoma
gentamicin	Gentak, Garamycin Ophthalmic	0.3%	Eye drop	Ophthalmic	Treatment of glaucoma
latanoprost	Xalatan	0.005%	Eye drop	Ophthalmic	Treatment of glaucoma
pilocarpine	Isopto Carpine	1%, 2%, 4%	Eye drop	Ophthalmic	Treatment of glaucoma
timolol	Timoptic	0.25%, 0.5%	Eye drop, gel	Ophthalmic	Treatment of glaucoma
travoprost	Travatan, Travatan Z	0.004%	Eye drop	Ophthalmic	Treatment of glaucoma
ciprofloxacin	Ciloxan	0.3%	Eye drop, ointment	Ophthalmic	Treatment of bacterial conjunctivitis
moxifloxacin	Moxeza, Vigamox	0.5%	Eye drop	Ophthalmic	Treatment of bacterial conjunctivitis
sulfacetamide	Bleph-10	10%	Eye drop	Ophthalmic	Treatment of bacterial conjunctivitis
tobramycin	Tobrex, AK-Tob	0.3%	Eye drop, ointment	Ophthalmic	Treatment of bacterial conjunctivitis
trimethoprim, polymyxin B	Polytrim Ophthalmic	1 mg/ 10,000 U	Eye drop	Ophthalmic	Treatment of bacterial conjunctivitis
neomycin, polymyxin B, dexamethasone	Dexasporin, Maxitrol	3.5 mg/ 10,000 U/0.1%	Eye drop, ointment	Ophthalmic	Treatment of ocular infections
fluorometholone	FML, FML Forte	0.1%	Eye drop, ointment	Ophthalmic	Treatment of ocular inflammation

Generic Name	Brand Name	Common Strengths/ Dosages	Dosage Forms	Route	Indication
prednisolone	Pred Forte, Pred Mild	0.12%, 1%	Eye drop	Ophthalmic	Treatment of ocular inflammation
ciprofloxacin, dexamethasone	Ciprodex	0.3%/0.1%	Ear drop	Otic	Treatment of acute otitis externa
ciprofloxacin, hydrocortisone	Cipro HC Otic	0.2%/0.1%	Ear drop	Otic	Treatment of acute otitis externa
ofloxacin	Floxin Otic	0.3%	Ear drop	Otic	Treatment of otitis media
acetic acid, hydrocortisone	Acetasol, VoSol HC	1%/2%	Ear drop	Otic	Treatment of external ear infections
hydrocortisone, neomycin, polymyxin B	Cortisporin Otic	3.5 mg/ 10,000 U/1 mg	Ear drop	Otic	Treatment of external ear infections
acetic acid	VoSol	2%	Ear drop	Otic	Removal of wax and debris from the ear
benzocaine	Anbesol, Orabase, Orajel *Available OTC	7.5%, 10%, 20%	Cream, gel	Oral mucosa	Treatment of pain
benzocaine, menthol	Cepacol *Available OTC	10%/2 mg	Lozenge	Throat	Treatment of pain and sore throat
phenol	Chloraseptic	1.4%	Spray	Throat	Treatment of pain and sore throat

ENDOCRINE AGENTS

Review endocrine USAN stems by looking at Table 5-26. These stems identify the most commonly prescribed medications used to treat diabetes mellitus.

NOTE

Insulin is stored in the pharmacy refrigerator prior to being dispensed.

Table 5-26. USAN Stems for Endocrine Agents

Stem	Description	Example
-formin	Hypoglycemic	metformin
-glinide	Meglitinide	repaglinide
-gliptin	Dipeptidyl peptidase-4 inhibitor	saxagliptin
-glitazone	Thiazolidine derivative	rosiglitazone

Diabetes mellitus is a chronic condition resulting from abnormally high levels of glucose. This may be due to an inadequate production of insulin by the pancreas or an inability for the cells to react to the activity of insulin. Diabetes mellitus can be further subdivided into two categories based on these mechanisms. **Type I diabetes** is an autoimmune disease that occurs when there is little to no production of insulin. Treatment for this type of diabetes is based solely on the use of exogenous insulin. In **type II diabetes**, insulin is present, but the cells are not sensitive to its action. This type of diabetes is treated with oral medications with insulin therapy and other injectables reserved for chronic resistance. Acute complications include hyperglycemia (high blood glucose levels) and hypoglycemia (low blood glucose levels). Patients should perform daily glucose testing. Their practitioner should also screen for **HbA1c** (a test to check for the presence of glycated hemoglobin) to assess average blood sugar over a period of three months.

Sulfonylureas, like glimepiride (Amaryl), are used to stimulate insulin secretion from beta cells. This class of medications is noted to cause hypoglycemia and weight gain. α-glucosidase inhibitors, including acarbose (Precose), prevent the digestion of carbohydrates that are turned into simple sugars. Serious side effects include severe stomach pain, constipation, and easy bruising. **Rapid insulin secretors**, such as repaglinide (Prandin), increase the sensitivity of beta cells to elevated blood glucose levels. This class of medications is taken immediately before a meal to reduce postprandial hyperglycemia. **Insulin-sensitizing agents**, such as the thiazolidinediones and biguanides, are also used in the treatment of type II diabetes. These include medications such as pioglitazone (Actos) and metformin (Glucophage), respectively. **Dipeptidyl peptidase-IV (DPP-IV) inhibitors**, such as saxagliptin (Onglyza), are used in addition to diet and exercise and have been shown to improve glucose tolerance and HbA1c. Canagliflozin (Invokana) belongs to a new class of **selective sodium-glucose transporter-2 (SGLT2) inhibitors** indicated as adjunct therapy to diet and exercise.

Hypothyroidism is an endocrine disorder resulting from a deficiency in the production of a thyroid hormone from the thyroid gland. Thyroid levels can be examined by checking T4 (thyroxine tetraiodothyronine) and T3 (triiodothyronine). T4 is actively converted to T3, which accounts for most of the metabolic activity. A deficiency in one or more of these hormones may warrant the initiation of medication. Medications used to treat hypothyroidism target either T4 (e.g., levothyroxine) or T3 (e.g., liothyronine sodium) production. Generally, medications targeting T4 are used because of their longer half-life, leading to once-a-day dosing and the conversion to T3 in the bloodstream. These medications are taken in the morning, 30 minutes before eating. Antacids and medications that contain iron should be avoided because they may interfere with absorption.

Hyperthyroidism is a result of an excess of thyroid hormones due to an overactive thyroid gland. TRH (thyrotropin-releasing hormone) is released from the hypothalamus, which in turn sends a signal to the pituitary gland to release TSH (thyroid-stimulating hormone). This, in turn, signals the thyroid gland to release thyroid hormones T4 and T3. Overactivity of these glands may result in an increase in and potential excessive production of thyroid hormones. The antithyroid medications methimazole (Tapazole) and propylthiouracil (PTU) are used to block the production of thyroid hormones. Patients are monitored for potential agranulocytosis, a condition that occurs due to the suppression of white blood cell production. Table 5-27 lists numerous endocrine agents.

Table 5-27. Endocrine Agents

Generic Name	Brand Name	Common Strengths/Dosages	Dosage Forms	Route	Indication
acarbose	Precose	25 mg, 50 mg, 100 mg	Tablet	PO	Treatment of diabetes mellitus
alogliptin	Nesina	25 mg	Tablet	PO	Treatment of diabetes mellitus
alogliptin, metformin	Kazano	12.5 mg/500 mg, 12.5 mg/1,000 mg	Tablet	PO	Treatment of diabetes mellitus
alogliptin, pioglitazone	Oseni	25 mg/15 mg, 25 mg/30 mg, 25 mg/45 mg	Tablet	PO	Treatment of diabetes mellitus
canagliflozin	Invokana	100 mg, 300 mg	Tablet	PO	Treatment of diabetes mellitus
exenatide	Byetta	5 mcg, 10 mcg	Parenteral	SQ	Treatment of diabetes mellitus
glimepiride	Amaryl	1 mg, 2 mg, 4 mg	Tablet	PO	Treatment of diabetes mellitus
glipizide	Glucotrol	2.5 mg, 5 mg, 10 mg	Tablet	PO	Treatment of diabetes mellitus
glyburide	DiaBeta, Micronase	1.25 mg, 1.5 mg, 2.5 mg, 3 mg, 5 mg, 6 mg	Tablet	PO	Treatment of diabetes mellitus
liraglutide	Victoza	0.6 mg, 1.2 mg, 1.8 mg	Parenteral	SQ	Treatment of diabetes mellitus
metformin	Glucophage	500 mg, 750 mg, 850 mg, 1,000 mg	Tablet	PO	Treatment of diabetes mellitus
metformin, glipizide	Metaglip	2.5 mg/250 mg, 2.5 mg/500 mg, 5 mg/500 mg	Tablet	PO	Treatment of diabetes mellitus
metformin, glyburide	Glucovance	1.25 mg/250 mg, 2.5 mg/500 mg, 5 mg/500 mg	Tablet	PO	Treatment of diabetes mellitus
miglitol	Glyset	25 mg, 50 mg, 100 mg	Tablet	PO	Treatment of diabetes mellitus
nateglinide	Starlix	60 mg, 120 mg	Tablet	PO	Treatment of diabetes mellitus
pioglitazone	Actos	15 mg, 30 mg, 45 mg	Tablet	PO	Treatment of diabetes mellitus
pramlintide	Symlin	60 mcg	Parenteral	SQ	Treatment of diabetes mellitus
repaglinide	Prandin	0.5 mg, 1 mg, 2 mg	Tablet	PO	Treatment of diabetes mellitus
rosiglitazone	Avandia	2 mg, 4 mg, 8 mg	Tablet	PO	Treatment of diabetes mellitus
rosiglitazone, metformin	Avandamet	1 mg/500 mg, 2 mg/500 mg, 4 mg/500 mg	Tablet	PO	Treatment of diabetes mellitus
saxagliptin	Onglyza	2.5 mg, 5 mg	Tablet	PO	Treatment of diabetes mellitus

Generic Name	Brand Name	Common Strengths/Dosages	Dosage Forms	Route	Indication
sitagliptin	Januvia	25 mg, 50 mg, 100 mg	Tablet	PO	Treatment of diabetes mellitus
sitagliptin, metformin	Janumet	50 mg/500 mg, 50 mg/1,000 mg	Tablet	PO	Treatment of diabetes mellitus
levothyroxine	Levoxyl, Synthroid, Tirosint	13 mcg, 25 mcg, 50 mcg, 75 mcg, 88 mcg, 100 mcg, 112 mcg, 125 mcg, 137 mcg, 150 mcg, 175 mcg, 200 mcg, 300 mcg, 500 mcg	Tablet, capsule, parenteral	PO, IV, IM	Treatment of hypothyroidism
liothyronine sodium	Cytomel	5 mcg, 10 mcg, 25 mcg, 50 mcg	Tablet, parenteral	PO, IV	Treatment of hypothyroidism
methimazole	Tapazole	5 mg, 10 mg	Tablet	PO	Treatment of hyperthyroidism
propylthiouracil	PTU	50 mg	Tablet	PO	Treatment of hyperthyroidism

Insulin is used in the treatment of diabetes. Patients with type I diabetes mellitus are unable to produce insulin due to the autoimmune destruction of beta cells in the pancreas. A lack of insulin production leads to a dangerous increase in glucose levels. Exogenous insulin is used to provide glycemic control, reducing microvascular complications and cardiovascular events and also decreasing mortality. A diagnosis of type II diabetes may also warrant the use of insulin to supplement oral antidiabetic therapy (see Table 5-28). Insulin regimens may include a basal (long-acting) insulin given with preprandial (premeal) short-acting or rapid-acting insulin.

Table 5-28. Insulin

Type	Generic Name	Brand Name	Dosage Form	Route
Rapid-acting	insulin aspart	Fiasp	Parenteral	SQ
	insulin aspart	NovoLog	Parenteral	SQ
	insulin glulisine	Apidra	Parenteral	SQ
	insulin human	Afrezza	Oral inhalation	Inhalation
	insulin lispro	Admelog	Parenteral	SQ
	insulin lispro	Humalog	Parenteral	SQ
Short-acting	regular insulin	Humulin R, Novolin R	Parenteral	SQ
Intermediate-acting	NPH insulin	Humulin N, Novolin N	Parenteral	SQ
Long-acting	insulin degludec	Tresiba	Parenteral	SQ
	insulin detemir	Levemir	Parenteral	SQ
	insulin glargine	Lantus, Toujeo	Parenteral	SQ

GASTROINTESTINAL AGENTS

Test yourself on gastrointestinal USAN stem names by covering the descriptions in Table 5-29 with your hand. Review the stems that you do not recognize right away before proceeding.

Table 5-29. USAN Stems for Gastrointestinal Agents

Stem	Description	Example
-prazole	Antiulcer agents (benzimidazole derivatives)	lansoprazole
-setron	Serotonin 5-HT3 antagonists	ondansetron
-tidine	H2-receptor antagonists	famotidine

Gastrointestinal agents are used to treat conditions of the GI tract, including constipation, diarrhea, gastroesophageal reflux (GERD), heartburn, indigestion, nausea, spasms, ulcers, and vomiting. Ulcers can be caused by excess acid production, chronic use of nonsteroidal anti-inflammatory agents, or by the bacteria *Helicobacter pylori*. The most effective way to treat ulcers caused by *H. pylori* is to use drug combinations that include acid-reducing agents and antibiotics. Although most of these medications can be taken orally, intravenous, topical, and rectal formulations are available for patients who require alternative routes (see Table 5-30). Common side effects of the gastrointestinal agents include upset stomach, nausea and vomiting, and headaches.

TIP

Some medications used to treat gastroesophageal reflux are available without a prescription. The pharmacy technician should inform the patient of any OTC medications as noted on his or her prescription. OTC medications may be covered by insurance; coverage should be verified before filling the prescription.

Table 5-30. Gastrointestinal Agents

Generic Name	Brand Name	Common Strengths/Dosages	Dosage Forms	Route	Indication
aluminum hydroxide, magnesium hydroxide	Maalox *Available OTC	200 mg/200 mg/ 5 mL	Liquid	PO	Treatment of heartburn and indigestion
aluminum hydroxide, magnesium hydroxide, simethicone	Maalox Advanced, Mylanta *Available OTC	200 mg/200 mg/ 20 mg/5 mL	Liquid	PO	Treatment of heartburn and indigestion
calcium carbonate	Tums *Available OTC	500 mg, 750 mg, 1,000 mg	Tablet	PO	Treatment of heartburn and indigestion
calcium carbonate, magnesium hydroxide	Rolaids *Available OTC	550 mg/110 mg	Tablet	PO	Treatment of heartburn and indigestion
cimetidine	Tagamet HB, Tagamet *Available OTC	200 mg, 300 mg, 400 mg, 800 mg, 300 mg/5 mL	Tablet, liquid	PO	Treatment of heartburn, indigestion, and ulcers
famotidine	Pepcid AC, Pepcid *OTC formulation available	10 mg, 20 mg, 40 mg	Tablet	PO	Treatment of heartburn, indigestion, and ulcers

Generic Name	Brand Name	Common Strengths/Dosages	Dosage Forms	Route	Indication
nizatidine	Axid AR, Axid *Available OTC	75 mg, 150 mg, 300 mg, 15 mg/mL	Tablet, capsule, liquid	PO	Treatment of heartburn, indigestion, and ulcers
ranitidine	Zantac-75, Zantac-150, Zantac *Available OTC	75 mg, 150 mg, 300 mg, 15 mg/mL, 25 mg/mL	Tablet, liquid, parenteral	PO	Treatment of heartburn, indigestion, and ulcers
metoclopramide	Reglan	5 mg, 10 mg, 5 mg/mL, 5 mg/5 mL	Tablet, solution, parenteral	PO, IV	Treatment of GERD and treatment of chemotherapy-induced nausea/vomiting
dexlansoprazole	Dexilant	30 mg, 60 mg	Tablet	PO	Treatment of GERD and ulcers
esomeprazole	Nexium 24 HR, Nexium *Available OTC	20 mg, 40 mg	Capsule, granule for oral suspension, powder for parenteral administration	PO	Treatment of GERD and ulcers
lansoprazole	Prevacid 24 HR, Prevacid *Available OTC	15 mg, 30 mg	Capsule, powder for parenteral administration	PO, IV	Treatment of GERD and ulcers
omeprazole	Prilosec OTC, Prilosec *Available OTC	20 mg, 40 mg	Tablet, capsule	PO	Treatment of GERD and ulcers
pantroprazole	Protonix	20 mg, 40 mg	Tablet, granule for oral suspension, powder for parenteral administration	PO, IV	Treatment of GERD and ulcers
rabeprazole	Aciphex	20 mg	Tablet	PO	Treatment of GERD and ulcers
sucralfate	Carafate	1 g, 1 g/10 mL	Tablet, liquid	PO	Treatment of active duodenal ulcer
mesalamine	Apriso, Asacol, Canasa, Pentasa, Rowasa	250 mg, 375 mg, 400 mg, 1,000 mg, 4 g/60 mL	Tablet, capsule, suppository	PO, rectal	Treatment of ulcerative colitis
sulfasalazine	Azulfidine	500 mg	Tablet	PO	Treatment of ulcerative colitis
bismuth subcitrate potassium, metronidazole, tetracycline	Pylera	140 mg/125 mg/ 125 mg	Capsule	PO	Treatment of ulcers due to the bacteria *H. pylori*

Generic Name	Brand Name	Common Strengths/Dosages	Dosage Forms	Route	Indication
bismuth subsalicylate, metronidazole, tetracycline	Helidac	262.4 mg/250 mg/ 500 mg	Tablet, capsule	PO	Treatment of ulcers due to the bacteria *H. pylori*
lansoprazole, amoxicillin, clarithromycin	Prevpac	30 mg/1 g/500 mg	Tablet, capsule	PO	Treatment of ulcers due to the bacteria *H. pylori*
misoprostol	Cytotec	100 mcg, 200 mcg	Tablet	PO	Treatment of NSAID-induced ulcers
dicyclomine	Bentyl	10 mg, 20 mg, 10 mg/mL, 10 mg/5 mL	Capsule, tablet, solution, parenteral	PO, IV	Treatment of irritable bowel syndrome
hyoscyamine	Levbid, Levsin, Anaspaz, Cystospaz, Nulev	0.125 mg, 0.375 mg, 0.125 mg/5 mL, 0.5 mg/mL	Tablet, elixir, parenteral	PO, IV	Treatment of gastrointestinal disorders, including spasms
meclizine	Antivert, Bonine *Available OTC	12.5 mg, 25 mg	Tablet	PO	Treatment of motion sickness
dolasetron	Anzemet	50 mg, 100 mg, 20 mg/mL	Tablet, parenteral	PO, IV	Treatment of nausea and vomiting
granisetron	Kytril, Sancuso	1 mg, 3.1 mg/24 hr, 2 mg/10 mL, 1 mg/mL	Tablet, solution, patch, parenteral	PO, topical, IV	Treatment of nausea and vomiting
ondansetron	Zofran, Zofran ODT	4 mg/8 mg	Tablet, film, parenteral	PO, IV	Treatment of nausea and vomiting
prochlorperazine	Compazine	5 mg, 10 mg, 25 mg	Tablet, suppository	PO, rectal	Treatment of nausea and vomiting
promethazine	Phenergan, Promethegan	12.5 mg, 25 mg, 50 mg, 6.25 mg/5 mL, 25 mg/mL, 50 mg/mL	Tablet, syrup, suppository, parenteral	PO, rectal, IV	Treatment of nausea and vomiting
polyethylene glycol 3350	MiraLAX *Available OTC	17 g	Powder for solution	PO	Osmotic laxative
polyethylene glycol electrolyte solution	GoLyte/ GoLytely	2 L, 4 L	Liquid	PO	Bowel preparation
polyethylene glycol electrolyte solution and bisacodyl	HalfLytely	2 L, 5 mg	Liquid	PO	Bowel preparation
docusate	Colace *Available OTC	50 mg, 100 mg	Tablet, capsule	PO	Stool softener
bisacodyl	Dulcolax *Available OTC	5 mg, 10 mg	Tablet, suppository	PO, rectal	Treatment of constipation

Generic Name	Brand Name	Common Strengths/Dosages	Dosage Forms	Route	Indication
lactulose	Enulose, Kristalose	10 mg/10 mg/15 mL	Powder packet, solution	PO	Treatment of constipation
psyllium	Metamucil *Available OTC	500 mg, 0.52 g, 3.5 g, 4.1 g	Capsule, powder	PO	Treatment of constipation
senna	Senokot, Senna-Gen *Available OTC	8.6 mg, 15 mg, 25 mg, 8.8 mg/5 mL	Tablet, syrup	PO	Treatment of constipation
attapulgite	Kaopectate	600 mg/15 mL, 750 mg/15 mL	Liquid	PO	Treatment of diarrhea
loperamide	Imodium, Imodium A-D *Available OTC	2 mg, 1 mg/5 mL	Tablet, caplet, liquid	PO	Treatment of diarrhea
loperamide, simethicone	Imodium Advanced *Available OTC	2 mg/125 mL	Tablet, caplet	PO	Treatment of diarrhea
diphenoxylate, atropine	Lomotil	2.5 mg/0.025 mg, 2.5 mg/0.025 mg/ 5 mL	Tablet, solution	PO	Treatment of diarrhea (C-V)

NOTE

Medications that are used to treat pain are highly regulated. Some states may require double counting procedures, and others may have restrictions on who may count narcotics. Check your state regulations to ensure that you are meeting all requirements.

MUSCULAR, SKELETAL, AND OSTEOPOROSIS MEDICATIONS

Use Table 5-31 to test your knowledge of the USAN stem names for common muscular, skeletal, and osteoporosis medications.

Table 5-31. USAN Stems for Muscular, Skeletal, and Osteoporosis Medications

Stem	Description	Example
-ac	Anti-inflammatory agents (acetic acid derivatives)	diclofenac
-caine	Local anesthetics	lidocaine
-coxib	COX-2 inhibitor	celecoxib
-dronate	Bisphosphonates	ibandronate
-icam	Anti-inflammatory agents (isoxicam type)	piroxicam

Medications in this group treat a wide range of symptoms and diseases (see Table 5-32). Medications for pain are grouped based on their ability to relieve pain, their abuse potential, and their effect (e.g., anti-inflammatory).

Opioid-based medications are scheduled under the Controlled Substances Act. Most of the controlled pain agents are C-II or C-V and are indicated for moderate-to-severe pain. These agents exert their action by binding and interacting with mu (μ) receptors. Dosing schedules for these medications vary and depend on the indication and duration of treatment. The opioid-based agents (e.g., oxycodone, hydrocodone) can cause CNS depression and constipation. The non-narcotic opioids are indicated for mild-to-moderate pain. They have anti-inflammatory effects like the NSAIDs. Non-selective COX inhibitors target COX-I and COX-II and include the drugs ibuprofen or naproxen. Selective COX inhibitors target COX-II and include the drug Celebrex. Adverse effects for these agents include gastrointestinal upset, cramping, ulcers, and headaches.

Medications for the treatment of rheumatoid arthritis can be taken daily, weekly, or monthly. They work by preventing synovial infection due to the inactivation of Tumor Necrosis Factor (TNF). A risk for serious infection is possible while taking agents with a parenteral formulation. Oral rheumatoid arthritis agents can cause gastrointestinal side effects such as nausea, cramping, and diarrhea. Muscle relaxants relieve local skeletal muscle spasms and, in return, can make the user feel drowsy, dizzy, or confused. Drugs that treat osteoporosis can cause stomach ulcers. Patients may be told to take their medication with a full glass of water and remain upright for 30 minutes to lessen the risk of developing a stomach ulcer.

Bisphosphonates are first-line pharmacological agents indicated for the treatment of osteoporosis due to osteoclast-mediated bone loss. They are also prescribed for conditions such as low bone density, multiple myeloma, and Paget's disease. These agents indirectly increase bone density by inhibiting bone resorption. Bisphosphonates should be taken in the morning, 60 minutes before eating or drinking. When taking these agents, the patient should sit in an upright position, drink a full glass of water, and remain in the upright position for 60 minutes as a precaution to avoid esophageal and gastrointestinal side effects. Bisphosphonates are available in daily, weekly, or monthly dosage regimens.

Table 5-32. Muscular, Skeletal, and Osteoporosis Medications

Generic Name	Brand Name	Common Strengths/Dosages	Dosage Forms	Routes	Indication
fentanyl	Actiq, Duragesic, Sublimaze, Onsolis, Fentora	400 mcg, 600 mcg, 800 mcg, 1,200 mcg, 1,600 mcg, 12.5 mcg/hr, 25 mcg/hr, 50 mcg/hr, 75 mcg/hr, 100 mcg/hr	Lozenge, patch, parenteral, buccal film, buccal tablet	PO, transdermal, IV, IM, buccal	Treatment of moderate to severe pain (C-II)
hydrocodone, acetaminophen	Vicodin, Lorcet, Lortab	5 mg/300 mg, 7.5 mg/300 mg, 10 mg/300 mg	Tablet	PO	Treatment of moderate to severe pain (C-II)
hydrocodone, ibuprofen	Vicoprofen	2.5 mg/200 mg, 5 mg/200 mg, 7.5 mg/200 mg, 10 mg/200 mg	Tablet	PO	Treatment of moderate to severe pain (C-II)
hydromorphone	Dilaudid	2 mg, 4 mg, 8 mg, 12 mg, 16 mg, 24 mg, 32 mg, 1 mg/mL, 2 mg/mL, 4 mg/mL, 10 mg/mL	Tablet, capsule, liquid, parenteral	PO, IV, IM	Treatment of moderate to severe pain (C-II)
meperidine	Demerol	50 mg, 100 mg, 50 mg/5 mL, 25 mg/mL, 50 mg/mL, 75 mg/mL, 100 mg/mL	Tablet, solution, parenteral	PO, IV, IM	Treatment of moderate to severe pain (C-II)

Generic Name	Brand Name	Common Strengths/Dosages	Dosage Forms	Routes	Indication
methadone	Dolophine	5 mg, 10 mg, 40 mg, 5 mg/5 mL, 10 mg/5 mL, 10 mg/mL	Tablet, solution, parenteral	PO, IV, IM	Treatment of moderate to severe pain (C-II)
morphine	Roxanol	15 mg, 30 mg, 10 mg/5 mL, 20 mg/5 mL, 1 mg/mL, 5 mg/mL, 10 mg/mL, 50 mg/mL	Tablet, solution, parenteral	PO, IV, IM	Treatment of moderate to severe pain (C-II)
morphine ER	MS Contin, Kadian, Avinza	15 mg, 30 mg, 50 mg, 60 mg, 90 mg, 100 mg, 120 mg, 200 mg	Tablet, capsule	PO	Treatment of moderate to severe pain (C-II)
oxycodone	Oxy IR	5 mg, 10 mg, 15 mg, 20 mg, 30 mg, 5 mg/5 mL	Tablet, capsule	PO	Treatment of moderate to severe pain (C-II)
oxycodone ER	OxyContin	10 mg, 15 mg, 20 mg, 30 mg, 40 mg, 60 mg, 80 mg	Tablet	PO	Treatment of moderate to severe pain (C-II)
oxycodone, acetaminophen	Percocet, Roxicet, Endocet	2.5 mg/325 mg, 5 mg/325 mg, 5 mg/500 mg, 7.4 mg/500 mg, 7.5 mg/325 mg, 10 mg/325 mg, 10 mg/650 mg	Tablet	PO	Treatment of moderate to severe pain (C-II)
oxycodone, aspirin	Percodan	4.8355 mg/325 mg	Tablet	PO	Treatment of moderate to severe pain (C-II)
butorphanol	Stadol	1 mg/mL, 2 mg/mL, 10 mg/mL	Nasal spray, parenteral	Nasal, IV, IM	Treatment of moderate to severe pain (C-IV)
pentazocine, naloxone	Talwin NX	50 mg/0.5 mg	Tablet	PO	Treatment of moderate to severe pain (C-IV)
tramadol	Ultram	50 mg, 100 mg, 200 mg, 300 mg	Tablet	PO	Treatment of moderate to severe pain (C-IV)
baclofen	Lioresal	10 mg, 20 mg	Tablet	PO	Muscle relaxant
cyclobenzaprine	Flexeril	5 mg, 7.5 mg, 10 mg, 15 mg	Tablet, capsule	PO	Muscle relaxant
metaxalone	Skelaxin	800 mg	Tablet	PO	Muscle relaxant

Generic Name	Brand Name	Common Strengths/Dosages	Dosage Forms	Routes	Indication
methocarbamol	Robaxin	500 mg, 750 mg, 100 mg/mL	Tablet, parenteral	PO, IV, IM	Muscle relaxant
orphenadrine	Norflex	100 mg, 30 mg/mL	Tablet, parenteral	PO, IV, IM	Muscle relaxant
tizanidine	Zanaflex	4 mg, 5 mg	Parenteral	IV	Muscle relaxant
carisoprodol	Soma	250 mg, 350 mg	Tablet	PO	Muscle relaxant (C-IV)
acetaminophen	Tylenol	80 mg, 120 mg, 160 mg, 325 mg, 500 mg, 650 mg, 160 mg/5 mL, 80 mg/0.8 mL	Tablet, capsule, suppository, solution	PO, rectal	Treatment of mild to moderate pain
celecoxib	Celebrex	100 mg, 200 mg	Tablet	PO	Treatment of pain and inflammation
diclofenac	Voltaren, Solaraze	25 mg, 50 mg, 75 mg, 100 mg, 1%, 3%	Tablet, gel	PO	Treatment of pain and inflammation
etodolac	Lodine	200 mg, 300 mg, 400 mg, 500 mg, 600 mg	Tablet	PO	Treatment of pain and inflammation
ibuprofen	Motrin, Aleve *OTC formulation available	200 mg, 400 mg, 600 mg, 800 mg, 100 mg/5 mL, 400 mg/5 mL	Tablet, capsule, liquid	PO	Treatment of pain and inflammation
indomethacin	Indocin	25 mg, 50 mg, 75 mg, 25 mg/5 mL	Capsule, suspension, suppository	PO, rectal	Treatment of pain and inflammation
ketorolac	Toradol	10 mg, 15 mg/mL, 30 mg/mL	Tablet, parenteral	PO, IV	Treatment of pain and inflammation
meloxicam	Mobic	7.5 mg, 15 mg, 7.5 mg/mL	Tablet, suspension	PO	Treatment of pain and inflammation
nabumetone	Relafen	500 mg, 750 mg	Tablet	PO	Treatment of mild to moderate pain and inflammation
naproxen	Aleve, Naprosyn *OTC formulation available	250 mg, 375 mg, 500 mg, 125 mg/5 mL	Tablet, suspension	PO	Treatment of mild to moderate pain and inflammation
piroxicam	Feldene	10 mg, 20 mg	Capsule	PO	Treatment of mild to moderate pain and inflammation

Generic Name	Brand Name	Common Strengths/Dosages	Dosage Forms	Routes	Indication
dexamethasone	Decadron	0.5 mg, 0.75 mg, 1 mg, 1.5 mg, 2 mg, 4 mg, 6 mg, 0.5 mg/5 mL	Tablet, suspension, elixir	PO	Treatment of inflammation
methylpredniso-lone	Medrol	2 mg, 4 mg, 8 mg, 16 mg, 32 mg	Tablet	PO	Treatment of inflammation
prednisone	Deltasone, Orasone	2.5 mg, 5 mg, 10 mg, 20 mg, 5 mg/5 mL	Tablet, solution	PO	Treatment of inflammation
adalimumab	Humira	40 mg	Parenteral	SQ	Treatment of rheumatoid arthritis
anakinra	Kineret	100 mg	Parenteral	SQ	Treatment of rheumatoid arthritis
etanercept	Enbrel	50 mg/mL	Parenteral	SQ	Treatment of rheumatoid arthritis
infliximab	Remicade	100 mg	Parenteral	SQ	Treatment of rheumatoid arthritis
leflunomide	Arava	10 mg, 20 mg	Tablet	PO	Treatment of rheumatoid arthritis
methotrexate	Rheumatrex	2.5 mg, 5 mg, 7.5 mg, 10 mg, 15 mg, 25 mg/mL	Tablet, parenteral	PO, IM	Treatment of rheumatoid arthritis
sulfasalazine	Azulfidine	500 mg	Tablet	PO	Treatment of rheumatoid arthritis
lidocaine	Lidoderm	5%	Patch	Topical	Treatment of pain
alendronate	Fosamax	5 mg, 10 mg, 35 mg, 70 mg, 70 mg/75 mL	Tablet, solution	PO	Treatment and prevention of osteoporosis
alendronate, vitamin D	Fosamax Plus D	70 mg/2,800 U, 70 mg/5,600 U	Tablet	PO	Treatment and prevention of osteoporosis
calcitonin	Fortical, Miacalcin	200 U	Nasal spray	Nasal	Treatment and prevention of osteoporosis
ibandronate	Boniva	2.5 mg, 150 mg	Tablet	PO	Treatment and prevention of osteoporosis
risedronate	Actonel	5 mg, 30 mg, 35 mg, 150 mg	Tablet	PO	Treatment and prevention of osteoporosis

Generic Name	Brand Name	Common Strengths/Dosages	Dosage Forms	Routes	Indication
raloxifene	Evista	60 mg	Tablet	PO	Treatment and prevention of osteoporosis in postmenopausal women
teriparatide	Forteo	20 mcg	Parenteral	SQ	Treatment of osteoporosis

REPRODUCTIVE AGENTS

Table 5-33 includes the most common USAN stem name used for reproductive agents. The USAN stem "estr-" indicates that the pharmaceutical agent contains the hormone estrogen. Recall this USAN stem name when identifying hormones used in reproductive agents.

Table 5-33. USAN Stem for Reproductive Agents

Stem	Description	Example
estr-	Estrogens	estradiol

Reproductive agents are most commonly associated with hormone therapy (see Table 5-34). Women are prescribed agents that contain a form of progestin (e.g., medroxyproges-terone) and estrogen (e.g., estradiol) or a combination of both. The progestins are used to treat conditions such as abnormal vaginal bleeding or an overgrowth of the uterus lining. Estrogens, on the other hand, are typically prescribed to regulate hormonal imbalances. Estrogens can be used to treat symptoms of menopause in the treatment of certain breast cancers. Testosterone is prescribed to men to treat symptoms of low testosterone. Typical side effects for reproductive agents include headaches, mood disorders, anxiety, fluid retention, weight gain, and menstrual irregularities.

NOTE

Oral contraceptives comes in quantities of 21 or 28 tablets. Typically, packages that have 21 tablets contain 21 active tablets. Packages that have 28 tablets contain 21 active tablets and 7 placebo tablets. The manufacturer adds the 7 placebo tablets so the consumer remembers to start a new pack after 28 days.

Table 5-34. Reproductive Agents

Generic Name	Brand Name	Common Strengths/Dosages	Dosage Forms	Route	Indication
conjugated equine estrogens	Premarin, Premarin Vaginal Cream, Premphase	0.3 mg, 0.45 mg, 0.625 mg, 0.9 mg, 1.25 mg, 0.625 mg/5 mg, 0.625 mg/g	Tablet, cream	PO, intravaginal	Hormone replacement
conjugated equine estrogens, medroxyprogesterone	Prempro	0.3 mg,/1.5 mg, 0.45 mg/1.5 mg, 0.625 mg/2.5 mg, 0.625 mg/5 mg	Tablet	PO	Hormone replacement
estradiol	Estrace Vaginal Cream, Estrace Vaginal Ring	0.1 mg/g, 2 mg	Cream, ring	PO, intravaginal	Hormone replacement
estradiol	Alora, Climara, Estraderm, Vivelle-Dot	0.025 mg/24 hr, 0.0375 mg/hr 0.05 mg/24 hr, 0.06 mg/hr, 0.075 mg/24 hr, 0.1 mg/24 hr	Patch	Transdermal	Hormone replacement
estradiol	Vagifem	10 mg, 25 mg	Tablet	Intravaginal	Hormone replacement
estradiol, norethindrone	Activella, CombiPatch	0.5 mg/0.1 mg, 1 mg/0.5 mg	Tablet, patch	PO, transdermal	Hormone replacement
estradiol, norgestimate	Ortho-Prefest	1 mg, 1 mg/0.09 mg	Tablet	PO	Hormone replacement
ethinyl estradiol, norethindrone	Femhrt	2.5 mcg, 0.5 mg, 5 mcg/1 mg	Tablet	PO	Hormone replacement
micronized estradiol	Estrace	0.5 mg, 1 mg, 2 mg	Tablet, solution, suspension	PO, IM, SC	Hormone replacement
synthetic conjugated estrogens	Cenestin	0.3 mg, 0.45 mg, 0.625 mg, 0.9 mg, 1.25 mg	Tablet	PO	Hormone replacement
testosterone	Testim, AndroGel, Depo-Testosterone	1%, 100 mg/mL	Gel, parenteral	Topical, IM	Hormone replacement
medroxyprogesterone	Depo-Provera, Depo-SubQ	2.5 mg, 5 mg, 10 mg, 104 mg/0.65 mL, 150 mg/mL	Tablet	PO	Contraceptive
estradiol, norelgestromin	Xulane	35 mcg/150 mcg	Patch	Transdermal	Combination hormonal contraceptive
etonogestrel and ethinyl estradiol vaginal ring	NuvaRing	0.12–0.15 mg/24 hr	Ring	Intravaginal	Combination hormonal contraceptive

Generic Name	Brand Name	Common Strengths/Dosages	Dosage Forms	Route	Indication
levonorgestrel	Kyleena	17.5 mcg	IUD	Intrauterine	Hormonal contraceptive
levonorgestrel	Liletta	20 mcg	IUD	Intrauterine	Hormonal contraceptive
levonorgestrel	Mirena	20 mcg	IUD	Intrauterine	Hormonal contraceptive
levonorgestrel	Skyla	13 mcg	IUD	Intrauterine	Hormonal contraceptive

Common Oral Contraceptives

Oral contraceptives contain varying amounts of estrogen and progestin. Use Table 5-35 below to familiarize yourself with these commonly prescribed agents.

Table 5-35. Common Oral Contraceptives

Active Ingredient(s)	Brand Name
ethinyl estradiol and desogestrel	Apri Cyred Desogen Emoquette Enskyce Isibloom Juleber Reclipsen
ethinyl estradiol and drospirenone	Ocella Syeda Yasmin Zarah
ethinyl estradiol and levonorgestrel	Altavera Aubra Aviane Chateal Falmina Kurvelo Larissia Lessina Levora Lillow Lutera Marlissa Orsythia Portia 28 Sronyx Vienva

Active Ingredient(s)	Brand Name
ethinyl estradiol and norethindrone	Aurovela, Aurovela Fe Blisovi Fe Estrostep Fe Generess Fe Junel, Junel Fe Larin, Larin Fe Layolis Fe Loestrin 21, Loestrin Fe Microgestin, Microgestin Fe Tarina Fe
ethinyl estradiol and norgestrel	Cryselle 28 Elinest Lo/Ovral 28 Low-Ogestrel 28
norethindrone	Camila Errin Heather Jencycla Jolivette Lyza Nora-BE Norlyda Ortho Micronor Sharobel

Emergency Contraceptives

Emergency contraception is a method of birth control that is used to prevent pregnancy after unprotected sex. Often called the morning after pill, an emergency contraceptive pill (ECP) must be taken within a designated period of time following intercourse. This form of contraception works by preventing fertilization due to the inhibition of ovulation.

There are two forms of ECPs available:

- Ella (ulipristal acetate): One pill is taken within five days after unprotected sex.
- Plan B One-Step, Next Choice One-Dose, My Way (levonorgestrel): One pill is taken within three days after unprotected sex.

NOTE

Cough medications that contain codeine are often scheduled as C-V and may have refill limitations, dispensing restrictions, and recordkeeping requirements. These laws vary by state.

RESPIRATORY AGENTS

Use Table 5-36 to review common USAN stems for respiratory agents.

Table 5-36. USAN Stems for Respiratory Agents

Stem	Description	Example
-ast	Antiasthmatics/antiallergics	montelukast
-astine	H_1 receptor antagonists	azelastine
-(a)tadine	H_1 receptor antagonists (loratadine derivatives)	loratadine
-terol	Bronchodilators	albuterol

Respiratory agents (see Table 5-37) are used to treat many conditions, including asthma, chronic obstructive pulmonary disease (COPD), emphysema, colds, and allergies. Medications associated with asthma are given via inhalation through an inhaler or nebulizer. Medications like albuterol work by causing **bronchodilation** (used to expand the airway). These inhalers may be used as "rescue inhalers" to treat acute respiratory distress. Other inhalers are used as maintenance medications to prevent breathing difficulties from occurring. **Leukotriene inhibitors**, like montelukast, stop inflammatory responses by blocking leukotrienes. **Corticosteroids** inhibit inflammatory mediators and are available in both oral and inhalation dosage forms. Inhaled corticosteroids may cause oral candidiasis (thrush), and patients should be instructed to swish and spit after inhaling the medication. Oral corticosteroids may cause weight gain, an increase in facial hair, or even breast development in men with chronic use. Cough and cold agents treat a variety of symptoms. **Expectorants** are used to thin mucus associated with coughs and colds. **Decongestants** are used to treat congestion. Antitussives are used in cough and cold products to relieve dry coughs. These agents are often used in combination to treat multi-cold symptoms.

Table 5-37. Respiratory Agents

Generic Name	Brand Name	Common Strengths/Dosages	Dosage Forms	Route	Indication
montelukast	Singulair	4 mg, 10 mg	Tablet	PO	Prophylaxis and long-term management of asthma
zafirlukast	Accolate	10 mg, 20 mg	Tablet	PO	Prophylaxis and long-term management of asthma
zileuton	Zyflo CR	600 mg	Tablet	PO	Prophylaxis and long-term management of asthma
beclomethasone	Beconase, Qvar	40 mcg, 80 mcg, 168 mcg	Nasal spray, inhaler	Nasal, inhalation	Treatment of allergies, including rhinitis and inflammation
budesonide	Rhinocort	32 mcg	Nasal spray	Nasal	Treatment of allergies, including rhinitis and inflammation
ciclesonide	Omnaris, Alvesco	37.50 mg, 50 mg, 80 mcg, 160 mcg	Nasal spray, inhaler	Nasal, inhalation	Treatment of allergies, including rhinitis and inflammation
fluticasone	Flonase, Veramyst *OTC formulation available	27.5 mcg, 50 mcg	Nasal spray	Nasal	Treatment of allergies, including rhinitis and inflammation
mometasone	Nasonex, Asmanex	100 mcg, 220 mcg	Nasal spray, inhaler	Nasal, inhalation	Treatment of allergies, including rhinitis and inflammation

Generic Name	Brand Name	Common Strengths/Dosages	Dosage Forms	Route	Indication
triamcinolone	Nasacort *OTC formulation available	110 mcg	Nasal spray	Nasal	Treatment of allergies, including rhinitis and inflammation
budesonide, formoterol	Symbicort	80 mcg, 160 mcg	Inhaler	Inhalation	Treatment of allergies and inflammation, bronchodilator
fluticasone, salmeterol	Advair Diskus	100-50 mcg, 250-50 mcg, 500-50 mcg	Inhaler	Inhalation	Treatment of allergies and inflammation, bronchodilator
dexamethasone	Decadron, Dexamethasone Intensol	0.5 mg, 0.75 mg, 1 mg, 1.5 mg, 4 mg, 6 mg, 0.5 mg/5 mL	Tablet	PO	Treatment of inflammation
methylprednisolone	Medrol	4 mg	Tablet	PO	Treatment of inflammation
prednisolone	Orapred, Pediapred	15 mg/5 mL	Solution	PO	Treatment of inflammation
prednisone	(The brand name for prednisone is no longer available in the U.S.)	1 mg, 2.5 mg, 5 mg, 10 mg, 20 mg, 5 mg/5 mL, 5 mg/mL	Tablet, solution	PO	Treatment of inflammation
azelastine	Astelin	137 mcg	Nasal spray	Nasal	Treatment of allergies, antihistamine
cetirizine	Zyrtec *OTC formulation available	10 mg, 1 mg/mL	Tablet, solution	PO	Treatment of allergies, antihistamine
chlorpheniramine	Chlor-Trimeton *OTC formulation available	4 mg	Tablet	PO	Treatment of allergies, antihistamine
desloratadine	Clarinex	5 mg	Tablet	PO	Treatment of allergies, antihistamine
diphenhydramine	Benadryl *OTC formulation available	25 mg	Capsule, tablet, solution, parenteral	PO, IV	Treatment of allergies, antihistamine
fexofenadine	Allegra *OTC formulation available	60 mg, 180 mg	Tablet	PO	Treatment of allergies, antihistamine
hydroxyzine	Vistaril	10 mg, 25 mg, 50 mg, 25 mg/mL, 50 mg/mL	Capsule, parenteral	PO, IV	Treatment of allergies, antihistamine
levocetirizine	Xyzal	5 mg	Tablet	PO	Treatment of allergies, antihistamine

Generic Name	Brand Name	Common Strengths/Dosages	Dosage Forms	Route	Indication
loratadine	Claritin, Alavert *OTC formulation available	10 mg	Tablet	PO	Treatment of allergies, antihistamine
epinephrine	EpiPen, Auvi-Q	0.15 mg/0.15 mL, 0.15 mg/0.3 mL, 0.3 mg/0.3 mL, 2.25%	Parenteral	IM, SQ	Treatment of anaphylactic shock, bronchodilator
aminophylline	Amoline, Aminophyllin	25 mg/mL, 50 mg/mL	Parenteral	IV	Treatment of asthma, bronchodilator
theophylline	Theo-24, Theophylline	100 mg, 200 mg, 300 mg, 400 mg, 800 mg	Capsule, parenteral	PO, IV	Treatment of asthma, bronchodilator
flunisolide	Aerospan HFA	80 mcg	Inhaler	Inhalation	Treatment of asthma, corticosteroid
albuterol	ProAir HFA, Proventil HFA, Ventolin HFA, AccuNeb	90 mcg, 0.63 mg, 1.25 mg	Inhaler, solution	Inhalation	Treatment of asthma, COPD, bronchodilator
formoterol	Foradil	12 mcg	Inhaler	Inhalation	Treatment of asthma, COPD, bronchodilator
levalbuterol	Xopenex, Xopenex HFA	0.31 mg, 0.63 mg, 1.25 mg, 45 mcg	Solution, inhaler	Inhalation	Treatment of asthma, COPD, bronchodilator
salmeterol	Serevent	50 mcg	Inhaler	Inhalation	Treatment of asthma, COPD, bronchodilator
ipratropium	Atrovent	18 mcg	Inhaler	Inhalation	Treatment of COPD, bronchodilator
ipratropium, albuterol	Combivent	103–18 mcg	Inhaler	Inhalation	Treatment of COPD, bronchodilator
tiotropium	Spiriva	18 mcg	Inhaler	Inhalation	Treatment of COPD, bronchodilator
guaifenesin	Robitussin, Mucinex *OTC formulation available	200 mg, 400 mg, 600 mg, 1,200 mg	Solution, tablet	PO	Treatment of cough, expectorant
benzonatate	Tessalon	100 mg, 200 mg	Capsule	PO	Treatment of cough, antitussive
dextromethorphan	Delsym *OTC formulation available	30 mg	Solution	PO	Treatment of cough, antitussive
oxymetazoline	Afrin	0.05%	Nasal spray	Nasal	Treatment of nasal decongestion

Generic Name	Brand Name	Common Strengths/Dosages	Dosage Forms	Route	Indication
phenylephrine	Sudafed PE *OTC formulation available	10 mg	Tablet	PO	Decongestant
pseudoephedrine	Sudafed *Available OTC **Kept behind the pharmacy counter	30 mg	Tablet	PO	Decongestant

NOTE

Women who are pregnant or are of childbearing age should not handle any testosterone reductase agents, including dutasteride and finasteride. Absorption of testosterone reductase agents through the skin may cause fetal abnormalities.

URINARY SYSTEM AGENTS

Urinary system agents are used to treat a variety of conditions ranging from painful urination to the treatment of benign prostatic hyperplasia (BPH). Use Table 5-38 to identify common USAN stem names used in treating these conditions.

Table 5-38. USAN Stems for Urinary Agents

Stem	Description	Example
-afil	PDE inhibitors	sildenafil
-steride	Testosterone reductase inhibitors	dutasteride

The urinary system performs functions related to the removal of waste products and fluid balance maintenance, including electrolyte and pH balances. Medications in this category can be prescribed to relieve urinary difficulty or to treat painful urination (see Table 5-39). Antimuscarinic agents (e.g., tolterodine) prevent bladder contractions and are used to treat overactive bladders and urinary incontinence. **Phosphodiesterase (PDE) inhibitors** (e.g., sildenafil) are used to treat male impotence. They increase blood flow to the penis following sexual stimulation. Patients on PDE inhibitors may experience headaches and should be cautioned of a potential adverse effect called priapism (painful and persistent erection), which constitutes a medical emergency. Men over the age of 50 may experience symptoms of an enlarged prostate, commonly known as **benign prostatic hyperplasia (BPH)**. Symptoms of BPH include painful or limited urination, incomplete bladder emptying, and urgency. Patients may be prescribed an alpha blocker (e.g., tamsulosin), which works by relaxing the muscles of the prostate and bladder.

Table 5-39. Urinary Agents

Generic Name	Brand Name	Common Strengths/Dosages	Dosage Forms	Route	Indication
avanafil	Stendra	50 mg, 100 mg, 200 mg	Tablet	PO	Erectile dysfunction
sildenafil	Viagra	25 mg, 50 mg, 100 mg	Tablet	PO	Erectile dysfunction
tadalafil	Cialis	5 mg, 10 mg, 20 mg	Tablet	PO	Erectile dysfunction
vardenafil	Levitra, Staxyn	2.5 mg, 5 mg, 10 mg, 20 mg	Tablet, orally disintegrating tablet	PO	Erectile dysfunction
alfuzosin	Uroxatral	10 mg	Tablet	PO	Treatment of benign prostatic hyperplasia (BPH)
doxazosin	Cardura	1 mg, 2 mg, 4 mg, 8 mg	Tablet	PO	Treatment of benign prostatic hyperplasia (BPH)
dutasteride	Avodart	0.5 mg	Capsule	PO	Treatment of benign prostatic hyperplasia (BPH)
finasteride	Proscar	5 mg	Tablet	PO	Treatment of benign prostatic hyperplasia (BPH)
tamsulosin	Flomax	0.4 mg	Capsule	PO	Treatment of benign prostatic hyperplasia (BPH)
terazosin	Hytrin	1 mg, 2 mg, 5 mg, 10 mg	Capsule	PO	Treatment of benign prostatic hyperplasia (BPH)
darifenacin	Enablex	7.5 mg, 15 mg	Tablet	PO	Treatment of overactive bladder
oxybutynin	Ditropan, Ditropan XL, Gelnique, Oxytrol	3.9 mg, 5 mg, 10 mg, 15 mg, 10%	Tablet, gel, transdermal patch	PO, transdermal, topical	Treatment of overactive bladder
solifenacin	VESIcare	5 mg, 10 mg	Tablet	PO	Treatment of overactive bladder
tolterodine	Detrol, Detrol LA	1 mg, 2 mg, 4 mg	Tablet, capsule	PO	Treatment of overactive bladder
phenazopyri-dine	AZO Standard, Pyridium *OTC formulation available	95 mg, 100 mg, 200 mg	Tablet	PO	Treatment of painful urination

MISCELLANEOUS MEDICATIONS

Table 5-40 provides additional information on the medications used to treat Alzheimer's disease and Parkinson's disease.

Alzheimer's disease is a progressive disorder that affects memory and cognition. Pharmaceutical drug therapy is focused on two main neurotransmitters: acetylcholine and glutamate, both of which are associated with memory and learning. Medications are aimed at inhibiting the breakdown of acetylcholine in order to improve patient symptoms and outcomes or are aimed at inhibiting the buildup of glutamate. The medications used to treat Alzheimer's disease exert their therapeutic effect by enhancing cholinergic activity (donepezil, rivastigmine, tacrine), by inhibiting acetylcholinesterase (galantamine), by acting as antagonists for the N-methyl-D-aspartate (NMDA) receptor associated with glutamate production (memantine), or by using a combination of pathways to improve cholinergic activity. Common side effects for these agents include dizziness, confusion, diarrhea or constipation, fatigue, and headaches. Alzheimer's medications are indicated for long-term control and treatment.

Parkinson's disease is a progressive neurological disorder that affects movement. Early symptoms include tremors, stiffness, and slowness of movement. They are due to inactivity or a decrease in the neurotransmitter dopamine. Medications used for Parkinson's are aimed at increasing the free levels of dopamine in the body by one of three mechanisms: acting as dopamine agonists (pramipexole, ropinirole), introducing exogenous dopamine (levodopa), or prolonging the effect of levodopa by acting as a catechol-O-methyltransferase (COMT) inhibitor (entacapone). Side effects of these agents may include nausea, orthostatic hypotension, and, in some cases, dyskinesia (involuntary movements resulting from the administration of large doses of levodopa). Patients are slowly weaned off these medications. Medication therapy is long-term.

Table 5-40. Alzheimer's Disease and Parkinson's Disease

Generic Name	Brand Name	Common Strengths/Dosages	Dosage Forms	Route	Indication
donepezil	Aricept	5 mg, 10 mg	Tablet	PO	Treatment of Alzheimer's disease
galantamine	Razadyne	4 mg, 8 mg, 12 mg, 16 mg, 24 mg	Tablet, capsule	PO	Treatment of Alzheimer's disease
memantine	Namenda	5 mg, 10 mg	Tablet	PO	Treatment of Alzheimer's disease
memantine extended-release, donepezil	Namzaric	14 mg/10 mg, 28 mg/10 mg	Capsule	PO	Treatment of Alzheimer's disease
rivastigmine	Exelon	1.5 mg, 2.5 mg, 3 mg, 6 mg, 4.6 mg/24 hr, 9.5 mg/24 hr	Capsule, patch	PO, transdermal	Treatment of Alzheimer's disease
tacrine	Cognex	10 mg, 20 mg, 30 mg, 40 mg	Capsule	PO	Treatment of Alzheimer's disease
benztropine	Cogentin	0.5 mg, 1 mg, 2 mg, 1 mg/mL	Tablet, parenteral	PO, IV	Treatment of Parkinson's disease
carbidopa, levodopa	Sinemet	10 mg/100 mg, 25 mg/100 mg, 25 mg/250 mg, 50 mg/200 mg	Tablet	PO	Treatment of Parkinson's disease

Generic Name	Brand Name	Common Strengths/Dosages	Dosage Forms	Route	Indication
entacapone	Comtan	200 mg	Tablet	PO	Treatment of Parkinson's disease
pramipexole	Mirapex	0.125 mg, 0.25 mg, 0.375 mg, 0.5 mg, 0.75 mg, 1 mg, 1.5 mg, 2.25 mg, 3.75 mg, 4.5 mg	Tablet	PO	Treatment of Parkinson's disease
ropinirole	Requip	0.25 mg, 0.5 mg, 1 mg, 2 mg, 3 mg, 4 mg, 5 mg	Tablet	PO	Treatment of Parkinson's disease
rotigotine	Neupro	1 mg/24 hr, 2 mg/24 hr, 3 mg/24 hr, 4 mg/24 hr, 6 mg/24 hr, 8 mg/24 hr	Patch	Transdermal	Treatment of Parkinson's disease

Attention-deficit hyperactivity disorder (ADHD), as discussed in Table 5-41, is a chronic condition that affects attention and results in hyperactivity and impulsivity. Medications in this category are either classified as stimulants or as nonstimulants. Stimulant drugs (e.g., lisdexamfetamine, dexmethylphenidate) increase the levels of dopamine, which is a neurotransmitter associated with mood, motivation, pleasure, and attention. These agents may cause restlessness, insomnia, loss of appetite, personality changes, and mood swings. There is also a potential for abuse and psychiatric problems, including depression and paranoia. Nonstimulant agents work to increase the levels of the neurotransmitter norepinephrine (atomoxetine). Atomoxetine (Strattera) may cause somnolence, mood swings, and, in some cases, suicidal ideations.

Table 5-41. Attention-Deficit Hyperactivity Disorder (ADHD)

Generic Name	Brand Name	Common Strengths/Dosages	Dosage Forms	Route	Indication
atomoxetine	Strattera	10 mg, 18 mg, 25 mg, 40 mg, 60 mg, 100 mg	Capsule	PO	Treatment of ADHD
guanfacine	Intuniv	1 mg, 2 mg, 3 mg, 4 mg	Tablet	PO	Treatment of ADHD
dexmethylphenidate	Focalin, Focalin XR	2.5 mg, 5 mg, 10 mg, 20 mg	Tablet, capsule	PO	Treatment of ADHD (C-II)
dextroamphetamine	Adderall, Adderall XR	5 mg, 7.5 mg, 10 mg, 12.5 mg, 15 mg, 20 mg, 30 mg	Tablet, capsule	PO	Treatment of ADHD (C-II)
lisdexamfetamine	Vyvanse	20 mg, 30 mg, 40 mg, 50 mg, 70 mg	Capsule	PO	Treatment of ADHD (C-II)
methylphenidate	Concerta, Daytrana, Focalin, Metadate CD, Ritalin, Ritalin LA, Ritalin SR	5 mg, 10 mg, 18 mg, 20 mg, 27 mg, 30 mg, 36 mg, 50 mg, 54 mg, 10 mg/9 hr, 15 mg/9 hr, 20 mg/9 hr, 30 mg/9 hr	Tablet, capsule, patch	PO, transdermal	Treatment of ADHD (C-II)

The treatment of **bipolar disorder** involves a combination of mood-stabilizing drugs (see Table 5-42) and psychotherapy. Several types of bipolar disorder exist. Treatment depends on the diagnosis as well as on the symptoms present. **Schizophrenia** is a complex brain disorder that often results in an altered perception of reality. The selection of appropriate medications is based on the symptoms present. Symptoms are often categorized as positive (symptoms shown in excess, like hallucinations or delusions) or as negative (symptoms that are deficient, like social withdrawal or flat affect). Traditional antipsychotics are an older class of medications that are used to treat only positive symptoms. This class includes medications like fluphenazine and haloperidol, which have a potential to cause tardive dyskinesia (involuntary, repetitive body movements) and extrapyramidal side effects (antipsychotic drug side effects resulting in parkinsonism and abnormal involuntary movement, often referred to as acute dyskinesia). Atypical antipsychotics are used to treat both positive and negative symptoms. Agents in this class include olanzapine and risperidone. These agents cause less extrapyramidal side effects and are generally used more often than traditional agents.

Table 5-42. Bipolar Disorder and Schizophrenia

Generic Name	Brand Name	Common Strengths/Dosages	Dosage Forms	Route	Indication
lithium	Lithobid	150 mg, 300 mg, 450 mg, 600 mg, 300 mg/5 mL	Tablet, capsule, oral solution	PO	Treatment of bipolar disorder
aripiprazole	Abilify	2 mg, 5 mg, 10 mg, 15 mg, 20 mg, 30 mg, 300 mg, 400 mg	Tablet, parenteral	PO, IM	Treatment of schizophrenia
chlorpromazine	Thorazine	10 mg, 25 mg, 50 mg, 100 mg, 200 mg, 25 mg/mL	Tablet, parenteral	PO, IV, IM	Treatment of schizophrenia
clozapine	Clozaril	25 mg, 50 mg, 100 mg, 150 mg, 200 mg	Tablet	PO	Treatment of schizophrenia
fluphenazine	Prolixin	1 mg, 2.5 mg, 5 mg, 10 mg, 25 mg/mL	Tablet, parenteral	PO, IM	Treatment of schizophrenia
haloperidol	Haldol	0.5 mg, 1 mg, 2 mg, 5 mg, 10 mg, 20 mg, 5 mg/mL	Tablet, parenteral	PO, IM	Treatment of schizophrenia
lurasidone	Latuda	20 mg, 40 mg, 60 mg	Tablet	PO	Treatment of schizophrenia
olanzapine	Zyprexa	2.5 mg, 5 mg, 7.5 mg, 10 mg, 15 mg, 20 mg	Tablet, parenteral	PO, IM	Treatment of schizophrenia
paliperidone	Invega	1.5 mg, 3 mg, 6 mg	Tablet	PO	Treatment of schizophrenia
quetiapine	Seroquel	25 mg, 100 mg, 200 mg, 300 mg	Tablet	PO	Treatment of schizophrenia
risperidone	Risperdal	0.25 mg, 0.5 mg, 1 mg, 2 mg, 3 mg, 4 mg, 1 mg/mL	Tablet, oral solution	PO	Treatment of schizophrenia
thiothixene	Navane	1 mg, 2 mg, 5 mg, 10 mg, 20 mg	Capsule	PO	Treatment of schizophrenia
ziprasidone	Geodon	20 mg, 40 mg, 60 mg, 80 mg	Capsule	PO	Treatment of schizophrenia

Gout, which is the focus of Table 5-43, is a form of arthritis caused by an excess of uric acid in the blood. Too much uric acid can cause the formation of crystals in joints, often presenting as pain, stiffness, and swelling. Medications in this category aim at reducing uric acid levels. Uricosuric agents, like probenecid, increase the elimination of uric acid by the kidneys. These agents are contraindicated in patients with uric acid kidney stones and hypersensitivities. The xanthine oxidase inhibitor allopurinol exerts its action by inhibiting the conversion of hypoxanthine to uric acid. Patients should be monitored for the presence of an allergic reaction and the potential for hepatotoxicity. Uricosuric agents and xanthine oxidase inhibitors are used long-term to reduce uric acid levels. Colchicine is indicated for acute flare-ups and may cause gastrointestinal upset.

Table 5-43. Gout

Generic Name	Brand Name	Common Strengths/Dosages	Dosage Forms	Route
allopurinol	Zyloprim	100 mg, 300 mg	Tablet	PO
colchicine	Colcrys	0.6 mg	Tablet, capsule	PO
febuxostat	Uloric	40 mg	Tablet	PO
probenecid*		0.5 g	Tablet	PO

*No brand name formulation is currently available.

The most common class of medications used to treat migraines, as shown in Table 5-44, is the 5-HT1 receptor agonists, often referred to as the "triptans" because they end in the USAN stem "triptan." These agents constrict blood vessels and reduce inflammation by targeting serotonin at the 5-HT1 receptor. These medications are used at the onset of symptoms and may cause asthenia (abnormal weakness), dizziness, and somnolence.

Table 5-44. Migraines

Generic Name	Brand Name	Common Strengths/Dosages	Dosage Forms	Route
acetaminophen, aspirin, caffeine	Excedrin Migraine *Available OTC	250 mg/250 mg/ 65 mg	Tablet, caplet	PO
almotriptan	Axert	6.25 mg, 12.5 mg	Tablet	PO
eletriptan	Relpax	20 mg, 40 mg	Tablet	PO
frovatriptan	Frova	2.5 mg	Tablet	PO
naratriptan	Amerge	1 mg, 2.5 mg	Tablet	PO
rizatriptan	Maxalt	5 mg, 10 mg	Tablet	PO
sumatriptan	Imitrex	5 mg, 20 mg, 25 mg, 50 mg, 100 mg, 6 mg/0.5 mL, 12 mg/mL	Tablet, spray, parenteral	PO, intranasal, SQ
zolmitriptan	Zomig	2.5 mg, 3 mg	Spray	Intranasal

Smoking cessation agents, as discussed in Table 5-45, are aimed at helping patients quit using tobacco. Bupropion exerts its primary effect by inhibiting dopamine reuptake by neuronal cells. The main side effects include insomnia and dry mouth. Bupropion may lower the seizure threshold and should be taken cautiously with other agents that may have similar effects. Varenicline is a nicotine agonist that prevents nicotine stimulation. Neuropsychiatric symptoms, such as depression and suicidal ideations, have been reported. A potential for nausea, seizures, and hypersensitivity is also possible while taking varenicline. Many nicotine replacement products are available over-the-counter. These agents are used to give the body nicotine, thus, reducing withdrawal symptoms. Side effects are usually mild and cease upon cessation of therapy. Pregnant patients and those with a history of cardiovascular disease should consult their physician before initiating therapy.

Table 5-45. Smoking Cessation

Generic Name	Brand Name	Common Strengths/Dosages	Dosage Forms	Route
bupropion	Zyban	75 mg, 100 mg, 150 mg, 200 mg, 300 mg	Tablet	PO
nicotine	NicoDerm CQ, Nicotrol, Nicotrol NS, Nicorette *OTC formulation available	7 mg, 14 mg, 21 mg, 10 mg/mL	Gum, patch, nasal spray	PO, nasal, transdermal
varenicline	Chantix	0.5 mg, 1 mg	Tablet	PO

SUMMARY

☐ Having an understanding of pharmacology is a fundamental component of pharmacy practice.

☐ Drug interactions can occur for a variety of reasons, including as a result of changes in metabolism, absorption, and excretion.

☐ Pharmacy technicians should be able to identify commonly prescribed medications, including the drug class, indication, common strengths, side effects, and duration of therapy.

☐ Drug endings may have similarities within a classification. Memorizing specific prefixes and suffixes may help you remember a drug class or an indication and is a great way to remember medications.

☐ Medication dosing parameters are based on the therapeutic index. Medications with a narrow therapeutic index will require frequent monitoring to ensure that blood concentrations are within therapeutic limits.

☐ Proper storage of medications is crucial to preserve the original potency, to advise about proper adherence, and to maintain safety.

MEDICATIONS PRACTICE QUESTIONS

1. Which of the following medications is a beta blocker used for the treatment of hypertension?

   (A) candesartan
   (B) diltiazem
   (C) lisinopril
   (D) metoprolol

2. Azithromycin is classified as a bacteriostatic anti-infective agent. Which of the following drugs also has bacteriostatic properties?

   (A) cephalexin
   (B) erythromycin
   (C) levofloxacin
   (D) penicillin

3. Medications ending in the USAN approved suffix "-afil" are used to treat _____.

   (A) gout
   (B) hyperlipidemia
   (C) impotence
   (D) osteoporosis

4. A suppository is a solid formulation used for what type of administration?

   (A) intravenous
   (B) oral
   (C) rectal
   (D) topical

5. A branch of pharmacology that refers to the biological and physical effects of the drug on the body is referred to as _____.

   (A) pharmacodynamics
   (B) pharmacokinetics
   (C) pharmacotherapeutics
   (D) pharmacophysiology

6. Which of the following medications does NOT have a formulation that is available over-the-counter?

   (A) acyclovir
   (B) fluticasone
   (C) loperamide
   (D) omeprazole

7. The Controlled Substances Act places medications into one of five schedules based on the drug's medical use, abuse potential, and likelihood to cause dependence. Which of the following medications is classified as a controlled substance under this federal act?

(A) omeprazole
(B) ondansetron
(C) oxazepam
(D) oxybutynin

8. *Helicobacter pylori* is a type of bacteria associated with the formation and/or exacerbation of which of the following disease states?

(A) acne vulgaris
(B) peptic ulcer disease
(C) oral thrush
(D) otitis media

9. Which of the following medications is indicated in the treatment of epilepsy?

(A) lansoprazole
(B) levetiracetam
(C) levofloxacin
(D) lovastatin

10. Antibiotics may have a duration of therapy lasting _____ days.

(A) 30
(B) 21
(C) 15
(D) 10

ANSWERS EXPLAINED

1. **(D)** Metoprolol is a beta blocker, which is indicated by the suffix "-olol." Candesartan is an angiotensin receptor blocker (ARB). Diltiazem is a calcium channel blocker (CCB). Lisinopril is an angiotensin-converting enzyme (ACE) inhibitor.

2. **(B)** Erythromycin is a macrolide antibiotic with bacteriostatic activity. Cephalexin is a cephalosporin antibiotic with bactericidal activity. Levofloxacin is a quinolone antibiotic with bactericidal activity. Penicillin is a bactericidal-type antibiotic in the penicillin class of antibiotics.

3. **(C)** Medications ending in the suffix "-afil" include the phosphodiesterase (PDE) inhibitors and are used to treat male impotence. Medications that treat gout, hyperlipidemia, and osteoporosis do not end in the suffix "-afil."

4. **(C)** A suppository is used for either rectal or vaginal administration. Suppositories may not be injected intravenously, taken orally, or placed topically onto the skin.

5. **(A)** Pharmacodynamics refers to the biological and physical effects of the drug on the body. Pharmacokinetics is a branch of pharmacology that refers to the rate of drug absorption, distribution, metabolism, and excretion. Pharmacotherapeutics is a branch of pharmacology that studies the therapeutic uses and effects of drugs. Pharmacophysiology is a branch of pharmacology that studies the actions of drugs upon living organisms.

6. **(A)** Acyclovir is an antiviral agent with no current over-the-counter formulation available. Fluticasone is available OTC as a nasal spray (Flonase). Loperamide has several oral formulations available OTC as Imodium. Omeprazole is available OTC as Prilosec in a tablet or capsule.

7. **(C)** Oxazepam (Serax) is a Schedule IV substance (in accordance with the Controlled Substances Act) used to treat anxiety. Omeprazole (Prilosec), ondansetron (Zofran), and oxybutynin (Ditropan XL) are not scheduled drugs under the Controlled Substances Act.

8. **(B)** *Helicobacter pylori* is associated with the formation and/or exacerbation of peptic ulcer disease. *H. pylori* is not associated with the formation of acne vulgaris, oral thrush, or otitis media.

9. **(B)** Epilepsy can be treated using levetiracetam (Keppra). Lansoprazole (Prevacid) is indicated for the treatment of gastroesophageal reflux disease (GERD). Levofloxacin (Levaquin) is an anti-infective quinolone-type antibiotic. Lovastatin (Mevacor) is indicated for the treatment of hypercholesterolemia.

10. **(D)** Typical antibiotic therapy lasts 7–10 days.

Federal Requirements

6

KNOWLEDGE DOMAIN 2.0

Federal Requirements **12.50%**

→ Knowledge Area 2.1: Federal requirements for handling and disposal of non-hazardous, hazardous, and pharmaceutical substances and waste

→ Knowledge Area 2.2: Federal requirements for controlled substance prescriptions (i.e., new, refill, transfer) and DEA controlled substance schedules

→ Knowledge Area 2.3: Federal requirements (e.g., DEA, FDA) for controlled substances (i.e., receiving, storing, ordering, labeling, dispensing, reverse distribution, take-back programs, and loss or theft of)

→ Knowledge Area 2.4: Federal requirements for restricted drug programs and related medication processing (e.g., pseudoephedrine, Risk Evaluation and Mitigation Strategies [REMS])

→ Knowledge Area 2.5: FDA recall requirements (e.g., medications, devices, supplies, supplements, classifications)

LEARNING OBJECTIVES

☐ Identify federal laws and regulations that affect pharmacy practice.

☐ Describe labeling requirements for both prescription and over-the-counter substances.

☐ Explain procedures that relate to the ordering, receiving, and documentation of non-controlled medications.

☐ Be familiar with federal guidelines for restricted drug programs and related medication processing.

☐ Describe restrictions placed on the sales of products containing pseudoephedrine.

☐ Understand federal guidelines that govern controlled prescriptions, including refill restrictions, prescription filling, DEA numbers, and transfers.

☐ Understand federal guidelines that surround the receipt, storage, ordering, disposal, removal, and transfer of controlled prescriptions.

PHARMACY LAW

The PTCE follows federal guidelines and regulations. Federal laws take precedence unless the state law is stricter, in which case the state law governs. Pharmacy technicians should check with their State Board of Pharmacy for additional laws that may apply.

Federal laws and regulations have impacted pharmacy practice by protecting patients' well-being and maintaining efforts to ensure the safety and health of all patients. Many of these laws originated from crisis events, which brought attention to the issues of safety and security. These crisis events led to the creation of legislation that would not only provide these safety measures but would also shape reform in pharmacy practice.

Pure Food and Drug Act of 1906

- This act prohibited interstate commerce of misbranded and adulterated drugs, foods, and drinks.
- The focus was on purity, not safety.
- This act did not protect false therapeutic claims.
- Legislation did not require manufacturer labels to list active ingredients, directions for use or warnings, and safety concerns.

Federal Food, Drug, and Cosmetic Act (FFDCA) of 1938

- This act was produced in response to shortfalls of the Pure Food and Drug Act of 1906.
- Enactment of this legislation was hastened in 1937 due to the deaths of over 100 individuals who had consumed a sulfa-based elixir that contained diethylene glycol, a chemical similar to ethylene glycol used in antifreeze.
- This act required drug labeling to include directions for use, warnings, and safety concerns.
- It provided mandates for premarketing approval of all drugs.
- This act ensured that the FDA oversees all provisions and classifies offenses as either misbranded or adulterated. A product may be labeled **misbranded** if it meets any of the following criteria:

  1. The product is misrepresented, which is often seen in labeling (e.g., the omission of important information on the label).
  2. The product does not comply with color additive provisions as established by the FFDCA.
  3. The product is dangerous when used "in the dosage or manner or with the frequency or duration prescribed, recommended, or suggested in the labeling" as per the U.S. Food and Drug Administration, 2017.
  4. The label fails to include the "name and place of business of the manufacturer, packer, or distributor and an accurate statement of the quantity of the contents in terms of weight, measure, or numerical count" as per the U.S. Food and Drug Administration, 2017.
  5. "Any required wording is not prominently displayed as compared with other wording on the device or is not clearly stated" as per the U.S. Food and Drug Administration, 2017.

A product may be labeled **adulterated** if the drug "fails to conform to compendial standards of quality, strength, or purity" as per the U.S. Food and Drug Administration, 1980.

Tables 6-1 and 6-2 list the current drug labeling requirements for prescription and over-the-counter (OTC) drugs, respectively. Figure 6-1 shows an example of an over-the-counter label.

Table 6-1. Prescription Drug Labeling Requirements*

- Highlights
- Limitations statement
- Product name and initial FDA approval date
- Boxed warning
- Recent major changes
- Indications and usage
- Dosage and administration
- Dosage form and strength
- Contraindications
- Warnings and precautions
- Adverse reactions
- Drug interactions
- Use in specialized populations
- Patient counseling information

*From the U.S. Food and Drug Administration, 2007

Drug Facts

Active ingredient (in each tablet)   **Purpose**
Chlorpheniramine maleate 2 mg...Antihistamine

Uses temporarily relieves these symptoms due to hay fever or other upper respiratory allergies: ■ sneezing   ■ runny nose   ■ itchy, watery eyes   ■ itchy throat

Warnings
Ask a doctor before use if you have
■ glaucoma   ■ a breathing problem such as emphysema or chronic bronchitis
■ trouble urinating due to an enlarged prostate gland
Ask a doctor or pharmacist before use if you are taking tranquilizers or sedatives
When using this product
■ drowsiness may occur   ■ avoid alcoholic drinks
■ alcohol, sedatives, and tranquilizers may increase drowsiness
■ be careful when driving a motor vehicle or operating machinery
■ excitability may occur, especially in children
If pregnant or breast-feeding, ask a health professional before use.
Keep out of reach of children. In case of overdose, get medical help or contact a Poison Control Center right away.

Directions

adults and children 12 years and over	take 2 tablets every 4 to 6 hours; not more than 12 tablets in 24 hours
children 6 years to under 12 years	take 1 tablet every 4 to 6 hours; not more than 6 tablets in 24 hours
children under 6 years	ask a doctor

▼

Drug Facts (continued)   ▲

Other information ■ store at 20-25°C (68-77°F)   ■ protect from excessive moisture

Inactive ingredients D&C yellow no. 10, lactose, magnesium stearate, microcrystalline cellulose, pregelatinized starch

*Image courtesy of the U.S. Food and Drug Administration

Figure 6-1. Over-the-counter (OTC) label example

Table 6-2. OTC Drug Labeling Requirements*

- Active drug
- Uses
- Warnings
- Inactive ingredients
- Purpose
- Directions
- Other information, such as storage requirements
- Expiration date
- Batch or NDC number
- Name and address of the manufacturer, packer, or distributor
- Quantity of the product in the package
- Instructions in case of an overdose

*From the U.S. Food and Drug Administration, 2017

The Comprehensive Drug Abuse Prevention and Control Act of 1970

- It is more commonly known as the Controlled Substances Act.
- This law requires registration, recordkeeping, and rules regarding dispensing of controlled drugs.
- Substances are placed into one of five categories called schedules. Table 6-3 lists these different schedules and what types of substances are placed into each.

Table 6-3. Controlled Substances Schedules

Schedule	Description	Example
Schedule I	– High potential for abuse – No legally accepted medical use in the U.S.	– heroin – LSD – peyote – methaqualone
Schedule II	– High potential for abuse – Substances may lead to severe psychological or physical dependence – Legally accepted medical use in the U.S.	– codeine – hydromorphone – methadone – meperidine – oxycodone – fentanyl – amphetamine – methylphenidate – hydrocodone (no more than 15 mg per dosage unit)
Schedule III	– Potential for abuse is less than that of Schedule II drugs – Substances may lead to moderate or low physical dependence and/or high psychological dependence	– buprenorphine – codeine (when used in combination products with no more than 90 mg of codeine per dosage unit) – ketamine – anabolic steroids

Schedule	Description	Example
Schedule IV	– Potential for abuse is less than that of Schedule III drugs	– alprazolam – diazepam – carisoprodol – midazolam – temazepam
Schedule V	– Potential for abuse is less than that of Schedule IV drugs – Contains limited quantities of narcotics	– cough medications with no more than 200 mg of codeine per 100 mL or per 100 g – Robitussin AC – diphenoxylate

REGISTRATION

New pharmacies must first obtain a state license. Facilities that dispense controlled substances register with the DEA by using a **DEA 224 form**. The form can be obtained online or a written form can be requested by contacting the DEA. The certificate of registration should be maintained at the registered location and kept in an accessible place for inspections. Registration is valid for 3 years and can be renewed using a **DEA 224a form** available online. This form can be completed 60 days prior to the expiration date. In the event that the pharmacy needed a duplicate Certificate of Registration form (**DEA 223 form**), the pharmacy can request a copy online, via phone, or via email.

ORDERING, RECEIVING, AND DOCUMENTING REQUIREMENTS

Pharmacies must maintain complete and accurate inventories for all controlled substances, including those purchased, received, dispensed, or otherwise disposed of.

- Schedule II medications may be ordered using a paper **DEA 222 form**, which is a triplicate form that must be handwritten or typed and then signed by the individual who is registered with the DEA. The DEA has also developed the Controlled Substance Ordering System (CSOS), which allows individuals who are registered with the DEA to electronically order controlled substances without using a paper DEA 222 form.
- A maximum of 10 items may be ordered per form. The number of items should match the quantity marked on the bottom of the form. Copy 1 (top copy) is retained by the supplier. Copy 2 (middle copy) is forwarded to the DEA. Copy 3 (bottom copy) is received by the purchaser.
- The DEA 222 form is valid for only 60 days.
- The DEA 222 form should contain the pharmacy's name and DEA number and must be signed by the person who receives and verifies the inventory.

Upon receipt, the purchaser must record the number of items received and the date that they were received. All DEA 222 forms, including those that are incomplete or illegible, should not be thrown away. Instead, they must be maintained in the pharmacy for a minimum of 2 years.

- Schedule II prescriptions should be maintained for a period of 2 years and are filed separately from Schedule III, IV, and V prescriptions.
- Schedule III, IV, and V prescriptions should be maintained for a period of 2 years.

- Schedule III, IV, and V prescriptions may be ordered online, over the phone, or via fax. All invoices should be maintained by the pharmacy, signed, dated, and stamped with a red "C." Invoices must be maintained for a minimum of 2 years.

Prescriptions containing controlled substances, and stock bottles containing controlled substances, may also have a red "C" stamp to visually note the presence of a controlled medication.

INVENTORY AND STORAGE REQUIREMENTS

All controlled substances should be inventoried upon the very first day that the pharmacy opens (the first day of business). Federal law requires a biennial inventory of controlled substances. The inventory record must be kept in a retrievable location and maintained for 2 years.

In regard to storage, federal requirements dictate that all controlled substances must be stored in a securely locked cabinet or dispersed on pharmacy shelves with non-controlled medications. However, many pharmacies will keep C-IIs in a locked cabinet. C-III, IV, and V medications may be placed on pharmacy shelves with other non-controlled medications, but federal law does state that the area must be secure. For this reason, pharmacy doors are locked and only approved personnel are allowed into the pharmacy.

- Inventory counts of Schedule II drugs should be kept separate in a separate file from inventory counts of Schedule III, IV, and V drugs.
- Schedule II drugs must be physically counted; Schedule III, IV, and V drugs can be estimated, unless the bottle contains more than 1,000 tablets or capsules, in which case a physical count is required.

PRESCRIPTION RESTRICTIONS

Schedule II prescriptions may be either written or computer generated, but they must be presented in person at the pharmacy. The prescription is to be signed in ink or should contain a digital signature by the prescribing authority. It must also contain a valid **DEA number**. Institutions are granted an institutional DEA number. Prescribers from that hospital are given an identifier number to be used with the institutional DEA number. DEA numbers are required on all controlled prescriptions.

- DEA numbers consist of 2 letters and 7 numbers.
- The first letter of the DEA number identifies the type of registrant.

  - A/B/F/G: Hospital, clinic, practitioner, teaching institution, pharmacy
  - M: Mid-level practitioner
  - P/R: Manufacturer, distributor, researcher, importer, exporter, reverse distributor, narcotic treatment program
  - G: Department of Defense (DoD) personal services contractor
  - X: Suboxone/Subutex prescribing program

- The second letter is the first letter of the prescribing individual's last name.

Schedule III or IV prescriptions may be handwritten or computer-generated, but they must be signed by the prescriber in ink or must contain a digital signature. They may also be sent electronically. Depending upon state law, they may also be faxed or phoned into the pharmacy.

The use of DEA numbers on non-controlled prescriptions is strongly opposed by the DEA. In 2007, all covered health care providers were required to obtain a unique 10-digit identifier, known as a **National Provider Identifier** or NPI. Covered health care providers and health plans must use the NPI on all administrative and financial transactions, as mandated by HIPAA. NPI numbers are used to process pharmacy claims and are often found on the prescription or prescriber profile.

REFILL RESTRICTIONS

Prescriptions for Schedule II drugs may not be refilled. Schedule III and IV drugs may be refilled up to 5 times within 6 months after the date of issue. Partial fills for Schedule III and IV drugs are irrelevant as long as the total quantity dispensed meets the total quantity prescribed within the 6 month time frame. Each partial fill is recorded in the same manner as a refill. Partial fills (emergency fills) for Schedule II drugs may be dispensed if the pharmacist cannot supply the full quantity for a written or an emergency oral prescription. The pharmacist must note the quantity supplied on the front of the prescription. The remaining quantity must be supplied within 72 hours of the partial dispensing date. A new prescription must be presented for the remaining quantity to be dispensed. The prescribing physician should be notified of any prescriptions not picked up within 72 hours. Prescriptions for Schedule V and non-controlled prescriptions may be refilled as authorized by the prescriber.

TRANSFER RESTRICTIONS

The original prescription for Schedule III, IV, and V drugs may be transferred one time between pharmacies. Pharmacies that share an online database may transfer a Schedule III, IV, or V prescription up to the maximum number of refills as stated on the original prescription.

- All transferred prescriptions must be communicated between pharmacists.
- The transferring pharmacist must write "void" on the front of the prescription and include the name, address, and DEA number of the receiving pharmacy on the back.
- The receiving pharmacist's name should also be noted on the back of the prescription.
- The receiving pharmacist should write "transfer" on the front of the prescription and record the following:

  ○ The original date of issuance for the prescription
  ○ The number of refills
  ○ The original dispensing date
  ○ The number of refills remaining
  ○ The name, address, and DEA number of the transferring pharmacy
  ○ The name of the pharmacist who is receiving the transferred prescription
  ○ The name, address, and DEA number of the pharmacy where the prescription was originally filled (including the original prescription number)

- Both the original and transferred prescription should be filed and maintained for a period of 2 years.

RETURN, DESTRUCTION, AND THEFT REGULATIONS

Controlled substances may be returned between DEA registrants using a DEA 222 form. Outdated or damaged controlled substances may be destroyed using a DEA 41 form. The registrant who is destroying the medication must provide the following:

- His/her DEA registration number, name, and address on the DEA registration, as well as a valid telephone number
- An inventory of the controlled substances that are to be destroyed, including NDC numbers, names, strengths, forms, and quantities
- The date, location, and method of destruction
- The signatures of two witnesses who are authorized employees

The pharmacy can also choose to transfer controlled substances to a DEA-registered reverse distributor who handles the disposal of controlled substances. In the case of a transfer to a reverse distributor, the reverse distributor must issue a DEA 222 form or an electronic equivalent to the pharmacy. If Schedule III–V medications are submitted to a reverse distributor for disposal, the pharmacy must maintain a record of distribution, listing the name, strength, dosage form, quantity, and date of the transfer. The reverse distributor will then complete and submit a DEA 41 form to the DEA.

Upon theft of a medication, the pharmacy must notify both the nearest DEA diversion office and the local police department and then fill out a **DEA 106 form**. The original form is sent to the DEA, and a copy of the form is retained by the pharmacy.

TAKE BACK EVENTS AND UNUSED PRESCRIPTION DISPOSAL

The DEA periodically hosts national prescription take back events in communities where temporary collection sites are set up for the safe disposal of prescription drugs. Additionally, permanent collection sites are also available to DEA-registered collectors. These collection sites are often found in retail pharmacies, hospitals, and law enforcement facilities. These sites may offer mail-back programs or collection receptacles to assist in the collection of unused medications.

Consumers can also read the patient package insert for specific disposal instructions. If disposal instructions are not available, and a collection site is also not available, the following steps are recommended:

- Mix unused medication with an inedible substance, such as coffee grounds, dirt, or cat litter.
- Place the mixture in a sealed container.
- Throw the container in the household trash.
- Delete all personal information on the prescription vial label, and dispose of the container.

The FDA has identified a series of medications that are considered to be potentially dangerous and recommends that they be immediately flushed down the toilet when a take back option is not available. These medications include buprenorphine, diazepam, fentanyl, hydrocodone, hydromorphone, meperidine, methadone, methylphenidate, morphine, oxycodone, and sodium oxybate.

Poison Prevention Packaging Act (PPPA) of 1970

This act was passed in response to a growing number of accidental poisonings involving children. The Poison Prevention Packaging Act approved the U.S. Consumer Product Safety Commission's (CPSC) authority to identify household products and drugs that require child-resistant containers. Tests were performed, and a childproof container was deemed to be acceptable if no more than 20% of children could open the container. Exceptions for child-proof containers were determined for certain products as outlined in Table 6-4.

Table 6-4. Childproof Container Exemptions*

- OTC products available in a single-sized package with the label "This Package for Households Without Young Children" or "Package Not Child-Resistant"
- Powdered, unflavored aspirin and effervescent aspirin
- Sublingual nitroglycerin
- Inhalation aerosols
- Hormone replacement therapy
- Oral contraceptives in the original manufacturer's dispensing package
- Isosorbide dinitrate in dosage strengths of 10 milligrams or less
- Erythromycin ethylsuccinate containing no more than 8 grams or the equivalent of erythromycin
- Erythromycin ethylsuccinate tablets in packages containing no more than the equivalent of 16 grams of erythromycin
- Anhydrous cholestyramine in powder form
- Potassium supplements in unit dose forms, including individually wrapped effervescent tablets, unit dose vials of liquid potassium, and powdered potassium in unit dose packets, containing no more than 50 milliequivalents per unit dose
- Sodium fluoride drug preparations, including liquid and tablet forms, containing no more than 264 milligrams of sodium fluoride per package
- Betamethasone tablets packaged in the manufacturers' dispenser packages containing no more than 12.6 milligrams of betamethasone
- Mebendazole in tablet form in packages containing no more than 600 milligrams of the drug
- Methylprednisolone in tablet form in packages containing no more than 84 milligrams of the drug
- Colestipol in powder form in packages containing no more than 5 grams of the drug
- Pancrelipase preparations in tablet, capsule, or powder form
- Prednisone in tablet form when dispensed in packages containing no more than 105 milligrams of the drug

*As per the U.S. Consumer Product Safety Commission, 2005

RESTRICTED DRUG PROGRAMS AND PROVISIONS

Some medications have special requirements, as mandated by the FDA, to improve patient safety and/or compliance. These requirements limit the way medications are dispensed, prescribed, or purchased. In 2007, the FDA established the Food and Drug Administration Amendments Act (FDAAA), which placed special requirements on identified medications.

The FDA also approved a special restricted distribution program called the **Risk Evaluation and Mitigation Strategies (REMS)** program. An REMS program encourages safe and effective medication use. Medications are selected based on adverse effects, teratogenicity, abuse potential, and the necessity for appropriate dosing to minimize patient risk. The FDA may require manufacturers to submit a REMS program upon drug approval. Selected medications that require a REMS program include buprenorphine, clozapine, fentanyl, hydromorphone, isotretinoin, naltrexone ER, oxycodone, pseudoephedrine, thalidomide, and vigabatrin. Nicotine-containing products and opioids also have REMS initiatives in place. Medications may also be part of a limited distribution program, which generally provides access to specialty medications, insurance assistance, and patient counseling services. REMS programs vary and may include the use of medication guides, communication plans, elements to assure safe use (ETASU), an implementation system, and a timetable for submission of assessments.

Pseudoephedrine-Containing Products

Ephedrine, pseudoephedrine, and phenylpropanolamine are described as "scheduled listed chemical products" under the Controlled Substances Act. This act places restrictions on products that contain ephedrine, pseudoephedrine, and phenylpropanolamine.

- **SALES RESTRICTIONS:** An individual may not purchase more than 3.6 g/day and 9 g/month (a 30-day period) of base product from a retail pharmacy or more than 7.5 g/month of base product from a mail-order pharmacy.
- **STORAGE REQUIREMENTS:** Products must be maintained behind the pharmacy.
- **RECORDKEEPING REQUIREMENTS:** A written or an electronic logbook must be maintained with information pertaining to the product name, quantities sold, patient identifying information (name and address of the purchaser), date, and time of the sale.

Isotretinoin (Absorica, Amnesteem, Claravis, Myorisan)

Isotretinoin is used to treat severe nodular acne and belongs to a class of drugs known as retinoids. Isotretinoin is not used as first-line therapy for the treatment of acne; conventional treatment, including systemic antibiotic therapy, should be initiated first. Isotretinoin is teratogenic and is associated with other potentially serious side effects, including psychiatric disorders. For these reasons, and to minimize fetal exposure, isotretinoin may only be prescribed using an REMS program known as iPLEDGE.

The goals of the iPLEDGE program are to prevent fetal exposure to isotretinoin and to inform prescribers, pharmacists, and patients about the serious risks and safe use conditions for isotretinoin. This program is a computer-based, risk management system that links all members of the health care team (the prescriber, the pharmacy, the patient, and the wholesaler). The key points to remember about the iPLEDGE program are:

- **REGISTRATION:** The prescriber, the pharmacy, the patient, and the wholesaler must be included in the iPLEDGE registry. Patients must complete a consent form that outlines the potential consequences of taking the drug, obtain counseling about the potential risks and requirements for safe use, and comply with all required pregnancy testing.
- **PRESCRIPTIONS:** All prescriptions must be written for 30-day allotments. Prescriptions cannot be faxed, sent electronically, or phoned in. There is a 7-day window, counting the date of a pregnancy test as day 1, to fill and pick up all prescriptions.
- **TESTING AND SAFETY:** Female patients of childbearing potential must have had two negative urine or serum pregnancy tests before they can receive the prescription. The patient must have also used two forms of birth control for at least one month prior to initiation of isotretinoin therapy, during isotretinoin therapy, and for one month after isotretinoin therapy.
- **REPORTING:** Mandatory quarterly reporting of all isotretinoin adverse side effects is required, including all deaths within 15 days of the incident.

PATIENT PACKAGE INSERTS AND MEDICATION GUIDES

Manufacturers must provide patient package inserts and medication guides for drugs deemed to have serious and significant risks. These written guides and inserts must be given to patients. They inform patients about the risks and benefits of the prescription medications.

Patient package inserts, or PPIs, are written summaries of patient information about specific risks and benefits. PPIs are based on the FDA-approved package insert. This insert provides clinical information about the drug and is written in consumer-friendly terminology. The FDA mandates that certain classes of medications, such as estrogen-containing medications and oral contraceptives, include PPIs. In 2006, the FDA made a revision stating that all PPIs must also include a table of contents and a summary section that highlights the benefits and risks.

Medication guides are another form of written patient information. Medication guides address issues specific to particular drugs and drug classes. They contain FDA-approved information that can help patients avoid serious adverse events.

RECALLS

The Food and Drug Administration defines a drug recall as either an involuntary or a voluntary effort to remove a product from the market. The recall may be conducted by the drug manufacturer, by request of the FDA, or by a regulatory agency authorized by the FDA.

Recalls are classified by severity into three groups as shown in Table 6-5.

Table 6-5. Recall Classifications

Recall Category	Description	Example
Class I Recall	Involves violative products that are likely to cause serious adverse health consequences or death	- Label mix-up on a life-saving medication - For example, in 2008, heparin was recalled due to heparin contamination with oversulfated chondroitin sulfate.
Class II Recall	Involves violative products that may cause temporary health issues or where the probability of serious adverse health consequences is remote	- The presence of particles in a medication container - For example, in 2010, ketorolac was recalled due to the presence of small particles in the medication vial.
Class III Recall	Involves violative products that are not likely to cause adverse health consequences	- Packaging issues or defective delivery devices - For example, in 2008, many fentanyl 75 mcg pain patches were recalled because the patch was leaking active drug.

The FDA may take other actions including an FDA market withdrawal or an FDA medical device safety alert. In an FDA market withdrawal, a withdrawal is issued for a product that has a minor violation that would not warrant legal action. For example, a product may be withdrawn due to tampering without proof of manufacturing or distribution problems. In contrast, an FDA medical device safety alert is when a recall is issued for a medical device that may present an unreasonable risk of substantial harm.

HANDLING AND DISPOSAL OF NON-HAZARDOUS, HAZARDOUS, AND PHARMACEUTICAL SUBSTANCES AND WASTE

Medications are made of chemical compounds that not only affect the patient when used or taken, but also can have effects on the people that handle them. Caution must be taken to avoid absorption of a liquid through the skin or inhalation of dust; hazardous compounds can burn through the skin, and some medications cause teratogenic effects when taken. Personnel handling hazardous substances should use a minimum of two pairs of gloves. In the pharmacy, medication waste consists of medications that are unused, expired, or can no longer be used for the intended purpose. Medications that are returned to stock and medications that are sent to a reverse distributor are not included in this definition.

Non-Hazardous Substances

Non-hazardous waste, which includes the majority of pharmacy substances and medications, can be disposed of in designated bins, usually those that are blue or white, or in regular trash if it will be incinerated. The removal of this waste is typically handled by using a reverse distributor. IV fluids, such as lactated Ringer's, dextrose, and saline, may be poured down the drain. However, this practice is widely dependent on state laws and hospital policies.

Hazardous Substances

Disposal of pharmaceutical waste must meet all state and federal guidelines according to the U.S. Environmental Protection Agency (EPA). Hazardous waste can either be categorized into one of four categories (P, U, K, or F)—as listed in the Resource Conservation and Recovery Act—or be categorized as meeting a hazardous waste characteristic. These characteristics include ignitability, corrosivity, reactivity, and toxicity. Pharmaceutical wastes can be found on both P and U lists, as well as on characteristic lists:

- **EXAMPLES OF P-LIST WASTE:** epinephrine, nicotine patches, nitroglycerin, phentermine, physostigmine, and warfarin >0.3%
- **EXAMPLES OF U-LIST WASTE:** chlorambucil, cyclophosphamide, lindane, mercury, reserpine, selenium sulfide, and warfarin < 0.3%
- **EXAMPLES OF CHARACTERISTIC WASTE:** erythromycin gel 2% (ignitable), lindane (toxic), paclitaxel injections (toxic), selenium sulfide (toxic), silver nitrate applicators (ignitable), and thiomersal-containing drugs (toxic)

Chemotherapy agents are not listed under the EPA category list of hazardous drugs but are typically disposed as such and placed in yellow bins.

Pharmacies that prepare hazardous drugs must have a negative pressure room to house engineering controls. These controls are to be used for hazardous preparations only and are separate from the controls used for non-hazardous preparations. Approved biological safety cabinets are used for the preparation of hazardous medications. The OSHA recommends using only vertical laminar flow hoods. Any items in a spill cleanup kit that come in contact with hazardous waste must also be considered hazardous and disposed of properly.

Safety data sheets (SDS), which are written by the manufacturer, provide information about hazardous chemicals, including the associated hazards, proper handling and cleanup procedures, and proper selection of personal protective equipment (PPE). The SDS are maintained near the designated compounding area, or near designated hazardous chemicals, and should be consulted in case of accidental exposure. An initial incident report (IIR) may be used by the facility to document the exposure. SDS information is classified into 16 universal categories, as shown in Table 6-6.

Table 6-6. Safety Data Sheet Components[*]

1. Identification
2. Hazard(s) Identification
3. Composition/Information on Ingredients
4. First-Aid Measures
5. Fire-Fighting Measures
6. Accidental Release Measures
7. Handling and Storage
8. Exposure Controls/Personal Protection
9. Physical and Chemical Properties
10. Stability and Reactivity
11. Toxicological Information
12. Ecological Information (non-mandatory)
13. Disposal Considerations (non-mandatory)
14. Transport Information (non-mandatory)
15. Regulatory Information (non-mandatory)
16. Other Information

[*]From the U.S. Department of Labor

Hospitals typically employ the use of an outside hazardous waste vendor to assist in managing waste generated in the pharmacy. The vendor must be licensed by the EPA to transport hazardous wastes. Hazardous wastes must be properly stored in black, or other designated, waste bins until the vendor arrives and picks the waste up for removal. If hazardous wastes are mixed, the most restrictive requirements must be followed for disposal. Hazardous waste vendors can also take controlled substances if the vendor is registered with the DEA. A DEA 222 form must be used to document the transfer of C-II substances, while a detailed inventory log is used to document the transfer of C-III–C-V substances.

SUMMARY

☐ Restrictions on the use of medications vary. Pharmacy personnel should check their pharmacy policies and procedures, SDS, and REMS for information about the proper usage and distribution of these medications.

☐ Controlled medications are regulated by the DEA, and, as such, there are strict guidelines for controlled prescriptions.

☐ Controlled substance schedules are based on the substance's abuse potential and legal status.

☐ The handling and disposal of pharmaceutical compounds is critical and may vary based on the classification of the substance.

☐ Pharmacy technicians should be aware of state regulations, pharmacy policies and procedures, EPA guidelines, and SDS provisions when handling hazardous chemicals.

FEDERAL REQUIREMENTS PRACTICE QUESTIONS

1. Which copy of the triplicate DEA 222 form does the purchaser retain?

    (A) copy 1 (top copy)
    (B) copy 2 (middle copy)
    (C) copy 3 (bottom copy)
    (D) All copies are forwarded to the DEA.

2. Which of the following statements is true regarding prescription refills?

    (A) Schedule II prescriptions can be refilled up to 5 times in 6 months.
    (B) Schedule III prescriptions can be refilled up to 5 times in 6 months.
    (C) Schedule II prescriptions can be refilled for up to 1 year.
    (D) Schedule III prescriptions can be refilled for up to 1 year.

3. According to federal law, how long must Schedule III, IV, and V invoices be maintained in the pharmacy?

    (A) 1 year
    (B) 2 years
    (C) 3 years
    (D) 4 years

4. Which of the following is an example of a misbranded drug?

    (A) The OTC product label is missing potential drug warnings.
    (B) The drug was manufactured in an unsanitary facility.
    (C) The drug leaves the pharmacy and is then redispensed.
    (D) The bottle contents are outdated.

5. Oxycodone is an example of a drug that falls into which of the following controlled substance schedules?

    (A) Schedule I
    (B) Schedule II
    (C) Schedule III
    (D) Schedule IV

6. Which regulation was prompted, in part, due to the deaths of over 100 individuals as a result of the addition of diethylene glycol to a sulfa-based elixir?

   (A) Federal Food, Drug, and Cosmetic Act of 1938
   (B) Health Insurance Portability and Accountability Act of 1996
   (C) Comprehensive Drug Abuse Prevention and Control Act of 1970
   (D) Poison Prevention Packaging Act of 1970

7. Which DEA form should be filled out in the event of a theft of a Schedule II substance?

   (A) DEA 222
   (B) DEA 41
   (C) DEA 106
   (D) No form is needed.

8. Schedule II substances may be ordered electronically using which DEA-based web system?

   (A) Controlled Substances Ordered Online (CSOO)
   (B) Controlled Substance Ordering System (CSOS)
   (C) Controlled Substance Ordered Direct (CSOD)
   (D) Controlled Substance Ordering Program (CSOP)

9. What does REMS stand for?

   (A) Risk Evaluation and Mitigation Strategies
   (B) Risk Effort and Medical Strategies
   (C) Return Effect and Manipulation Systems
   (D) Recovery Evaluation and Master Strategies

10. Which of the following drugs is identified as a P-list substance by the EPA?

   (A) normal saline
   (B) metoprolol (Toprol XL)
   (C) warfarin (Coumadin)
   (D) amoxicillin (Amoxil)

ANSWERS EXPLAINED

1. **(C)** Copy 3 (bottom copy) is retained by the purchaser. The only copy that is forwarded to the DEA is copy 2.

2. **(B)** Schedule III prescriptions may be refilled up to 5 times in 6 months. Schedule II prescriptions cannot be refilled.

3. **(B)** Federal law mandates that Schedule III, IV, and V invoices be maintained in the pharmacy for a minimum of 2 years.

4. **(A)** The omission of potential drug warnings is an example of misbranding. The production of a drug in unsanitary conditions is an example of adulteration. Drugs that are redispensed after leaving the pharmacy or are outdated are considered adulterated.

5. **(B)** Oxycodone is classified as a Schedule II drug as defined by the Controlled Substances Act. Schedule I drugs do not have any legal medical use in the United States.

6. **(A)** The Federal Food, Drug, and Cosmetic Act of 1938 was prompted, in part, by the deaths of over 100 individuals who took a sulfa-based elixir that contained diethylene glycol, an ingredient found in antifreeze. The Health Insurance Portability and Accountability Act of 1996 was enacted to place privacy safeguards on all protected health information (PHI). The Comprehensive Drug Abuse Prevention and Control Act of 1970 placed controlled substances into one of five schedules based on each substance's abuse potential and legal status. The Poison Prevention Packaging Act of 1970 was enacted in response to a growing number of accidental poisonings in children.

7. **(C)** A DEA 106 form must be filled out in the event of a theft of a Schedule II substance. Schedule II substances are controlled. Therefore, the DEA must be alerted using a DEA 106 form. A DEA 222 form is used to purchase or transfer Schedule II medications. A DEA 41 form is filled out for any outdated or damaged controlled substances.

8. **(B)** The Controlled Substance Ordering System (CSOS) is a program that is run by the DEA and allows for secure electronic submissions of controlled substances without using the paper DEA 222 form.

9. **(A)** REMS is the abbreviation for Risk Evaluation and Mitigation Strategies.

10. **(C)** The EPA places hazardous waste into two separate categories. Warfarin is identified as both a P-list and U-list drug based on the strength in question. Normal saline, metoprolol, and amoxicillin are not identified as hazardous waste by the EPA.

Patient Safety and Quality Assurance

7

KNOWLEDGE DOMAIN 3.0

Patient Safety and Quality Assurance   **26.25%**

→ Knowledge Area 3.1: High-alert/risk medications and look-alike/sound-alike [LASA] medications

→ Knowledge Area 3.2: Error prevention strategies (e.g., prescription or medication order to correct patient, Tall Man lettering, separating inventory, leading and trailing zeros, bar code usage, limit use of error-prone abbreviations)

→ Knowledge Area 3.3: Issues that require pharmacist intervention (e.g., drug utilization review [DUR], adverse drug event [ADE], OTC recommendation, therapeutic substitution, misuse, adherence, post-immunization follow-up, allergies, drug interactions)

→ Knowledge Area 3.4: Event reporting procedures (e.g., medication errors, adverse effects, and product integrity, MedWatch, near miss, root-cause analysis [RCA])

→ Knowledge Area 3.5: Types of prescription errors (e.g., abnormal doses, early refill, incorrect quantity, incorrect patient, incorrect drug)

→ Knowledge Area 3.6: Hygiene and cleaning standards (e.g., handwashing, personal protective equipment [PPE], cleaning counting trays, countertop, and equipment)

LEARNING OBJECTIVES

☐ Describe safety procedures, including infection control standards and handling and disposal requirements.

☐ Identify possible sources of medication errors, including the role of each party in reducing errors.

☐ Compare and contrast knowledge deficit vs. performance deficit.

☐ Identify common look-alike/sound-alike [LASA] drug names.

☐ Identify common high-alert/high-risk medications.

☐ Be familiar with common safety strategies that are used to limit potential errors.

The Food and Drug Administration has received over 95,000 reports of medication errors since 2000. These reports were voluntarily made through an adverse event reporting system called MedWatch. Why do medication errors occur? Are they due to patient misuse, practitioner error, or even an error in the pharmacy? All of these can be true. In 2019, the National Coordinating Council for Medication Error Reporting and Prevention (NCCMERP) defined a medication error as "any preventable event that may cause or lead to inappropriate medication use or patient harm while the medication is in the control of the health care professional, patient, or consumer." (© 2019 National Coordinating Council for Medication Error Reporting and Prevention. All Rights Reserved.)

An awareness of the existence of medication errors is the first step in preventing these errors from happening in the future. Fortunately, medication errors are preventable, and health care is in a constant state of advancement, with patient safety at the forefront. Health care professionals, patients, and their families are all responsible for identifying and preventing errors when possible.

Potential errors may include:

- Wrong patient
- Wrong route
- Wrong drug
- Wrong dosage form
- Wrong strength
- Wrong rate of administration
- Wrong time
- Wrong technique
- Wrong doctor
- Wrong preparation of dose
- Skipped dose
- Patient is not informed that the prescription has been called in

CAUSES OF MEDICATION ERRORS

Medication error sources may include deficits in the following categories as outlined in Table 7-1.

Table 7-1. Knowledge Deficit vs. Performance Deficit

Knowledge Deficit	Performance Deficit
■ Lack of knowledge or training ■ Employee may not have been given the information needed to perform the task	■ Employee has the knowledge, but the knowledge is not applied to the situation ■ Lack of sleep or illness ■ Personal problems ■ Employee is not paying attention to his or her job and/or may be distracted by background noises, such as talking, radio, phone ringing, etc.

A thorough evaluation of a medication error will discover why an error occurred and work toward preventing similar errors in the future. Did the practitioner make a mistake when writing the prescription? Did he or she select the wrong drug when typing out the electronic script? What errors were made when the pharmacy technician entered the script into the computer? Did the pharmacist perform a drug utilization review when checking the script for errors?

ERROR PREVENTION STRATEGIES

In order to implement medication error prevention strategies, you must identify possible sources for medication errors. Errors do not just occur from one source. In fact, the causes of errors can be quite complex. Possible sources for medication errors include doctors, nurses, the pharmacy, and patients and their family members.

Tables 7-2, 7-3, 7-4, and 7-5 are categorized by the individual(s) responsible for the error. Each table lists potential causes of errors and their respective solutions.

Table 7-2. Causes of Errors and Solutions—Prescribers

Error	Solution
Illegible handwriting	Use a computer to type the prescription or write legibly.
Ambiguous orders	Write specific instructions. Do not use the phrase "as directed."
Incomplete orders	Write complete instructions indicating the drug name, route, strength, frequency, quantity, and directions for use.
Verbal orders	Repeat the order to the pharmacist. Use written or faxed orders.
Inappropriate use of decimal points	Always include a zero before a decimal point.
Unapproved abbreviations	Avoid using abbreviations.
Dosage calculations	Require an independent double check.

Table 7-3. Causes of Errors and Solutions—Nurses

Error	Solution
Poor labeling	Read the label 3 times.
Patient identifiers	Use the barcoding system to identify the patient and the medication.
Borrowing medications	Avoid borrowing medications.
Unit dose vs. floor stock	Use unit dose medications when available.

Table 7-4. Causes of Errors and Solutions—The Pharmacy

Error	Solution
Labeling orders	Use standard format.
Misinterpretation	Avoid distractions. Verify patient information, including date of birth.
Calculations	Require an independent double check.
Sound-alike drugs	Require indications for all high-risk drugs.
Transcription	Repeat back all phone orders.

Table 7-5. Causes of Errors and Solutions—Patients and Family Members

Error	Solution
Patients bringing medications from home	Bring a list of medications, and leave the medications themselves at home.
Family members bringing medications from home	Bring a list of medications, and leave the medications themselves at home.
Family members pushing button on the PCA pump	Explain tolerance considerations to family members.

As a pharmacy technician, your role in preventing medication errors is crucial. There are several points in the dispensing process when you can help stop a medication error from occurring:

- **PRESCRIPTION DROP-OFF:** Communication here is key! Always obtain the patient's name, date of birth, and allergy information. If you work in a hospital, verify the patient's name, medical record number (MRN), and date of birth. You do not want to rely on the patient's room number as an identifier because rooms are subject to change. Be sure that you have current allergy information, including the specific reaction in your file. You may also want to consider asking for food allergies, especially in a hospital setting, to help avoid any potential food-drug allergies or possible interactions. Pediatric patients should have an updated weight on file with each new prescription. This is necessary to verify that the medication is accurate, since pediatric doses are usually based on both weight and age.
- **ORDER ENTRY:** Always minimize any distractions, which can be tough! Personal business should be left at home, and your focus always needs to be on the task at hand. Medication familiarity is a top priority. You should keep up with new drugs that are being launched on the market, and you should also familiarize yourself with common look-alike/sound-alike (LASA) drugs and high-alert medications.

One type of error is a potential 10-fold dosing error, which can occur with medications that come in similar-looking strengths. A good example of this is prednisone 5 mg and 50 mg. Another type of error occurs when drug names end with the letter "l," which can be deceiving. The "l" can be misread as the number "1." For example, the pharmacy technician may misread enalapril 2.5 mg tablets as enalapril 12.5 mg tablets. In addition, drug suffixes can pose potential errors. Some medications end in CR, XL, SR, etc. Common drug errors include an omission of a suffix or an incorrect dosing interval. A great example of this is the antidepressant Wellbutrin, which is available in three different variations: Wellbutrin, Wellbutrin SR, and Wellbutrin XL. Pay close attention to medications with a suffix to ensure that you are selecting the correct drug. Also, be on the lookout for ambiguous abbreviations. Alert the pharmacist if you see an ambiguous abbreviation used on a prescription, and be cautious of prescriptions that are written for more than three or four dosing units. For example, if a prescription is written for six tablets in one dose, ask the pharmacist to double check the dose.

Finally, be cautious of any prescriptions that require a patient to split, crush, or break a tablet. Many tablets cannot be tampered with and may contain an extended-release mechanism or a coating to protect the integrity of the tablet as it moves through the GI tract. Tablets may also taste bad or can be harmful to the patient if not taken intact.

- **FILLING:** Keep medications that look-alike/sound-alike away from each other on the pharmacy shelf. The use of tall man lettering can help bring attention to similar looking or similar sounding drug name bottles. Shelf tags or labels may also be used to emphasize product details, warnings, or other concerns. You can also place a marker, or an empty bottle, to indicate that a medication has been moved. If you work in a hospital, pay extra attention to unit dose medications and vials. The use of barcoding technology has significantly improved medication safety. Be sure to troubleshoot any problems to avoid rescanning medications multiple times.
- **PRESCRIPTION DISPENSING:** To avoid giving a medication to the wrong patient, always ask for a second identifier, such as the patient's date of birth or address. If you work in a hospital, you can verify the patient's MRN or date of birth. Barcoding technology can

also be used at pick up to verify that a prescription has been picked up. If the patient is picking up more than one prescription, and they are in separate bags, be sure to match the name and address on each bag to the patient. Pediatric suspensions are not reconstituted until the patient is at the pharmacy in order to avoid degradation. Be sure that there is a double-check procedure in place to ensure that medications that require reconstitution are not sold to a patient without being reconstituted. Some pharmacies will add a brightly colored note or sticker on the prescription receipt to alert the technician that the product needs to be reconstituted prior to dispensing. The reconstituted medications and other oral medications will also require the use of a calibrated measuring device. Keep a bucket with various calibrated spoons, cups, and syringes next to the out-window, and select the appropriate device based on the dose and the patient's age.

CONTINUOUS QUALITY IMPROVEMENT (CQI)

Pharmacies have an obligation to uphold high standards of quality, safety, and efficacy in order to avoid medication errors and provide superior health care. Quality is an implication of worth, a standard of excellence. While the pharmacist oversees the prevention and management of medication errors, it is the responsibility of all pharmacy team members to ensure safety in the health system. Many pharmacies have implemented **continuous quality improvement (CQI)** programs to ensure that these standards are met. CQI programs can improve outcomes and customer satisfaction while decreasing costs and liability. The basic outline for this process is "detect and document-evaluate-report-prevent."

Pharmacy CQI plans should include the following:

- An evaluation of the medication use process
- A process for identifying and tracking medication errors
- Definitions of medication error categories
- An increase in awareness and reporting of medication errors by involving health care professionals, patients, and caregivers
- Systems to detect errors and the development of interventions to correct the deficiency
- A focus on improvements rather than on punitive aspects of medication error reporting
- A respect for the confidentiality of all parties involved in the medication error

Continuous quality improvement methods institute a process of review, assessment, and implementation. The American Society of Consultant Pharmacists have indicated that assessments should include an evaluation of the cause(s) of error(s), as well as a review of data to determine potential trends, frequency, significance, and outcomes of medication errors. **Prevention strategies** should include interventions for reducing errors. These may include the following:

- **Fail-safes** and **constraints**, which include a change in the system itself or in the individual's interaction with the system, may be implemented. An example of this is the integration of the register with the computer system to block a prescription from being rung up unless it was verified by the pharmacist.
- The use of **forcing functions**, often referred to as a "lock and key," provides a stop in the system, requiring important information to be provided before proceeding. Medications must be scanned using a barcode that will match the NDC of the selected drug to the profiled medication. Pharmacies commonly use this function to insert a notation before overriding a high-alert medication.

- Pharmacies are implementing **automation** and **computerization** through medication use processes that are designed to assist in filling prescriptions and can lessen the fallibility of human memory reliance. Common examples of this include the use of electronic processing software with clinical decision support systems, the use of e-prescribing or CPOE to avoid transcription or misinterpreting errors, the assistance of robots and dispensing technology to count or fill prescriptions, and the use of warnings, alerts, and flags in computer systems.
- **Standardization** is also integrated to provide a uniform approach to avoid variation or complexity. This is accomplished through the use of preprinted prescription blanks that contain either common medication protocols (e.g., corticosteroid tapering) or lists of other frequently prescribed medications to reduce the potential for errors due to confusing or missing directions or even due to illegible handwriting.
- **Redundancies**, **reminders**, and **checklists** are also used as an intervention strategy by incorporating duplicate checks, audits, or verifications to provide information in an accessible format. This includes having more than one person verify the prescription, using independent double checks for high-alert medications, using the brand and generic names of medications when communicating about a prescription, counseling patients about medications, using auxiliary labels to provide warnings and alerts, and using preprinted prescription blanks with prompts for pertinent information like allergies, indication, or date of birth.
- **Education standards** and **information technology** are used to convey a level of knowledge and understanding in pharmacy practice. Pharmacy personnel may be required to complete continuing education (CE) hours or certification in advanced areas of practice. Proper training procedures, including infection control procedures, may also need to be renewed as required by law.
- **Pharmacy policies** and **procedures** should be maintained and followed, and protocols must be in place for the recording and transcription of prescriptions. CQI initiatives should incorporate goals and measurable standards. Any interventions should be analyzed and assessed frequently, allowing for changes to be made as needed; management of these initiatives requires the understanding of two key terms:
  - **Quality control:** identifying areas that require change due to inconsistency
  - **Quality assurance:** implementing a systematic review of quality-related events (QRE) to uphold the quality of care standards and their review over time

QUALITY-RELATED EVENTS (QRE)

A **quality-related event** is the inappropriate dispensing or administration of a prescribed medication. These events include, but are not limited to, variations or the failure to identify or manage:

- Clinical abuse/misuse
- Drug-allergy interactions
- Drug-disease contraindications
- Drug-drug interactions
- Inadequate or incorrect packaging, labeling, or directions
- Incorrect dosage or duration of treatment
- Incorrect drug

- Incorrect drug strength
- Incorrect patient
- Overutilization or underutilization
- Therapeutic duplication

The occurrence of a QRE should be documented and maintained as required by the corresponding State Board of Pharmacy (see Figure 7-1). Documentation must be completed the same day that the incident occurred. Documentation must include a description and an analysis of the event and the actions taken.

Quality-Related Event Documentation

I. QRE Prescription Data Prescription No.: _____

Attach copy of: ☐ prescription   ☐ label   ☐ photo copy of vial (mark all available)

II. QRE Data
QRE Type: (select all that apply)

A. Prescription processing error:

☐ (1) Incorrect drug
☐ (2) Incorrect strength
☐ (3) Incorrect dosage form
☐ (4) Incorrect patient
☐ (5) Inaccurate or incorrect packaging, labeling, or directions
☐ (6) Other: _____

B. A failure to identify and manage

☐ (1) Over/under utilization
☐ (2) Therapeutic duplication
☐ (3) Drug-disease contraindication
☐ (4) Drug-drug interactions
☐ (5) Incorrect duration of treatment
☐ (6) Incorrect dosage
☐ (7) Drug-allergy interaction
☐ (8) Clinical abuse/misuse

Prescription was received by the pharmacy via: ☐ telephone   ☐ written   ☐ computer   ☐ fax

Prescription was: ☐ new   ☐ refill

III. QRE Contributing Factors

Day of the week and time of QRE: _____

# of new prescriptions: _____   # of refill prescriptions: _____   RPh to tech ratio: _____

RPh staff status: ☐ regular staff   ☐ occasional/substitute staff

# of hours RPh on duty: _____   Average # of prescriptions filled per hour: _____

# of other RPhs on duty: _____   # of support staff on duty: _____

Describe preliminary root contributors:

_____
_____
_____
_____

Describe remedial action taken:

_____
_____
_____

Name and title of preparer of this report: _____

Date: _____

Figure 7-1. Sample Quality-Related Event (QRE) Documentation

ISSUES THAT REQUIRE PHARMACIST INTERVENTION

Multiple situations require pharmacist intervention. **Drug utilization review (DUR)** is a structured, comprehensive review strategy that is employed by pharmacists to review a patient's prescriptions, health history, and medication data. Changes in drug therapy may be necessary based on results of the DUR. According to the Academy of Managed Care Pharmacy, these reviews are performed on every prescription, help maintain accuracy in drug therapy, and improve patient outcomes.

Adverse drug events (ADE) are checked during the DUR process. During a prospective DUR, the patient's therapy is checked for accuracy and optimal care. Part of this process includes verifying that drug-drug interactions are not present. Drug-drug interactions can occur between prescription drugs or even between prescription and over-the-counter medications. It is important to resolve any ADE because drug-drug interactions can result in a change in the effect of the drug.

Over-the-counter (OTC) recommendations should never be made by a pharmacy technician. Pharmacy personnel should take a thorough patient history at the in-window. This should include the patient's medication history, as well as both the prescription and over-the-counter medications that he or she is taking. All medications should be reviewed. The pharmacist on duty should handle any requests for over-the-counter medication recommendations. Pharmacists should select a proper medication and strength based on the patient's allergies and prescription drug profile.

Therapeutic interchanges allow for the substitution of a medication to an alternative, usually from a non-preferred drug to one that is preferred. Many factors help determine the need for a therapeutic substitution, including cost. It is important to recognize that the patient needs to be informed of the therapeutic substitution.

Misuse of a medication is taking a medication for any reason other than the one for which it was prescribed. A misuse could be intentional or unintentional. Pharmacy personnel should be observant and proactive when dealing with patients who exhibit misuse or abuse tendencies. Misuse and abuse can be differentiated by looking at the patient's intentions and motivations.

According to the Substance Abuse and Mental Health Services Administration's Center for Behavioral Health Statistics and Quality, in 2011, drug misuse and abuse resulted in more than 1.4 million cases or emergency department (ED) visits. Figure 7-2 shows the spectrum of prescription drug abuse.

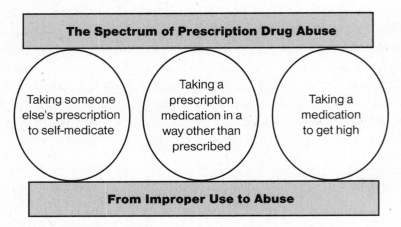

Figure 7-2. The spectrum of prescription drug abuse

With **intentional misuse**, the patient is dependent upon the medication and requires a larger dose than prescribed.

- The patient may take his or her medication inappropriately, including taking the prescription medication more often than prescribed.
- The patient may be taking someone else's prescription, often to self-medicate.
- The patient may take the prescription medication after it's no longer needed.

With **unintentional misuse**, the patient may or may not be dependent upon the medication.

- The patient may use his or her asthma inhaler all day long, even though it is meant for emergencies.
- The patient may take double the dose to relieve urgent pain. As time goes on, he or she becomes addicted to or reliant on increased doses due to tolerance issues.

Missed or skipped doses can occur for many reasons. The patient may have forgotten to take the dose or may have even run out of the medication. The caregiver could have failed to give the patient his or her medication on time, or the caregiver may have forgotten to give the patient the dose altogether. These situations require counseling from the pharmacist because patients should not assume that the missed dose can simply be taken with the next dose. Pharmacists can help identify and resolve situations that may be affecting optimal drug therapy. If a patient continues to miss doses, it can ultimately affect his or her health.

Adherence, specifically medication adherence, can be defined as the extent to which a patient takes a medication as prescribed. This includes multiple factors, such as getting prescriptions filled, picking up medications, remembering to take the medication, and following directions. Poor adherence can interfere with the ability to treat the disease and can result in complications. The consequences of non-adherence can involve both human lives and money. Up to two-thirds of all medication-related hospitalizations are attributed to non-adherence. Other complications of non-adherence include withdrawal syndromes, clotting, hypertension, return of an infection, or retitration. Pay particular attention to patients who are consistently late getting refills and/or have difficulty paying for medications. Also, patients on specialized medications that use devices, such as inhalers or insulin pens, should receive counseling on proper techniques.

Post-immunization follow-up can help prevent and manage immunization-related adverse effects. Adverse effects may be classified as local (redness or swelling) or systemic (fever, muscle pain, headache), frequent or rare, or they may be classified by severity of reaction with anaphylaxis and shoulder injury related to vaccine administration (SIRVA) as an adverse outcome. Protocols vary, but generally patients should be observed for 15 minutes post-immunization for signs of weakness, dizziness, or paleness that may result in syncope. Patients, pharmacists, or other immunizers can report any adverse events to the Vaccine Adverse Event Reporting System (VAERS). Pharmacists should be trained in basic life support (BLS) in the event of anaphylaxis. Shoulder injuries can also be prevented by employing proper administration techniques for all IM injections. Many states require pharmacists to complete training in immunization delivery and may also require the pharmacist to notify the patient's primary physician of the immunization.

SENTINEL EVENT

The Joint Commission defines a sentinel event as an "unexpected occurrence involving death or serious physical or psychological injury, or the risk thereof." The term "sentinel" is used to describe these events because they require immediate attention, investigation, and response. Sentinel events include a patient's suicide, an unanticipated death of a full-term infant, the abduction of a patient, the discharge of an infant to the wrong family, a rape, assault, or homicide of a patient, and a rape, assault, or homicide of a staff member, licensed independent practitioner, visitor, or vendor. Hospitals are expected to identify and respond appropriately to all sentinel events. Appropriate responses include conducting a root-cause analysis (RCA), developing an action plan to implement improvements in order to reduce risks, implementing improvements, and monitoring the effectiveness of those improvements.

HIGH-ALERT MEDICATIONS

The Institute for Safe Medication Practices (ISMP) defines high-alert medications as "drugs that bear a heightened risk of causing significant patient harm when they are used in error." Safeguards—including DUR reviews, pharmacist checks, and patient education—are all important steps in reducing errors and minimizing harm. Refer to Figures 7-3 and 7-4.

LOOK-ALIKE/SOUND-ALIKE [LASA] MEDICATIONS

These medications may look similar when written and/or tend to sound the same when spoken. Ultimately, these medications require pharmacists and pharmacy technicians to take extra precautions. The Institute for Safe Medication Practices (ISMP) maintains a list of common look-alike/sound-alike drugs.

In order to avoid errors, these drugs should be separated on the pharmacy shelf. Other strategies include the use of tall man lettering. This tactic requires the use of capital letters to designate areas of words that are dissimilar. For example, the insulin drugs NovoLog and Novolin may look or sound the same. The use of tall man lettering highlights the differences between these drug names: NovoLOG and NovoLIN.

ISMP List of High-Alert Medications
in Acute Care Settings

H igh-alert medications are drugs that bear a heightened risk of causing significant patient harm when they are used in error. Although mistakes may or may not be more common with these drugs, the consequences of an error are clearly more devastating to patients. We hope you will use this list to determine which medications require special safeguards to reduce the risk of errors. This may include strategies such as standardizing the ordering, storage, preparation, and administration of these products; improving access to information about these drugs; limiting access to high-alert medications; using auxiliary labels; employing clinical decision support and automated alerts; and using redundancies such as automated or independent double checks when necessary. (Note: manual independent double checks are not always the optimal error-reduction strategy and may not be practical for all of the medications on the list.)

Classes/Categories of Medications

adrenergic agonists, IV (e.g., **EPINEPH**rine, phenylephrine, norepinephrine)

adrenergic antagonists, IV (e.g., propranolol, metoprolol, labetalol)

anesthetic agents, general, inhaled and IV (e.g., propofol, ketamine)

antiarrhythmics, IV (e.g., lidocaine, amiodarone)

antithrombotic agents, including:

- anticoagulants (e.g., warfarin, low molecular weight heparin, unfractionated heparin)
- direct oral anticoagulants and factor Xa inhibitors (e.g., dabigatran, rivaroxaban, apixaban, edoxaban, betrixaban, fondaparinux)
- direct thrombin inhibitors (e.g., argatroban, bivalirudin, dabigatran)
- glycoprotein IIb/IIIa inhibitors (e.g., eptifibatide)
- thrombolytics (e.g., alteplase, reteplase, tenecteplase)

cardioplegic solutions

chemotherapeutic agents, parenteral and oral

dextrose, hypertonic, 20% or greater

dialysis solutions, peritoneal and hemodialysis

epidural and intrathecal medications

inotropic medications, IV (e.g., digoxin, milrinone)

insulin, subcutaneous and IV

liposomal forms of drugs (e.g., liposomal amphotericin B) and conventional counterparts (e.g., amphotericin B desoxycholate)

moderate sedation agents, IV (e.g., dexmedetomidine, midazolam, **LOR**azepam)

moderate and minimal sedation agents, oral, for children (e.g., chloral hydrate, midazolam, ketamine [using the parenteral form])

opioids, including:

- IV
- oral (including liquid concentrates, immediate- and sustained-release formulations)
- transdermal

neuromuscular blocking agents (e.g., succinylcholine, rocuronium, vecuronium)

parenteral nutrition preparations

sodium chloride for injection, hypertonic, greater than 0.9% concentration

sterile water for injection, inhalation and irrigation (excluding pour bottles) in containers of 100 mL or more

sulfonylurea hypoglycemics, oral (e.g., chlorpro**PAMIDE**, glimepiride, gly**BURIDE**, glipi**ZIDE**, **TOLBUT**amide)

Specific Medications

EPINEPHrine, IM, subcutaneous

epoprostenol (e.g., Flolan), IV

insulin U-500 (special emphasis*)

magnesium sulfate injection

methotrexate, oral, nononcologic use

nitroprusside sodium for injection

opium tincture

oxytocin, IV

potassium chloride for injection concentrate

potassium phosphates injection

promethazine injection

vasopressin, IV and intraosseous

All forms of insulin, subcutaneous and IV, are considered a class of high-alert medications. Insulin U-500 has been singled out for special emphasis to bring attention to the need for distinct strategies to prevent the types of errors that occur with this concentrated form of insulin.

Background

Based on error reports submitted to the ISMP National Medication Errors Reporting Program (ISMP MERP), reports of harmful errors in the literature, studies that identify the drugs most often involved in harmful errors, and input from practitioners and safety experts, ISMP created and periodically updates a list of potential high-alert medications. During June and July 2018, practitioners responded to an ISMP survey designed to identify which medications were most frequently considered high-alert medications. Further, to assure relevance and completeness, the clinical staff at ISMP and members of the ISMP advisory board were asked to review the potential list. This list of medications and medication categories reflects the collective thinking of all who provided input.

Abbreviation definitions: IV—intravenous IM—intramuscular

©ISMP 2018. Permission is granted to reproduce material with proper attribution for internal use within healthcare organizations. Other reproduction is prohibited without written permission from ISMP. Report medication errors to the ISMP National Medication Errors Reporting Program (ISMP MERP) at www.ismp.org/MERP.

*Copyright 2018 Institute for Safe Medication Practices (ISMP)

Figure 7-3. ISMP's list of high-alert medications in acute care settings

ISMP List of *High-Alert Medications* in Community/Ambulatory Healthcare

High-alert medications are drugs that bear a heightened risk of causing significant patient harm when they are used in error. Although mistakes may or may not be more common with these drugs, the consequences of an error are clearly more devastating to patients. We hope you will use this list to determine which medications require special safeguards to reduce the risk of errors and minimize harm.

This may include strategies like providing mandatory patient education; improving access to information about these drugs; using auxiliary labels and automated alerts; employing automated or independent double checks when necessary; and standardizing the prescribing, storage, dispensing, and administration of these products.

Classes/Categories of Medications
antiretroviral agents (e.g., efavirenz, lamiVUDine, raltegravir, ritonavir, combination antiretroviral products)
chemotherapeutic agents, oral (excluding hormonal agents) (e.g., cyclophosphamide, mercaptopurine, temozolomide)
hypoglycemic agents, oral
immunosuppressant agents (e.g., azaTHIOprine, cycloSPORINE, tacrolimus)
insulin, all formulations
opioids, all formulations
pediatric liquid medications that require measurement
pregnancy category X drugs (e.g., bosentan, ISOtretinoin)

Specific Medications
carBAMazepine
chloral hydrate liquid, for sedation of children
heparin, including unfractionated and low molecular weight heparin
metFORMIN
methotrexate, non-oncologic use
midazolam liquid, for sedation of children
propylthiouracil
warfarin

Background
Based on error reports submitted to the ISMP Medication Errors Reporting Program (ISMP MERP), reports of harmful errors in the literature, and input from practitioners and safety experts, ISMP created a list of potential high-alert medications. During June-August 2006, 463 practitioners responded to an ISMP survey designed to identify which medications were most frequently considered high-alert drugs by individuals and organizations. In 2008, the preliminary list and survey data as well as data about preventable adverse drug events from the ISMP MERP, the Pennsylvania Patient Safety Reporting System, the FDA MedWatch database, databases from participating pharmacies, public litigation data, literature review, and a small focus group of ambulatory care pharmacists and medication safety experts were evaluated as part of a research study funded by an Agency for Healthcare Research and Quality (AHRQ) grant. This list of drugs and drug categories reflects the collective thinking of all who provided input. This list was created as part of the AHRQ funded project "Using risk models to identify and prioritize outpatient high-alert medications" (Grant # 1P20HS017107-01).

Copyright 2011 Institute for Safe Medication Practices (ISMP). This document may be freely redistributed without charge in its entirety provided that this copyright notice is not removed. It may not be sold or distributed for a charge or for profit or used in commercial documents without the written permission of ISMP. Any quotes or references to this document must be properly cited. This document is provided "as is" without any express or implied warranty. This document is for educational purposes only and does not constitute legal advice. If you require legal advice, you should consult with an attorney.

ISMP
INSTITUTE FOR SAFE MEDICATION PRACTICES
www.ismp.org

*Copyright 2011 Institute for Safe Medication Practices (ISMP)

Figure 7-4. ISMP's list of high-alert medications in community/ambulatory health care

REDUCING ERRORS USING SAFETY STRATEGIES

Errors can occur anywhere and at any time. Pharmacies take many measures to eliminate errors, including separating inventory, using tall man lettering, educating their staff on the use of leading or trailing zeros, and limiting the use of error-prone abbreviations. (Note that a list of error-prone abbreviations can be found in Appendix J.)

Separating inventory is an important step in eliminating errors. Medications with similar names should be separated on the pharmacy shelf. High-risk medications should be stored separately from regular stock medications. Similar medication formulations should be placed together (e.g., liquid medications should be placed together, IV medications should be placed together, and ointments and creams should be placed together). This strategy allows the medication seeker to look only in the specific area of the formulation needed, resulting in less chance of an error.

Tall man lettering highlights areas of similar-sounding or similar-looking words to emphasize the dissimilarities. In addition to being used as a technique to limit errors when identifying look-alike/sound-alike drug names, manufacturers have even adapted this technique and often use it on the medication bottle to bring attention to the drug name. The technician should consult with the pharmacist on any look-alike/sound-alike medications.

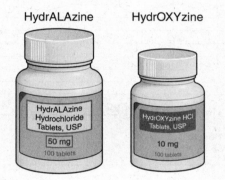

Figure 7-5. HydrALAzine/HydrOXYzine tall man lettering

Another way to eliminate medication errors is to avoid the use of error-prone abbreviations. Many abbreviations may be misinterpreted. The abbreviation "QID" may be misinterpreted as "QD." "D/C" may be interpreted as either "discharge" or "discontinue" depending upon the circumstance. A complete list of error-prone abbreviations can be found in Appendix J of this book.

Mathematics and calculations are an imperative part of the pharmacy. Errors can occur when pharmacy personnel do not follow the same techniques when writing numbers with decimal points. Writing decimals incorrectly can lead to medication errors. Two common errors are trailing zeros and naked decimal points. To avoid trailing zeros, write 5 instead of 5.0. To avoid naked decimal points, write 0.5 instead of .5.

Remember, periods are sometimes difficult to see. This can lead to a 10-fold error. Be sure to be as clear as possible!

Can you read the prescription shown in Figure 7-6?

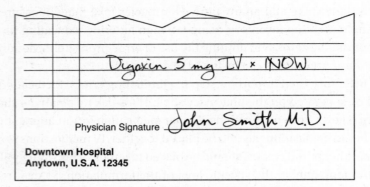

Figure 7-6. Sample Digoxin medication order

This prescription should read "Digoxin 0.5 mg." A dose of 5 mg would have resulted in the patient receiving 10× the prescribed dose.

How about Figure 7-7? Can you read it?

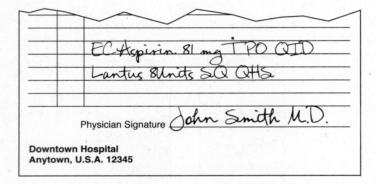

Figure 7-7. Sample insulin medication order

Lantus is long-acting insulin. In this particular prescription, the amount of Lantus may be misread and interpreted as 80 units instead of 8 units.

EVENT REPORTING PROCEDURES

Medication error reporting, review, and information dissemination are essential tools for improving processes in pharmacy services. Pharmacies should strive to be proactive in their approach at identifying areas of improvement and ultimately preventing more serious events. Some pharmacies assemble an adverse drug event committee to review and analyze medication errors, whereas others may utilize a leadership team to review errors.

A **root-cause analysis (RCA)** analytically identifies the underlying reasons for the occurrence of an adverse drug event or a near miss error for the purpose of identifying preventable measures. Evaluating root causes can lead to changes that can break the chain of events that would normally lead to an error. A root-cause analysis answers the following questions:

- What happened?
- Why did it happen?
- Who was involved?

- What typically happens?
- What should have happened according to policies and procedures?
- What was the missing or weak step in the process?
- What caused the missing or weak step?
- What is currently being done to prevent future failures during this step?
- What will prevent these failures from happening again?
- What actions need to be taken?
- How will outcomes be measured?

A RCA can apply to one event or to a series of events and involves collecting data, developing recommendations, implementing corrective action, and establishing systemic controls to avoid a recurrence of that event.

Near miss errors are medication errors that are identified before the patient receives the medication. Typically, these errors are identified during the final pharmacist check. The identification of near miss errors allows for these occurrences to be reviewed and action to be taken to prevent potential errors from occurring in the future. A near miss log can be maintained to document the error, identify causes and trends, and develop an action plan.

Medication errors, adverse drug effects, product quality problems, and therapeutic failures can be reported directly to the FDA through a monitoring system called **MedWatch**. This voluntary reporting system is available online and allows both health professionals and consumers to report issues with prescription and OTC medications, biologics, medical devices, combination products, special nutritional products, cosmetics, foods, and beverages. The Institute for Safe Medication Practices has a similar reporting system called the **Medication Errors Reporting Program (MERP)**, which is open to health care professionals to report medication errors that have occurred in the workplace.

HYGIENE AND CLEANING STANDARDS

Infection control is a process that is used to prevent nosocomial, or health care-associated, infections. Increasing antimicrobial resistance and the emergence of new pathogens prompted concerns for new standards of infection control. Hazardous materials and drugs produce adverse effects for the preparer.

The Occupational Safety and Health Administration (OSHA) requires employees to be protected from hazardous chemicals through handwashing and through the use of **personal protective equipment (PPE)**, including gowns, gloves, goggles, feet and hair covers, and masks. Glove selection depends upon the type of preparation being compounded and the presence of allergies, which may adversely affect the employee or the patient. Non-powdered gloves may be used when handling hazardous drugs, waste, or contaminants. Non-latex gloves may be used by preparers and/or patients who are allergic to latex.

Facilities are expected to implement infection prevention and control processes. Hands should be appropriately washed and decontaminated before and after patient interactions, prior to the production of any aseptic compounds, and upon contact with blood or other infectious materials. Proper handwashing procedures can be completed by using the following steps. First, remove debris from under your fingernails using nail cleaner and water. Then, wash your hands vigorously, making sure to include the forearm up to the elbow for a minimum of 30 seconds using antimicrobial soap and water. Scrubbing brushes should not be used on the skin as they can damage the skin or cause shedding. Last, completely dry the skin using lint-free wipes or an electronic hand dryer.

The use of appropriate PPE must be based on the risk of contamination and the type of compounded preparation. All equipment should be cleaned and disinfected before and after the preparation of medications. Counting trays and spatulas must be disinfected using 70% isopropyl alcohol. Additional caution should be given to the preparation of antibiotics, including penicillins and sulfonamides that have allergy potential. The use of a designated counting tray and a spatula for these types of medications is appropriate and should be labeled as such. Laminar flow hoods should be cleaned before and after batch preparations and maintained as required by law. Counters should be clutter free and clean of any debris. Non-sterile compounding areas and sterile compounding areas should be cleaned and maintained as described in *USP <795>* and *USP <797>*.

SUMMARY

☐ Errors may occur due to actions of the prescribers, administrators, pharmacy personnel, or even patients or their family members.

☐ It is important to determine the source of the error and then come up with a plan to resolve the situation and eliminate future errors.

☐ The pharmacist should always review look-alike/sound-alike and high-risk drugs before having the technician fill a prescription.

☐ Pharmacists should perform a drug utilization review (DUR) for each prescription to determine if any potential changes need to be made.

☐ Prescriptions should be screened for potential adverse drug events (ADE). Therapeutic substitutions can also be made to help patients with cost savings.

☐ Pharmacy personnel must understand when to use leading and trailing zeros.

☐ Pharmacy inventory should be separated by formulation as well as by usage. Medications with similar names should be separated on pharmacy shelves.

☐ Abbreviations on ISMP's list of error-prone abbreviations should not be used.

☐ Event reporting procedures are used to identify areas for improvement and prevent the occurrence of future adverse drug events.

PATIENT SAFETY AND QUALITY ASSURANCE PRACTICE QUESTIONS

1. A medication error may be the result of the wrong _____.

   (A) prescriber
   (B) dosage form
   (C) days supply
   (D) All of the above

2. The drugs Zyrtec 10 mg and Zoloft 10 mg are examples of _____.

   (A) over-the-counter (OTC) medications
   (B) look-alike names
   (C) therapeutic substitutions
   (D) tall man lettering

3. Pharmacy technicians who are interpreting unclear prescriptions should _____.

   (A) not request assistance and just fill the prescription
   (B) check with the pharmacist
   (C) call the doctor
   (D) All of the above

4. "AlprazOLam" is an example of a medication with _____.

   (A) tall man lettering
   (B) a look-alike/sound-alike name
   (C) a drug utilization review
   (D) HIPAA

5. Which of the following is an example of a knowledge deficit?

   (A) The employee is distracted by noise.
   (B) The employee comes into work with a fever and a cough.
   (C) The employee lacks training.
   (D) The employee is going through a difficult time in his/her personal life.

6. Which of the following is an example of an error caused by the prescriber?

   (A) illegible handwriting
   (B) family members bringing in medications for the patient without staff approval
   (C) borrowing medications from another patient
   (D) labeling error

7. True or False: Abuse and/or misuse of medications may be unintentional or intentional.

8. Error prevention strategies in the pharmacy setting include _____.

   (A) separating the inventory of medications with similar names
   (B) avoiding the use of error-prone abbreviations
   (C) organizing medications by formulation
   (D) All of the above

9. True or False: Medication guides contain FDA-approved information that can help patients avoid serious adverse effects.

10. Medication errors can occur for many reasons. Which of the following is a reason why a patient may miss or skip a dose?

   (A) The patient forgot to take the medication.
   (B) The patient's caregiver did not give the medication to the patient.
   (C) The patient ran out of the medication.
   (D) All of the above

ANSWERS EXPLAINED

1. **(D)** A medication error can occur due to any, or all, of these reasons.

2. **(B)** These drugs are among many on ISMP's list of common look-alike/sound-alike drug names.

3. **(B)** Pharmacy technicians should check with the pharmacist before proceeding to fill the prescription.

4. **(A)** Tall man lettering is used to distinguish dissimilarities and differentiate similar-looking drug names.

5. **(C)** The other choices are examples of performance deficits.

6. **(A)** Choice (B) is an error caused by family members. Choice (C) describes an error that could be caused by a nurse using another patient's medication for her current patient. Choice (D) describes an error that could be caused by a pharmacist, a pharmacy technician, or a nurse in a hospital setting.

7. **True** Abuse and/or misuse of medications may be unintentional or intentional. Pharmacy personnel should be cautious and examine a patient's medical history to evaluate for any potential dependency or abuse issues.

8. **(D)** Error prevention strategies include all of these choices.

9. **True** Medication guides address medication issues, adverse effects, or warnings for groups of medications. The patient can read the information in the medication guide to avoid serious adverse effects.

10. **(D)** A patient may skip or miss a dose due to any, or all, of these reasons.

Order Entry and Processing

8

KNOWLEDGE DOMAIN 4.0

Order Entry and Processing   **21.25%**

➜ Knowledge Area 4.1: Procedures to compound non-sterile products (e.g., ointments, mixtures, liquids, emulsions, suppositories, enemas)

➜ Knowledge Area 4.2: Formulas, calculations, ratios, proportions, alligations, conversions, Sig codes (e.g., b.i.d., t.i.d., Roman numerals), abbreviations, medical terminology, and symbols for days supply, quantity, dose, concentration, dilutions

➜ Knowledge Area 4.3: Equipment/supplies required for drug administration (e.g., package size, unit dose, diabetic supplies, spacers, oral and injectable syringes)

➜ Knowledge Area 4.4: Lot numbers, expiration dates, and National Drug Code (NDC) numbers

➜ Knowledge Area 4.5: Procedures for identifying and returning dispensable, non-dispensable, and expired medications and supplies (e.g., credit return, return to stock, reverse distribution)

LEARNING OBJECTIVES

☐ Define the term compounding, describe common situations in which compounding is required, and identify examples of non-sterile compounding.

☐ Identify the steps that are necessary in the compounding process.

☐ Understand the techniques by which solutions, suspensions, ointments, creams, powders, suppositories, and capsules are prepared.

☐ Understand the intake process, including prescription interpretation and data entry.

☐ Calculate doses that are required in order to process prescriptions, including days supply, quantity, dose, volume, etc.

☐ Perform pharmacy calculations.

☐ Learn commonly used formulas that are needed to fill prescriptions.

☐ Interpret commonly used abbreviations.

☐ Learn commonly used medical terminology.

☐ Be familiar with the equipment/supplies that are needed for drug administration.

☐ Understand the procedures that are used to identify medications that are returned to the pharmacy for credit, that are to be returned to stock, or that are using reverse distribution.

Manufacturers supply dosage forms to meet the needs of a majority of their patients. Sometimes a dosage form is unavailable, not currently on the market for that drug, or not carried by the pharmacy. In these cases, the pharmacist uses his or her chemistry background and knowledge of medications in order to make a special preparation. This process of mixing and preparing drug components to meet a patient's needs is called **extemporaneous compounding**. Technicians may be called upon to assist the pharmacist with these preparations. Compounded preparations can be made to adjust a dose, flavor a medication, reformulate the drug to remove an ingredient that a patient is allergic to (such as gluten), or even change a dosage form to one that is more suitable for the patient (e.g., changing from a tablet to a suspension).

> **Compounding vs. Manufacturing:** Compounding is the formulation of an individual compound that is made specifically to meet a patient's needs. It is not commercially available, and it is not available to be resold by the patient or the prescriber. Manufacturing involves batch compounding of FDA-approved compounds that are then sold to pharmacies or health care practitioners.

Extemporaneous compounding can be broken down into two categories: sterile compounding and non-sterile compounding. **Sterile compounding** is used for intravenous solutions, parenteral nutrition, and ophthalmic formulations. **Non-sterile compounding** is used for tablets, capsules, creams, ointments, suspensions, suppositories, transdermal applications, and troches.

The United States Pharmacopeial Convention is the leading authority in setting standards for product safety and purity. This nonprofit organization publishes a compendium called the *USP-NF (National Formulary)* with standards for chemical substances, compounded products, dosage forms, medical supplies, and dietary supplements. *USP <795>* (**Chapter 795**) describes compounding practices and procedures that are used for non-sterile preparations. *USP <797>* (**Chapter 797**) provides specific procedures and methods that are used for compounding sterile preparations.

NON-STERILE COMPOUNDING

Non-sterile compounding refers to any oral, transdermal, vaginal, or rectal medicinal preparations formulated using strict quality control standards. The use of high-grade pharmaceutical ingredients, along with training of personnel, safeguards against calculation errors, and documentation, certify the preparation's stability and consistency. *USP <795>*, the first set of enforceable standards that guide non-sterile compounding preparations, provides both guidelines and procedures for compounding with the intent of protecting both the patient and the preparer. These standards include:

- Ensuring pharmaceutical ingredient purity and potency
- Maintaining accuracy when mixing compounds in order to make customized medications
- Providing proper documentation on compounding procedures
- Maintaining and supplying acceptable packing, storing, and labeling
- Keeping all surfaces and equipment clean
- Using purified water when mixing compounds or when cleaning surfaces and equipment

Compounds may be prepared for specialty practices, including dermatology, home care, hormone replacement therapy, hospices, men's health, pediatrics, podiatry, veterinary medicine, and women's health. Pharmacy technicians may be required to obtain special certification and training to work in a designated compounding pharmacy. The Professional Compounding Centers of America (PCCA) offer certification and training for compounding professionals.

Non-sterile compounding can be divided into three distinct categories. Table 8-1 provides information about each of these categories.

Table 8-1. Non-Sterile Compounding Categories

Category	Description	Examples
Simple non-sterile compounding	Preparations are made according to standard formulas or recipes	■ alprazolam oral suspension ■ captopril oral solution
Moderate non-sterile compounding	Preparations are made using ingredients that require special handling	■ fentanyl patch ■ morphine sulfate suppository
Complex non-sterile compounding	Complex preparations require additional training and equipment	■ extended-release tablets ■ transdermal dosage forms

A proper environment with adequate space designated for compounding is required. The compounding facility should have an abundant supply of both clean hot and cold water. This supply should include purified water for washing equipment and supplies, as well as for compounding prescriptions that require the addition of water. Controlled lighting and temperature are necessary to avoid contamination and decomposition. The designated area should also be free of dust and contain an eye wash station.

Product Inventory

All bulk products are typically stored in tight, light-resistant containers at room temperature. Expiration dates, sources of ingredients, and NDC numbers are commonly checked to ensure accuracy and purity. Safety data sheets (SDS) for all non-sterile compounding procedures should be kept in the designated compounding area. Schedule II controlled substances should be locked in a designated area that is accessible to the pharmacist. Beyond-use dating (BUD) is often used for compounded products and indicates the expiration date of compounded preparations based on their stability and temperature storage conditions. Beyond-use dating is initiated at the time of compounding. As stated in Chapter 7, non-aqueous solutions have a BUD of no later than 6 months or a BUD equal to the earliest expiration date of any active pharmaceutical ingredient (API). Oral solutions that contain water have a BUD of no later than 14 days post reconstitution. Topical solutions and semisolid formulations that contain water have a BUD of no later than 30 days.

Equipment and Supplies

Compounding equipment may vary based on the pharmacy practice specialty. Pharmacy technicians need to be familiar with this equipment (its uses and maintenance).

- **MORTAR AND PESTLE:** These can be used to compound liquid or solid preparations.

  ○ Glass, with its smooth surface, is ideal for suspensions, oily agents, and chemotherapeutic agents.

  ○ Porcelain and Wedgwood provide a coarse-grained surface that is ideal for triturating.

- **SPATULA:** These instruments are made of stainless steel, hard rubber, or plastic and are used to prepare ointments and creams, loosen material from the surface of a mortar and pestle, and transfer ingredients.

- **OINTMENT SLAB:** This is a compounding slab made of ground glass. As an alternative, disposable non-absorbent parchment paper may also be used.

- **WEIGHING PAPERS AND CUPS:** These are disposable plastic or paper containers that are used to weigh powder or solid substances. The weight of the container must be tared out prior to weighing the substance. A tare weight is the weight of the empty container.

- **GRADUATED CYLINDER:** This is a cylindrical piece of laboratory glassware that is made of glass or polypropylene and is used to measure the volume of a liquid. Capacities range from 10 mL to 1,000 mL. The amount measured should be no less than 20% of the cylinder's capacity.

  ○ Liquid measurements are observed at eye level by verifying the volume at the bottom of a meniscus, which is the curved surface that appears due to surface tension. Refer to Figure 8-1.

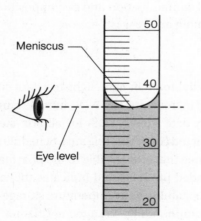

Figure 8-1. Reading a meniscus

- **PIPETTE:** This is a long, thin, calibrated, narrow glass tube that is used to measure and transfer small volumes of liquid.

- **CLASS III PRESCRIPTION BALANCE:** This is a two-pan balance system that is used to determine the weight of the material that is being compounded. It is required to have a class III prescription balance present in all pharmacies.

  ○ The balance must be calibrated; this process involves using a known weight and properly assessing the scale for accuracy.

○ This device can measure compounds that range in weight from 120 mg to 120 g.

○ This device has a sensitivity read of 6 mg, meaning that 6 mg of a substance will move the pointer of the balance one division off equilibrium.

○ The weights are cylindrical in shape, are often made of brass or polished metal, and range from 1–5 grams, with fractional weights ranging from 10–500 mg.

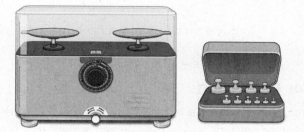

Figure 8-2. Class III prescription balance and brass weights

When weighing ingredients using the class III prescription balance, the following steps should be used:

1. Lock the balance by turning the arrest knob.
2. Verify that the internal weights are set to zero.
3. Unlock the balance, level the weights, and then relock the balance.
4. Place a weigh boat or weighing paper onto each pan.
5. Place the desired weight onto the right pan and the material that is to be weighed onto the left pan.
6. Unlock the balance, and observe the indicator arrow.
7. Lock the balance, and place the weights onto the right pan. Place the material that is to be weighed onto the left pan.
8. Release the balance, and note the shift on the pointer. If the pointer shifts to the right, there is not enough of the substance and more should be added. If the pointer shifts to the left, there is too much of the substance and some should be removed.
9. Arrest the balance each time before a substance is removed or added in Step 8 (if needed).
10. Write down the final measurement with the top down, and check your work.
11. Return the weights and supplies, clean the balance, close the lid, and verify that the balance is locked.

■ **REFRIGERATOR AND FREEZER:** These devices are used to store supplies.

○ Temperatures should be checked and logged in accordance with the law and pharmacy standards.

○ Refrigerator temperatures range from 2°C to 8°C (36°F to 46°F).

○ Freezer temperatures range from –20°C to –10°C (–4°F to 14°F).

■ **ELECTRONIC BALANCE:** This is a single-pan balance that is used to determine the weight of substances used in compounded prescriptions. This system provides a digital reading and has a sensitivity of 0.1 mg.

■ **FORCEPS:** This is an instrument that is used to grasp or hold small objects. It may also be used to transfer weights.

- **MOLDS AND PRESSES:** These are reusable trays that are used to prepare rectal and vaginal suppositories, oral rapid-dissolving tablets, troches, and lollipops.
- **STIR ROD:** This is a glass rod that is usually the thickness of a drinking straw and is used to mix liquids.
- **FUNNEL:** This is a tube that is made of glass, plastic, rubber, or stainless steel and is wide at the top and narrow at the bottom. It is used to transfer liquids or powders into small openings.
- **BEAKER:** This is a cylindrical container with a flat bottom that is used to store, mix, or heat liquids.

Containers for Packaging

Compounded products are stored in a variety of packages that range from amber-colored vials or bottles, to ointment jars, and to capsule and suppository boxes or containers. The selection is dependent upon the type of compound that is being prepared. Liquids are housed in amber-colored bottles while ointments and creams are placed into jars. The Topi-CLICK, a type of specialized topical packaging system, is a topical metered-dosing dispenser that provides consistent automated dosing throughout the patient's treatment. The Topi-CLICK system can house one to three months' worth of medication, and this system is primarily used for the delivery of topical creams.

Techniques Used to Prepare Prescriptions

The preparation of non-sterile prescriptions is customized according to industry and legal standards to maintain potency and purity. Compounding pharmacists will ensure that the final preparation is pure and accurate, properly labeled, and stored. The following are techniques used to produce compounded preparations:

- **TRITURATION** reduces the particle size of an ingredient by grinding it into a powder (e.g., by using a mortar and pestle).
- **SPATULATION** uses a spatula to mix ingredients in a plastic bag, on ointment paper, or via another medium.
- **LEVIGATION** grinds a powder by incorporating a liquid.
- **PULVERIZATION** is the process of reducing particle size in a solid by using a substance in which the particle is soluble (e.g., camphor, alcohol).
- **GEOMETRIC DILUTION** is a technique used when mixing different quantities of two or more ingredients to achieve a homogeneous mixture.

  ○ First, the smaller-quantity ingredient is mixed with an equal part of diluent (base) until the ingredient is incorporated in the diluent.
  ○ The diluent is continually added in small amounts until all of it has been incorporated and a homogeneous mixture has been formed.

- **SIFTING** is a process that is used to blend or combine powders by using a wire mesh sieve.
- **BLENDING** is general term that is used to describe the act of combining two substances.
- **TUMBLING** is a process that is used to mix powders in a bag or container and "tumble" or rotate the container to mix the ingredients thoroughly.
- **COMMINUTION** is the act of reducing a substance to fine particles.

Non-Sterile Compounding Process

Many different prescriptions can be made using non-sterile techniques. The pharmacist will evaluate the appropriateness of the order and determine product selection. Ingredient selection should be based on National Formulary (NF) or USP guidelines and should meet safety and purity standards. Table 8-2 contains a list of commonly made compounds.

Table 8-2. Compounded Preparations

Compound	Description
Capsules	Active drug is contained in a cylinder-shaped shell that is made of gelatin or methylcellulose
Creams	Oil in water (o/w) emulsion
Emulsions	A mixture of two or more liquids that are immiscible
Gels	A suspension of a solid in a liquid medium
Lozenge/troche	A tablet that is designed to be dissolved in the mouth
Ointment	Water in oil (w/o) emulsion
Paste	Formed by mixing a solid with a small amount of a liquid levigating agent
Powder	A finely ground mixture of an active and/or an inactive drug
Solution	A liquid dosage form where the active ingredient is dissolved in the liquid vehicle
Suppository	A solid dosage form that contains a base ingredient (e.g., cocoa butter) that is inserted into the vagina, rectum, or urethra
Suspension	A liquid dosage form where the active ingredient is dispersed in the liquid vehicle; must be shaken prior to use
Tablet	A solid dosage form made by compression or molding

Compounded preparations may include one, two, or multiple ingredients. Active ingredients produce a pharmacological response or change. Inactive ingredients are needed to fill prescriptions but do not produce a pharmacological response. A list of common inactive ingredients is displayed in Table 8-3.

Table 8-3. Commonly Used Inactive Ingredients

Inactive Ingredients	Description	Example
Acidifying agents	Provide acidic medium; bring stability to the formulation	citric acid
Alkalinizing agents	Provide alkalinizing medium; bring stability to the formulation	ammonia solution
Colorants	Provide color to preparations	FD&C Red 3
Emulsifying agents	Maintain dispersion of fine particles of liquid in vehicles	benzalkonium chloride
Flavorants	Provide flavor or odor to a preparation	menthol
Gelling agents	Used to increase viscosity by thickening and stabilizing the preparation	Carbopol 940
Levigating agents	Help reduce particle size	mineral oil
Lubricants	Prevent ingredients from clumping	magnesium stearate
Preservatives	Protect the formulation from microbial growth	methylparaben
Suspending agents	Increase viscosity to prevent sedimentation of powder in liquid	sodium lauryl sulfate
Sweeteners	Colorless, odorless agents that bring sweetness to a preparation	sorbitol
Wetting agents	Disperse air on the surface of drug molecules with liquid	betadex sulfobutyl ether sodium

NON-STERILE COMPOUNDING PROCEDURES

The steps for compounding non-sterile formulations are as follows:

1. Obtain the prescription.
2. Calculate the quantity of ingredients needed to make the preparation.
3. Wash your hands.
4. Document the ingredients needed to fill the prescription.
5. Obtain the equipment, ingredients, and materials needed to fill the prescription.
6. Clean the compounding area and equipment.
7. Obtain verification of the ingredients used and the quantities calculated prior to compounding.
8. Compound the preparation using the calculated formula.
9. Label the preparation.
10. Document the preparation on the compounding log.
11. Clean and store all equipment and materials.

The pharmacist then performs another check, termed the "final check," where he or she will verify the ingredients used, the calculations performed, the weight of the ingredients, the color, the odor (if present), and the pH (if needed). Auxiliary labels may be added as warranted. The pharmacist then signs off on the compound; this ensures consistency and accuracy.

Batch orders are prepared in anticipation of medication orders. These preparations may be determined based on need, and they should maintain similar standards. All batch orders should maintain consistency of ingredients. Labels for batch orders must contain a lot number, and extra labels should be tossed after a batch has been completed. Labeling requirements should be consistent with the formatting presented on the master formulation record.

COMPOUNDING A SPECIFIC FORMULATION

- **CAPSULE:** This is a solid dosage form that consists of a gelatin shell that encloses the active ingredient, typically a powder.

  - The powder that is used to fill a capsule is mixed using geometric dilution, and the particle size is grinded to a fine powder using trituration.
  - The **punch filling method** is when the powder is gathered together and compressed to form a dense cake. The capsule components are separated and then held vertically, and the open end of the base is punched in the powder until it is filled. Each capsule is then weighed to ensure an appropriate fill weight.
  - The **capsule machine method** is when a capsule machine, made of metal plates, is used to make up to 100 capsules at one time.
  - Capsule sizes vary, with the smallest size being 000 and the largest size being 5. The size of the capsule and the approximate amount contained within are inversely proportionate. The largest size, 000, can hold an average of 1,000 mg of powder, whereas the smallest size, 5, holds an average of 100 mg of powder.

- **SOLUTION:** This is a liquid dosage form in which the active ingredients are completely dissolved in a liquid vehicle.

  - The solvent is a substance, typically a liquid, that dissolves the solute, resulting in a solution.

○ The solute is the active ingredient that is dissolved in the solution.

○ The active ingredient should be triturated in order to reduce the particle size and to ensure an even distribution of particles.

- **SUSPENSION:** This is a coarse dispersion in which the internal phase (the active ingredient) is dispersed in the external phase (a suspending medium). The internal phase consists of insoluble solid particles that are dispersed in a suspending agent.

  ○ Physical stability and sedimentation, or the settling of particles, are common problems that exist with this formulation. Patients must shake the formulation well before using it.

  ○ To prepare a suspension, the active ingredient is triturated or levigated with a vehicle containing a wetting agent used to reduce the particle size of the insoluble internal phase and form a smooth paste. The soluble ingredients are dissolved in a vehicle and added to the paste to form a slurry. At this point, a flocculating agent can be added to form loose aggregates (called flocs) that increase the sedimentation rate, and a suspending agent is used to thicken the suspending medium, reducing sedimentation of the suspended particles and stabilizing the end product.

- **OINTMENT:** This is a preparation that contains an oil base, sometimes referred to as "water in oil." A base is selected, and then the product is prepared using one of two methods: incorporation or fusion.

  ○ Incorporation is a technique in which the components are mixed until a uniform preparation is attained. A mortar and pestle, spatula, or ointment mill may be used depending upon the scale of the product that is being produced.

  ○ Fusion utilizes heat to melt part of the entire individual ointment components. These components are then cooled with constant stirring until they are congealed. The congealed ointment can then be passed through an ointment mill or rubbed with a spatula in a mortar to ensure uniform texture throughout.

- **SUPPOSITORY:** This is a solid dosage form that uses oleaginous (fatty) or water-soluble bases to prepare a formulation that is used rectally or vaginally. The base maintains its solid, hard shape at room temperature. However, at body temperature, it will melt to a nonirritating oil. Suppositories are placed in aluminum wrappers and kept in a refrigerator to avoid melting. Suppositories are generally prepared three different ways: via hand rolling, using a compression mold, or through the use of a fusion mold.

  ○ Hand rolling is the oldest and simplest method of preparation. Grated cocoa butter and active ingredients are triturated in a mortar. The mass is formed into a ball in the palm of the hands and then rolled into a cylinder with a spatula or a small board. The cylinder is then cut into small uniform pieces, and one end is rolled to produce a conical shape.

  ○ Compression molding uses a special mold to compress the mixed mass ball of base and active ingredients into the cylinder, which is then closed. Pressure is applied at one end to release the mass from the other end of the mold. A moveable end plate is then removed, additional pressure is applied to the mass in the cylinder, and the formed suppository is ejected. The suppository can then be weighed to ensure accuracy.

○ Fusion molding is similar to compression molding but involves the use of heat to melt the suppository base. The active drug is then dispersed or dissolved into the melted base. The mixture is poured into the mold and allowed to congeal, and then the formed suppositories are removed and weighed for accuracy.

> **NOTE:** Any time a drug is added to a suppository base, it will displace an amount of the base as a function of its density. Density is considered in suppositories because the components are measured by weight but are compounded by volume. For example, if the drug has the same density as the base, the drug will displace an equivalent weight of the base. If the density of the drug is greater than that of the base, it will displace a proportionally smaller weight of the base.

- **ENEMA:** This is a liquid formulation that is inserted into the rectum to relieve constipation and for bowel cleansing. Water-based solutions, like Castile soap, sodium phosphate, and normal saline, are used to irritate the colon lining, draw water from the bloodstream into the colon, or expand the colon and prompt evacuation.

MEDICAL DEVICES AND EQUIPMENT USED FOR ADMINISTRATION

Dosage delivery devices are intended to facilitate proper dispensing of the product by the patient, the parent, or the caregiver. These devices are calibrated to ensure proper measurement of the appropriate dose. These devices contain markings at designated intervals, and the most common units are teaspoons, tablespoons, or milliliters.

Oral Devices

Oral pediatric medications are dispensed with an administration device that is suitable for the child's age. Medication cups, droppers, calibrated spoons, and oral syringes are used to accurately measure and dispense medications. Oral cups may contain measurements for teaspoons, tablespoons, and milliliters. The liquid is poured into the cup and measured to the bottom of the meniscus to maintain accuracy. Oral cups are reserved for volumes that are greater than 5 mL, and droppers, calibrated spoons, and oral syringes are used for volumes that are less than 5 mL. Oral droppers are used to administer small amounts of liquid medication to the eyes, ears, and, in rare cases, the mouth. They are calibrated by the manufacturer and should not be interchanged or used to administer other products. Oral droppers are not commonly used anymore for oral administration due to safety concerns and difficulty maintaining consistency while using the device. Calibrated spoons are hollowed spoons that allow for volumetric measurements up to 5 mL. The medication is poured into the hollow inside and measured in teaspoons or milliliters. The most commonly used delivery device is the oral syringe. Pharmacies generally carry 1, 3, 5, and 10 mL oral syringes, and a selection is based on the volume of medication to be given in one dose. Oral syringes provide precise and accurate measurements of medications. Depending upon the size of the syringe, the amount that is dispensed on each line varies. Table 8-4 demonstrates the calibration markings on various oral syringes.

Table 8-4. Oral Syringe Calibration

Syringe Size	mL Dispensed per Calibration Mark
1 mL	0.01
3 mL	0.1
5 mL	0.2
10 mL	0.5

Oral syringes may also be used with bottle adapters, small plastic inserts that fit into the bottle opening, to draw out liquid from the inverted bottle. One must be cautious when purchasing bottle adapters that are not provided by the medication manufacturer, as they may not fit well and can lead to spillage and inaccuracies in dosing.

To draw up a medication with an oral syringe, follow these steps:

1. Unscrew the cap that is located on the medication bottle.
2. Check for the clear syringe bottle adapter in the bottle, or attach an adapter cap that was sent with the syringe. If an adapter cap is used, screw the cap onto the medication bottle opening.
3. Insert the syringe into the bottle adapter, and press down until the syringe is snug. The plunger should be fully depressed to avoid withdrawing any liquid.
4. Invert the bottle with the attached syringe so that the bottle is upside down.
5. Draw up the prescribed amount of medication into the syringe by pulling back on the plunger to the prescribed medication dose.
6. Turn the bottle upright, remove the syringe, and administer the prescribed dose.

Injectable Syringes

Injectable syringes are also used to administer medications. Figure 8-3 depicts the parts of a syringe and a needle.

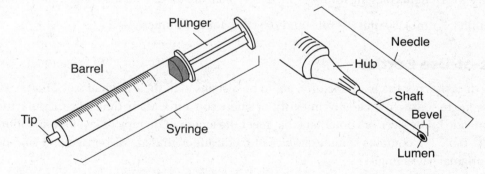

Figure 8-3. Parts of a syringe and a needle

A **needle** has two parts: the shaft and the hub. The shaft is the stem and has a bevel (diagonal point) on one end. The hub is the other end of the needle and attaches to the syringe. Also, note that the shaft contains a hollow bore, referred to as the lumen. Needles are referred to by their size. Needle lengths vary from $\frac{3}{8}$ inch to $3\frac{1}{2}$ inches. Another way to designate size is by referring to the needle's gauge. This refers to the size of the lumen, measured inversely, with sizes measuring from 13 (largest-size lumen) to 32 (smallest-size lumen). Some needles come attached to the syringe, while others are available in individual packaging. Selecting the appropriate needle is determined by the viscosity of the solution and the vial in which it is to be administered. Used needles should be discarded into a sharps container. Some needles contain a safety cap that automatically locks to protect the user from finger pricks. **Filter needles** are specialized needles that contain a filter that is used to catch any particles that may be present in an ampule. The filter needle is used to withdraw solution from the ampule. Then, an unfiltered needle can be attached to add the medication to the bag of solution.

Syringes have two main components: the barrel and the plunger. The barrel is a hollow tube with an open end on one side. Within the barrel is a plunger, which is a piston-type rod that moves within the barrel and is used both to draw and to release fluid. The tip of the syringe contains a point of attachment that is used to attach a needle. Some syringes contain a tapered tip that allows the needle to be held on by friction. Other needles have a locking device that allows the needle to be secured by turning and locking the needle in place. Graduation lines indicate the volume of solution. Capacity varies with syringes and ranges in size from 1 mL to 60 mL. Syringes are also disposable and should not be reused.

Diabetic Administration Supplies

Many injectable diabetes medications come in prefilled insulin pens. Those pens will require needles for administration. Insulin is injected subcutaneously and requires a thin, short needle for comfort and to avoid reaching muscles. The most common sites that are used are the abdomen, thighs, buttocks, and upper arms. The best technique to avoid injecting muscles is gather the skin and fat between the fingers and inject the folds. Typically, 29-gauge to 32-gauge needles with lengths ranging from $\frac{5}{32}$ inch to $\frac{1}{2}$ inch are used. Insulin syringes are available in 30 unit ($\frac{3}{10}$ mL), 50 unit ($\frac{1}{2}$ mL), and 100 unit (1 mL) volumes.

Unit-of-Use Bottles

Some drugs, as per the manufacturer, are to be dispensed in their original stock bottle container due to sensitivity, stability, integrity, or safety concerns. Many times the manufacturer will provide bottle sizes or containers that meet the length of therapy or last for one month's supply. Table 8-5 contains some examples of medications that are dispensed and stored in their original packaging:

Table 8-5. Examples of Medications That Are Dispensed in Their Original Packaging

Format	Medications
Tablets	■ Abilify (aripiprazole) 30 tablets/bottle ■ Accolate (zafirlukast) 60 tablets/bottle ■ Atripla (efavirenz, emtricitabine, tenofovir) 30 tablets/bottle ■ Latuda (lurasidone) 30 tablets/bottle ■ Medrol Dosepak (methylprednisolone) 21 tablets/blister pack ■ Micardis (telmisartan) 30 tablets/blister pack ■ Nitrostat (nitroglycerin) 25 tablets/bottle ■ Pristiq (desvenlafaxine) 30 tablets/bottle ■ Proscar, Propecia (finasteride) 30 tablets/bottle ■ Remeron (mirtazapine) 30 tablets/bottle ■ Suboxone, Zubsolv (buprenorphine and naloxone) 30 tablets/bottle ■ Tekturna (aliskiren) 30 tablets/bottle ■ Treximet (naproxen and sumatriptan) 9 tablets/round container ■ Wellbutrin XL (bupropion Hcl) 30 tablets/bottle ■ Z-Pak (azithromycin) 6 tablets/blister pack ■ Zofran (ondansetron) 30 tablets/bottle ■ Zoloft (sertraline) 30 tablets/bottle
Capsules	■ Aggrenox (aspirin and dipyridamole) 60 capsules/bottle ■ Avodart (dutasteride) 30 capsules/blister pack ■ Gengraf, Neoral (cyclosporine) 30 capsules/blister pack ■ Pradaxa (dabigatran) 60 capsules/bottle ■ Prevpac (lansoprazole, amoxicillin, clarithromycin) 8 capsules/daily administration card ■ Pylera (bismuth subcitrate potassium, metronidazole, tetracycline) 120 capsules/blister card
Orally Disintegrating Tablets	■ Zyprexa (olanzapine) 30 sachets/box
Films	■ Suboxone (buprenorphine and naloxone) 30 pouches/box
Liquids	■ Neoral (cyclosporine) oral solution 50 mL/bottle ■ Pediatric suspensions (amoxicillin, amoxicillin and clavulanate, cefdinir, etc.) ■ Trileptal (oxcarbazepine) 250 mL/bottle

Unit Dose Systems

Unit dose systems are medications that are prepackaged for single administration. These medications may come already prepackaged from the manufacturer or may be packaged by the pharmacy into unit dose systems. Hospitals commonly use unit dose systems because they are safer for the patient, more efficient and economical for the institution, and a more efficient use of personnel. Unit dose systems contain the medication name, strength, manufacturer name, lot number, NDC number, expiration date, and barcode. Long-term care pharmacies use blister card unit dose systems that provide 30 to 90 doses of medication at one time. Each card contains the medication name, strength, manufacturer name, expiration date, and lot number. A barcode and an NDC number may also be used to identify the medication.

Spacers

Spacers are devices that attach to an inhaler and hold medication until it is breathed in. A tube-based spacer is a device that is placed between the mouth and the inhaler. A valved holding chamber (VHC) is a type of spacer that has a one-way valve at the mouthpiece that is used to trap and hold the medication until the patient is ready to take a slow, deep breath. The valve stops the patient from accidently exhaling into the tube. Spacer devices may also have antistatic coatings (to prevent the medication from sticking to the inside of the spacer), compact sizes, whistles (that sound when the medication is inhaled too fast), flaps (to indicate the number of breaths taken), and various size masks.

MEDICATION-SPECIFIC NUMBERS

The **National Drug Code** number, most commonly referred to as the **NDC**, is a 10-digit, 3-segment number that identifies the labeler (manufacturer), product, and package.

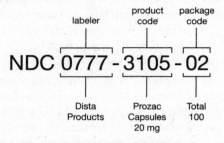

Figure 8-4. National Drug Code

The NDC consists of three segments:

- **FIRST SEGMENT:** This sequence of four or five numbers identifies the labeler (manufacturer or distributor). The Food and Drug Administration (FDA) assigns this segment.
- **SECOND SEGMENT:** These three or four middle digits refer to the product strength, dosage form, and formulation.
- **THIRD SEGMENT:** The final one or two digits identify the package form and size.

The NDC is used to verify product selections when filling a prescription. Pharmacy technicians can also scan the NDC barcode when ordering or to verify counts.

Medications also contain a second set of numbers called a **lot number**. This is a unique number that is issued by the manufacturer. It is assigned to a batch of medications during production. This number helps to identify and, in the event of a problem, isolate any medications with potential problems that occurred during production. It is usually stamped on the side of the packaging. Recalls will always state the lot number(s) involved for consumer verification. When a pharmacy receives a recall notice, they will pull the medication from shelves, medication carts, and storage areas to return it to the manufacturer.

The third set of numbers that is found on medications is the **product expiration date**. This set of numbers can be found on over-the-counter (OTC) medications, as well as on prescription medications. OTC medications and stock prescription medications receive an expiration date as determined by the manufacturer. Prescription medications that are repackaged and placed into vials for patient use also receive a beyond-use date. Typically, the expiration date for a prescription medication is set for one year from the date the medication was repackaged unless the manufacturer's expiration date comes before that. Medications that are reconstituted (e.g., children's antibiotics) and intravenous (IV) medications also have a beyond-use date.

Expired medications may be returned to the distributor for reimbursement. Each distributor determines its own return policy and may require authorization before returns are accepted and reimbursement is granted. When Schedule II medications are beyond their expiration date, a DEA 41 form must be completed, and the destruction of the expired drug must be witnessed. Some strategies that are used to decrease the amount of expired drugs in the pharmacy include using colored stickers to designate the month of expiration, writing the number associated with the month of expiration on the bottle in a visible area, and placing new products behind old products on the shelf (i.e., rotating stock).

Medications that are returned to the pharmacy cannot be sold. These medications are placed in a separate waste bin until they are removed by a reverse distributor. Medications that are filled but are not picked up by the patient can be returned to stock. These medications should not be added to the original stock container. Instead, these medications are kept in the original vial and all patient-specific information is removed. These medications can then be recounted into a new bottle and used again for another patient. This rule also applies to pharmacies that deliver medications. Medications that never leave the possession of the driver may be returned to stock. In the hospital setting, unit dose medications may be returned to stock. However, the storage condition of the product should be considered. For example, if a medication that requires refrigeration is found on the countertop, it may need to be discarded.

MEDICAL TERMINOLOGY

Health care professionals use medical terms to describe the human body, including its components. These terms are also used to describe any procedures that are performed, any conditions that affect the body, and any diagnoses that are made. Each medical term is made of three distinct parts: the prefix, the root word, and the suffix. The **prefix** is placed at the front of a word and is used to describe or change its meaning. It can also be used to indicate a location, a time, or a number. "Pre" means "before." The **root word** gives the word its meaning and often indicates an organ, a tissue, or a condition. The **suffix** is located at the end of a word and is used to change the meaning. Medical terms can contain multiple root words and often use **combining vowels**, like "i" and/or "o," to ease pronunciation. The combining vowel(s) can be found between root words or when a suffix begins with a consonant. A root word plus a vowel equals a **combining form**. For example, "micr" + "o" = "micr/o." Table 8-6 provides examples of how these components are used together to form medical terms.

Table 8-6. Examples of How Combining Forms and Suffixes Are Used to Form Medical Terms

Medical Term	Combining Form	Suffix	Meaning of the Suffix	Meaning of the Word
Dermatology	Dermat/o	-logy	The study of	The study of the skin
Dermatologist	Dermat/o	-logist	One who studies	One who studies the skin
Dermatopathy	Dermat/o	-pathy	Suffering or disease	Any disease of the skin

Additional examples of common prefixes and suffixes can be found in Appendix I.

PHARMACY CALCULATIONS

Calculations are a critical component of pharmacy practice. Pharmacy technicians should have an understanding of how to determine quantities of ingredients accurately. Having a working knowledge of the metric system, as well as familiarity with percentages, proportions, dilutions, and alligations, is crucial. In addition, a working knowledge of Roman numerals, system conversions, and metric and temperature conversions is strongly advised. More details to help you develop this working knowledge are available in Appendix K.

Calculating Days Supply

TIP

When calculating days supply, make sure to convert both the prescribed dose and the total amount of the drug in the container to the same unit.

Days supply is the amount of time that the medication will last. Prescriptions do not always last 30 or 90 days and often require simple calculations in order to determine the days supply. An incorrect days supply can result in the patient receiving too much or too little of the medication, as well as insurance claim rejections on future refills. Days supply can be determined by dividing the total number of doses to be dispensed by the number of doses taken per day. Hospital pharmacies supply medications based on units or singular doses.

Note that calculations are necessary when quantities are not written on prescriptions.

➥ Example 1—Capsules/Tablets

A prescription is written for cephalexin 250 mg #30 1 cap PO TID. What is the days supply?

Answer:

$$\frac{1 \text{ day}}{3 \text{ caps}} = \frac{x \text{ days}}{30 \text{ caps}}$$

Cross multiply and solve for x.

$$x = 10 \text{ days}$$

The next example is a bit trickier and requires some investigation. In order to calculate the days supply, you will need to know how many "puffs" are in one inhaler. This information can be found by looking at the inhaler package.

➥ Example 2—Inhalers

A prescription is written for ProAir inhaler 2 puffs QID. A ProAir inhaler has 200 puffs. What is the days supply?

Answer: First, determine the number of puffs in one day. 2 puffs QID is the same as 2 puffs, 4 times a day, or 8 puffs a day. Then, move on to calculating the days supply.

$$\frac{8 \text{ puffs}}{1 \text{ day}} = \frac{200 \text{ puffs}}{x \text{ days}}$$

Cross multiply and solve for x.

$$x = 25 \text{ days}$$

Example 3 deals with oral liquids. Oral liquids are generally not dispensed in the original container unless the amount to be dispensed is equivalent to the stock bottle amount or if the prescription is written for a complete bottle to be dispensed. Calculations are needed in order to determine the total amount, in mL, to be dispensed.

> **NOTE:** In order to determine what size bottle is needed for the volume of medication prescribed, take the total volume in mL (if not already given in oz) and divide it by 30. For example, a 120 mL prescription would be dispensed in a 4 oz bottle.

➡ Example 3—Oral Liquids

A prescription is written for Dilantin 125 mg/5 mL # 8 oz, 1 tsp PO BID. What is the days supply?

Answer: First, convert oz to mL.

$$\frac{x \text{ mL}}{8 \text{ oz}} = \frac{30 \text{ mL}}{1 \text{ oz}}$$

Cross multiply and solve for x.

$$x = 240 \text{ mL}$$

Now look at the total quantity that is to be taken in one day.

$$5 \text{ mL} \times 2 = 10 \text{ mL/day}$$

Finally, determine the days supply.

$$\frac{x \text{ days}}{240 \text{ mL}} = \frac{1 \text{ day}}{10 \text{ mL}}$$

Cross multiply and solve for x.

$$x = 24 \text{ days}$$

Many times, the prescription will specify an amount of time that the patient should take the medication for. It is best to determine the appropriate days supply based on the amount of drops the patient will use daily. The pharmacy technician should check the amount of mL that is contained in one bottle and select the appropriate size that will maintain the course of therapy as prescribed. In addition, it is customary to assume a conversion factor of 20 drops/mL (typically used for ophthalmic and otic solutions) when determining the total amount of drops per bottle. Some pharmacies may be conservative and use a conversion factor of 15 drops/mL (typically reserved for ophthalmic and otic suspensions). Third-party payers may also require a conversion factor of 16 drops/mL when determining days supply. Check with the pharmacist before proceeding.

➡ Example 4—Eye Drops and Ear Drops _____

A prescription is written for Cipro HC Otic suspension, 4 gtts ad BID × 7 days # 10 mL. What is the days supply?

Answer: Calculate the actual days supply based on a conversion factor of 20 drops/mL. First, determine the number of drops contained in the bottle.

$$x \text{ drops/bottle} = 10 \text{ mL} \times 20 \text{ drops/mL}$$
$$x = 200 \text{ drops/bottle}$$

Next, determine the volume of drops that a patient will use per day, and calculate the number of days this prescription will last. The script states: 4 gtts ad BID. This means that the patient will use 4 drops in the right ear twice a day for a total of 8 drops a day.

$$\frac{1 \text{ day}}{8 \text{ drops}} = \frac{x \text{ days}}{200 \text{ drops}}$$

Cross multiply and solve for x.

$$x = 25 \text{ days}$$

Insulin prescriptions are written in units. Days supply calculations are determined based on 1 mL = 100 units. Insulin may also be referred to as U-100, meaning that each mL contains 100 units. Typical sizing for insulin includes both 10 mL vials (1,000 units) and 3 mL syringes (available as a quantity of 5 syringes for a total quantity of 15 mL or 1,500 units).

➡ Example 5—Insulin _____

A prescription is written for Humulin-N U-100 insulin 10 mL vial, 35 U SC QD. What is the days supply?

Answer: There are 100 units/mL. First, determine the total number of units in the 10 mL vial of insulin.

$$\frac{100 \text{ U}}{1 \text{ mL}} = \frac{x \text{ U}}{10 \text{ mL}}$$

TIP

Labels for inhaler, liquid, and insulin preparations should include a beyond-use date when appropriate.

Cross multiply and solve for x.

$$x = 1,000 \text{ U}$$

Then, solve for the total days supply of this prescription.

$$\frac{35 \text{ U}}{1 \text{ day}} = \frac{1,000 \text{ U}}{x \text{ days}}$$

Cross multiply and solve for x.

$$x = 28.57 \text{ days} \approx 28 \text{ days}$$

Do not round up because the patient will not have enough to last until the next day.

Days supply calculations for ointment/cream prescriptions are not as concrete and require some additional information. It is important to note that ointments/creams vary in size. The days supply depends upon how often the patient will use the medication and how large of an area the patient will use the ointment or cream on. If an amount is not specified, err on the side of caution and use 1 g/dose to calculate days supply.

➥ Example 6—Ointments/Creams

A prescription is written for hydrocortisone 2.5% cream, 30 g tube, apply once daily to the affected area. What is the days supply?

Answer: For this example, we will use 1 g/dose to calculate the days supply. First, determine the total number of doses available in a 30 g tube.

$$\frac{1 \text{ gram}}{1 \text{ dose}} = \frac{30 \text{ g}}{x \text{ doses}}$$

Cross multiply and solve for x.

$$x = 30 \text{ doses}$$

Now solve for the total days supply for this prescription.

$$\frac{1 \text{ dose}}{1 \text{ day}} = \frac{30 \text{ doses}}{x \text{ days}}$$

Cross multiply and solve for x.

$$x = 30 \text{ days}$$

Now practice days supply using the following community and hospital pharmacy prescriptions.

➡ Prescription 1

John Smith M.D.
Family Practice
1234 Main Street
Anytown, OH 12345   DEA# AS7654321
(555) 555-5555   NPI# 789456123

Patient Name _Ava Thomas_

Address_____ Date _08/01/15_

℞

Robitussin #120

Sig: 1 tsp PO q4-6H PRN

Refill _0_ Times

_____   _John Smith M.D._
Dispense as Written   Substitution Permitted

🔒 Security features are listed on back. *Prescription is void if more than one controlled prescription is written on Rx.

TIP

Remember, one teaspoonful is equivalent to 5 mL.

1. What is the total quantity of this medication that is to be dispensed to the patient?

2. What is the minimum days supply for this prescription?

3. How many refills are on this prescription?

Answers:

1. The total is 120 mL. This can also be interpreted as 4 oz.

2. The minimum day's supply is 4 days.

1 teaspoonful by mouth every 4–6 hours as needed.

$$5 \text{ mL} \times 6 \text{ doses/day} = 30 \text{ mL/day}$$

$$\frac{30 \text{ mL}}{1 \text{ day}} = \frac{120 \text{ mL}}{x \text{ days}}$$

Cross multiply and solve for x.

$$x = 4 \text{ days}$$

3. There are no refills on this prescription.

John Smith M.D.
Family Practice
1234 Main Street
Anytown, OH 12345   DEA# AS7654321
(555) 555-5555   NPI# 789456123

Patient Name _Philip Johns_

Address_____ Date _08/01/15_

℞

    Xalatan #2.5

    Sig: 1 gtt OU QD

Refill _2_ Times

_____   _John Smith M.D._
Dispense as Written   Substitution Permitted

🔒 Security features are listed on back. *Prescription is void if more than one controlled prescription is written on Rx.

1. Translate the sig code into plain English.

2. Is this prescription written for an ear drop or an eye drop?

3. What is the days supply?

Answers:

1. Instill 1 drop in each eye every day.

2. This prescription is written for an eye drop.

3. The day's supply is 18 days.

$$2.5 \text{ mL} \times 20 \text{ gtts/mL} = 50 \text{ gtts}$$

$$\frac{2 \text{ gtts}}{1 \text{ day}} = \frac{50 \text{ gtts}}{x \text{ days}}$$

Cross multiply and solve for x.

$$x = 25 \text{ days}$$

Calculations for Dispensing Fees, Copays, and Cash Register Calculations

Dispensing fees are costs that are associated with filling the prescription. They are determined by a contractual agreement between a third party and the pharmacy. Dispensing fees for prescriptions include the cost of labor, equipment, medications, and rent.

Copays are determined by a contractual agreement between a third party and the patient. They are fixed dollar amounts that may reflect a percentage of the medication cost.

Cash register calculations require the technician to give the correct change to the patient. In addition, patients who pay cash for their prescriptions are charged a **usual and customary price** (U&C). These prices reflect the medication's cost (average wholesale price or AWP) and a professional fee. Some pharmacies also provide discounts to patients without insurance coverage.

➡ Example 1

What is the copay for a prescription of prednisone 20 mg # 10 if the copay is 20% of the U&C price of the prescription? The U&C price for prednisone 20 mg #10 is $4.76.

Answer: 20% is the same as saying $\frac{20}{100}$ or 0.2. To determine the co-pay, multiply the percentage by the U&C price.

$$0.2 \times \$4.76 = \$0.95$$

The copay for this prescription is $0.95.

➡ Example 2

A third-party contract allows for pharmacy reimbursement of prescription "X" based on the following formula: 80% of AWP + $1.65 dispensing fee. The AWP for prescription "X" is $34.20. Determine the pharmacy reimbursement for prescription "X."

Answer: 80% is the same as saying $\frac{80}{100}$ or 0.8. Pharmacy reimbursement can be determined by multiplying the AWP by 0.8 and adding the dispensing fee.

(0.8	×	$34.20)	+	$1.65	=	$29.01
percentage	×	AWP	+	dispensing fee	=	pharmacy reimbursement

The pharmacy reimbursement is $29.01.

➥ Example 3 _____

A patient's prescription costs $75.25, and a patient gives you $80.00. How much change should the patient receive?

Answer: There are multiple ways of counting out change, and the currency you provide to the patient can vary based on how you count out change. Here is one method you can use. Start counting out the currency using the smallest denomination of money that will get you to the next coin or bill size. Start with the purchase price of $75.25, and count to the amount given to you ($80.00).

>   3 quarters (75¢) will make $76.00
>   4 dollars ($4.00) will make $80.00

Therefore, the patient should receive $4.75 in change.

➥ Example 4 _____

A patient qualifies for a pharmacy discount of 5% on her prescription costs. What is the cost that the patient will pay if the retail price of her prescription is $6.15?

Answer: 5% is the same as saying $\frac{5}{100}$ or 0.05. To determine the amount the patient will pay, multiply the percentage by the prescription cost.

$$0.05 \times \$6.15 = \$0.31$$

This is the discount that the patient will receive. Subtract this amount from the prescription cost to determine the discounted amount to be paid by the patient.

$$\$6.15 - \$0.31 = \$5.84$$

The patient will pay a discounted amount of $5.84.

Percentages and Strengths

Percentages refer to a quantity out 100. Percentages can be considered to be a fraction. For example, the quantity 75% means $\frac{75}{100}$. Interpreting percentages can be tricky, especially when determining the units involved. Remember the following facts:

- Volume/volume percent (v/v%) is measured in mL/100 mL. This is used for liquids.
- Weight/weight percent (w/w%) is measured in g/100 g. This is used for ointments and creams.
- Weight/volume percent (w/v%) is measured in g/100 mL. This is used for drugs that are dissolved in solutions.

When converting a percentage to a fraction, the denominator is always 100. Review the following examples.

Make sure you are using the correct conversion factor and units when you set up proportions. Always double check your answer!

➡ Example 1

20 mL of glycerin is dissolved in water to make 80 mL of final solution. What is the percent strength of glycerin?

Answer: Calculate the percent strength by dividing the amount of active ingredient by the total weight or volume of the product. Then, multiply the result by 100 and add a percent sign (%). The active ingredient is glycerin, and the final volume is 80 mL.

$$\frac{20 \text{ mL}}{80 \text{ mL}} \times 100 = x$$
$$0.25 \times 100 = x$$
$$25\% = x$$

➡ Example 2

A prescription is written for ibuprofen 15% cream. How much ibuprofen powder is needed to prepare 30 grams of the compound?

Answer: First, set up your proportion. A proportion is a statement of equality between two ratios. Make sure to put what you want on the left side and what you need on the right side: WANT = NEED.

The prescription is written for 15% strength; this is what we want. 15% means $\frac{15 \text{ g}}{100 \text{ g}}$. The question also tells us that we need 30 g of the cream.

$$\frac{15 \text{ g}}{100 \text{ g}} = \frac{x}{30 \text{ g}}$$

Cross multiply and solve for x.

$$(15 \text{ g})(30 \text{ g}) = (x)(100 \text{ g})$$
$$450 \text{ g} = (x)(100 \text{ g})$$
$$x = \frac{450 \text{ g}}{100 \text{ g}}$$
$$x = 4.5 \text{ g}$$

This means that 4.5 g of ibuprofen powder is needed to prepare this prescription.

➡ Example 3

The prescription below is written for benzocaine gel 240 g:

benzocaine USP 2%

carbopol 940 NF 2%

alcohol USP 90%

distilled water 6%

How much benzocaine and carbopol are needed to prepare this prescription?

Answer: To solve this problem, you must determine the amount of each individual ingredient needed to make this preparation. The question does not ask for the amount of alcohol or distilled water needed to formulate this preparation, so only calculate the amount of benzocaine and carbopol. Set up a proportion for each ingredient using 240 g as the total amount of the final preparation.

$$\text{benzocaine:} \quad \frac{2\text{ g}}{100\text{ g}} = \frac{x}{240\text{ g}}$$

$$100x = 480\text{ g}$$

$$x = 4.8\text{ g}$$

$$\text{carbopol:} \quad \frac{2\text{ g}}{100\text{ g}} = \frac{x}{240\text{ g}}$$

$$100x = 480\text{ g}$$

$$x = 4.8\text{ g}$$

You will need 4.8 g of benzocaine and 4.8 g of carbopol to fill this prescription.

Diluting Stock Solutions

The concentration of a medication is the amount of drug (e.g., mg, g) given in a specified volume (e.g., mL). Concentrations may be expressed as a percent, fraction, or ratio. Stock solutions are concentrated solutions that are used to prepare less concentrated solutions. These less concentrated solutions (dilutions) are prepared by adding a diluent, such as sterile water.

Remember the following formula when solving these sorts of problems:

$$C1 \times V1 = C2 \times V2$$

where C1 is the initial concentration, V1 is the initial volume, C2 is the final concentration, and V2 is the final volume.

➡ Example 1 _____

400 mL of a 40% solution is diluted to 500 mL. What is the percent strength of the resulting solution?

Answer: To solve this problem, determine which components are given in the question. This question gives us a final volume of 500 mL with an initial volume of 400 mL. We are also given an initial concentration of 40%. An equation must be set up to determine the final concentration.

$$40\% \times 400\text{ mL} = x \times 500\text{ mL}$$

$$16{,}000\%\text{ mL} = x \times 500\text{ mL}$$

Divide both sides by 500 mL to solve for x. Make sure to cancel units.

$$\frac{16{,}000\%\ \text{mL}}{500\ \text{mL}} = x$$

$$32\% = x$$

The resulting solution will have a percent strength of 32%.

This problem can also be solved using the ratio and proportion method.

First, calculate the number of grams that are contained in 400 mL of the 40% solution.

$$\frac{40 \text{ g}}{100 \text{ mL}} = \frac{x}{400 \text{ mL}}$$

$$x = \frac{400 \text{ mL} \times 40 \text{ g}}{100 \text{ mL}}$$

$$x = 160 \text{ g}$$

This tells us that 160 g is diluted in 500 mL. The percent strength can be determined by calculating the number of grams in 100 mL.

$$\frac{160 \text{ g}}{500 \text{ mL}} = \frac{x}{100 \text{ mL}}$$

$$x = \frac{160 \text{ g} \times 100 \text{ mL}}{500 \text{ mL}}$$

$$x = 32 \text{ g} = 32\%$$

(Remember that percent is g per 100 mL.)

Alligations

Alligations are used to prepare a concentration of solution that is not commercially available. These solutions are made by mixing together two solutions when one solution contains a stronger concentration and the other contains a weaker concentration. The solutions must be expressed in percentages with the desired solution strength lying between the stronger and weaker concentrations.

Alligations can be solved using a table that looks similar to a tic-tac-toe board. See Table 8-7 below.

Table 8-7. Setting Up an Alligation Problem

Higher % strength solution (H)		Number of parts in higher % strength solution (P – L)
	Desired (product) % strength solution (P)	
Lower % strength solution (L)		Number of parts in lower % strength solution (H – P)

➥ Example 1 _____

How many mL of a 50% solution and of a 25% solution are needed to prepare 2 liters of a 40% solution?

Answer: First, set up a tic-tac-toe layout using the information provided, and solve for the number of parts of each solution.

Number of parts in higher % strength solution = (P − L)
Number of parts in lower % strength solution = (H − P)

50%		15 parts
	40%	
25%		10 parts

Next, determine the total number of parts by adding them together.

$$15 + 10 = 25 \text{ total parts}$$

Then, set up a proportion using the parts of each concentration. Remember to convert liters to milliliters (1 L = 1,000 mL, so 2 L = 2,000 mL).

$$\frac{15}{25} \times 2,000 \text{ mL} = 1,200 \text{ mL of 50\% solution}$$

$$\frac{10}{25} \times 2,000 \text{ mL} = 800 \text{ mL of 25\% solution}$$

Check your work by adding the total amounts of each concentration and comparing your answer to the total volume of the preparation, which in this case is 2,000 mL.

$$1,200 \text{ mL} + 800 \text{ mL} = 2,000 \text{ mL}$$

Infusion Rates and Drip Rates

Orders that are written for the rate at which an IV is infused are called infusion rates. These rates are expressed in mL/min, mL/hour, or amount of drug/time.

➡ **Example 1** _____

$$\text{rate of infusion} = \frac{\text{volume of fluid}}{\text{time of infusion}}$$

What is the rate of infusion in mL/hour of 1,000 mL of drug "X" to be infused over 8 hours?

Answer: Using the formula given:

$$\text{rate of infusion} = \frac{1,000 \text{ mL}}{8 \text{ hrs}}$$

$$\text{rate of infusion} = 125 \text{ mL/hr}$$

This equation can also be manipulated to solve for time.

➡ **Example 2** _____

$$\text{time of infusion} = \frac{\text{volume of fluid}}{\text{rate of infusion}}$$

The rate of infusion is 125 mL/hr, and the volume of fluid is 500 mL. How long will the IV bag last?

Answer: Using the formula above:

$$\text{time of infusion} = \frac{500 \text{ mL}}{125 \text{ mL/hr}}$$

$$\text{time of infusion} = 4 \text{ hours}$$

IV sets are used to deliver IVs to patients. These sets are calibrated for a specific number of drops per mL. Pharmacy technicians are expected to calculate the rate of infusion in drops per minute.

Common drop (gtts) factors are 10 gtts/mL (macro sets), 15 gtts/mL, and 60 gtts/mL (micro sets).

Use the following formula to solve for the infusion flow rate:

$$\text{infusion flow rate (gtts/min)} = \frac{\text{volume (mL)}}{\text{time (min)}} \times \text{drop factor (gtts/mL)}$$

➡ **Example 3** _____

What is the infusion rate of a 1 L lactated Ringer's solution with a flow rate of 125 mL/hr and a drop factor of 15 gtts/mL?

Answer: Recognize that 1 L = 1,000 mL.

$$\text{infusion flow rate (gtts/min)} = \frac{125 \text{ mL}}{60 \text{ min}} \times \frac{15 \text{ gtts}}{1 \text{ mL}}$$

$$\text{infusion flow rate (gtts/min)} = 31.25 \approx 31 \text{ gtts/min}$$

TIP

Drop factors can be found on the IV administration package.

Other Calculations/Doses Based on Body Weight, Age, and Body Surface Area

Many pediatric, geriatric, oncology, corticosteroid, and antibiotic medications are dosed based on body weight (usually mg/kg). Questions that involve doses based on body weight may require conversions from pounds to kilograms (1 kg = 2.2 lb).

➡ **Example 1** _____

The prescriber orders a drug to be dosed at 15 mg/kg/day. What is the daily dose for a 132 lb patient?

Answer:

$$132 \text{ lbs} \times \frac{1 \text{ kg}}{2.2 \text{ lbs}} = 60 \text{ kg}$$

Then, set up a ratio and proportion using the given dosing regimen.

$$\frac{15 \text{ mg}}{1 \text{ kg}} = \frac{x}{60 \text{ kg}}$$

$$(15 \text{ mg})(60 \text{ kg}) = (1 \text{ kg})(x)$$

$$900 \text{ mg per day} = x$$

Doses based on body weight can be determined using a nomogram, which is a chart that is used to determine body surface area (BSA) based on the patient's height and weight. Nomograms may be used if the BSA is not given in the question. The BSA is used to calculate doses for patients who are receiving chemotherapeutic agents and is measured in m^2.

➡ **Example 2** _____

A patient has a BSA of 1.54 m^2. Calculate the dose of fluorouracil, in mg, for the patient if the doctor has ordered 400 mg/m^2 daily.

Answer: Set up a proportion.

$$\frac{400 \text{ mg}}{1 \text{ m}^2} = \frac{x}{1.54 \text{ m}^2}$$

$$(400 \text{ mg})(1.54 \text{ m}^2) = (1 \text{ m}^2)(x)$$

$$616 \text{ mg} = x$$

One other way to calculate the BSA is to use the Mosteller formula. This formula can be adapted to calculate the BSA based on weight in kilograms and height in centimeters or based on weight in pounds and height in inches.

$$\text{BSA m}^2 = \sqrt{\frac{\text{height (cm)} \times \text{weight (kg)}}{3600}}$$

OR

$$\text{BSA m}^2 = \sqrt{\frac{\text{height (in)} \times \text{weight (lb)}}{3131}}$$

➡ Example 3

A patient weighs 27 lbs and is 30 inches tall. Calculate the patient's BSA using the Mosteller formula.

Answer:

$$\text{BSA m}^2 = \sqrt{\frac{\text{height (in)} \times \text{weight (lb)}}{3131}}$$

$$\text{BSA m}^2 = \sqrt{\frac{30 \text{ in} \times 27 \text{ lbs}}{3131}}$$

$$\text{BSA m}^2 = 0.51 \text{ m}^2$$

In the event that the manufacturer's recommended dose is not available, two alternative methods can be used to determine the pediatric dose. Clark's rule uses the child's weight in pounds and assumes an average adult weight of 150 pounds. This formula is valid for patients who weigh less than 150 pounds. Young's rule, on the other hand, uses the patient's age (under 12 years old) to determine the recommended dose. You can differentiate between the two formulas by remembering that Young's rule uses the age; this is even implied in the name (since "Young" implies age, not weight).

Clark's rule:

$$\text{Adult dose} \times \left(\frac{\text{Weight (lbs)}}{\text{Average adult weight of 150 lbs}} \right) = \text{Child's dose}$$

Young's rule:

$$\text{Adult dose} \times \left(\frac{\text{Age}}{\text{Age} + 12} \right) = \text{Child's dose}$$

➡ Example 4

Using Clark's rule, determine the dose that is required for an 11-year-old child, who weighs 75 pounds, if the average adult dose is 500 mg.

$$\text{Adult dose} \times \left(\frac{\text{Weight (lbs)}}{\text{Average adult weight of 150 lbs}} \right) = \text{Child's dose}$$

$$500 \text{ mg} \times \left(\frac{75 \text{ lbs}}{150 \text{ lbs}} \right) = \text{Child's dose} = 250 \text{ mg}$$

➡ Example 5

Using Young's rule, determine the dose that is required for an 11-year-old child, who weighs 75 pounds, if the average adult dose is 500 mg.

Answer:

$$\text{Adult dose} \times \left(\frac{\text{Age}}{\text{Age} + 12} \right) = \text{Child's dose}$$

$$500 \text{ mg} \times \left(\frac{11}{11 + 12} \right) = \text{Child's dose} = 239 \text{ mg}$$

SUMMARY

☐ Pharmacy personnel prepare non-sterile compounded medications according to standards of purity in order to maintain product sterility and accuracy.

☐ Proper selection of materials for non-sterile compounding formulations is determined based on the prescription, common practices, and current guidelines.

☐ Non-sterile compounding procedures are based on the standards set by the United States Pharmacopeia (USP <795>).

☐ Beyond-use dates are determined by the manufacturer and are used to identify the medication's expiration date.

☐ Each medication receives an associated lot number that indicates where and when the medication was processed. This lot number is an important tool that is used to identify a medication that has been affected by a recall.

☐ The National Drug Code (NDC) is a 10-digit sequence of numbers that identifies the labeler, product, and package size of the medication.

☐ Medication returns are identified as dispensable or non-dispensable. They may be eligible for credit, or they will either be returned to stock or returned using a reverse distributor.

☐ Pharmacy technicians should be familiar with common medical terminology, pharmacy abbreviations, Sig codes, and symbols used in pharmacy practice.

☐ Familiarity with pharmacy calculations is a necessary component of pharmacy practice.

ORDER ENTRY AND PROCESSING PRACTICE QUESTIONS

1. Which of the following equipment is NOT used in non-sterile compounding procedures?

   (A) graduated cylinder
   (B) mortar and pestle
   (C) prescription vial
   (D) laminar flow hood

2. Pharmacy personnel use various techniques when compounding preparations. Which of the following best describes levigation?

   (A) the process of grinding a powder by incorporating a liquid
   (B) the process of reducing a particle's size by incorporating a substance in which that particle is soluble
   (C) the process of reducing the particle size of an ingredient by grinding it into a powder
   (D) the process of using a spatula to mix ingredients

3. In the NDC number 0415-5258-26, the last two numbers indicate the _____.

    (A) dosage form
    (B) manufacturer
    (C) package size
    (D) drug strength

4. How many tablets should be dispensed given the following order?

    amoxicillin 250 mg tabs; sig 1 tab po BID × 10 days

    (A) 10
    (B) 20
    (C) 30
    (D) 40

5. A drug container has an expiration date of 07/2021. On which of the following days does this bottle's contents actually expire?

    (A) 06/30/2021
    (B) 07/01/2021
    (C) 07/31/2021
    (D) 08/01/2021

6. Which of the following units are used when interpreting an expression of a percentage (e.g., 10%)?

    (A) mg/mL
    (B) mg/L
    (C) g/mL
    (D) g/L

7. A patient returns a medication vial to your pharmacy, stating that he picked up the prescription in error and does not need it. What should you do with the medication?

    (A) Return the medication to stock since the patient did not use it.
    (B) Dispose of the medication in the pharmacy waste bin.
    (C) Tell the patient to throw out the medication in his home.
    (D) Place the medication in a designated bin for disposal via a reverse distributor.

8. Which of the following devices should be calibrated prior to use?

    (A) Class III prescription balance
    (B) graduated cylinder
    (C) laminar flow hood
    (D) mortar and pestle

9. What type of medication is dosed based on BSA?

   (A) antihistamines
   (B) corticosteroids
   (C) chemotherapeutic agents
   (D) antibiotics

10. Valproic acid syrup is available as 250 mg/5 mL. A patient is taking 500 mg qam and 250 qpm. How many milliliters are required for a 30 days supply?

   (A) 250 mL
   (B) 350 mL
   (C) 450 mL
   (D) 550 mL

ANSWERS EXPLAINED

1. **(D)** Laminar flow hoods are used in sterile compounding procedures. Graduated cylinders, mortars and pestles, and prescription vials are all examples of equipment used in non-sterile compounding procedures.

2. **(A)** Levigation is the process of grinding a powder by incorporating a liquid. Pulverization is the process of reducing a particle's size by incorporating a substance in which that particle is soluble. Trituration is the process of reducing the particle size of an ingredient by grinding it into a powder. Spatulation is the process of using a spatula to mix ingredients.

3. **(C)** The last two numbers of a product's National Drug Code (NDC) indicate the package size of the product.

4. **(B)** 1 tablet × twice a day = 2 tablets a day × 10 days = 20 total tablets dispensed.

5. **(C)** Unless a product has a clear expiration date (month, day, year), it is assumed that an expiration date with a month and year format does not expire until the last day of that month.

6. **(C)** Percentages may be expressed as g/mL, mL/mL, and g/g.

7. **(D)** Once a medication has left the pharmacy, it cannot be returned to stock and sold again. These medications are placed in a designated bin for removal via a reverse distributor.

8. **(A)** The Class III prescription balance must be calibrated prior to use. Graduated cylinders, as well as mortars and pestles, are supplies that are used in non-sterile compounding. Laminar flow hoods are used in the preparation of sterile compounded products.

9. **(C)** Chemotherapeutic agents are dosed based on body surface area (BSA). Antihistamines, corticosteroids, and antibiotics are based on weight.

10. **(C)** Determine the number of milliliters that are required for each dose (morning and evening).

Morning dose:

$$\frac{250 \text{ mg}}{5 \text{ mL}} = \frac{500 \text{ mg}}{x \text{ mL}}$$

$$x = 10 \text{ mL}$$

Evening dose:

$$\frac{250 \text{ mg}}{5 \text{ mL}} = \frac{250 \text{ mg}}{x \text{ mL}}$$

$$x = 5 \text{ mL}$$

Therefore, the patient is taking 15 mL/day. Thus:

$$\frac{15 \text{ mL}}{1 \text{ day}} = \frac{x \text{ mL}}{30 \text{ days}}$$

$$x = 450 \text{ mL for a 30 days supply}$$

Practice Tests

NOTE

Don't forget that in addition to the pretest and the following two practice tests, Barron's *PTCE: Pharmacy Technician Certification Exam, Second Edition* also includes a full-length online practice test, which you can take at any time on your computer, tablet, or smartphone.

Visit *http://bit.ly/Barrons-PTCE* to access the online PTCE exam.

*Be sure to have your copy of *PTCE: Pharmacy Technician Certification Exam, Second Edition* on hand to complete the registration process.

ANSWER SHEET
Practice Test 1

1. Ⓐ Ⓑ Ⓒ Ⓓ
2. Ⓐ Ⓑ Ⓒ Ⓓ
3. Ⓐ Ⓑ Ⓒ Ⓓ
4. Ⓐ Ⓑ Ⓒ Ⓓ
5. Ⓐ Ⓑ Ⓒ Ⓓ
6. Ⓐ Ⓑ Ⓒ Ⓓ
7. Ⓐ Ⓑ Ⓒ Ⓓ
8. Ⓐ Ⓑ Ⓒ Ⓓ
9. Ⓐ Ⓑ Ⓒ Ⓓ
10. Ⓐ Ⓑ Ⓒ Ⓓ
11. Ⓐ Ⓑ Ⓒ Ⓓ
12. Ⓐ Ⓑ Ⓒ Ⓓ
13. Ⓐ Ⓑ Ⓒ Ⓓ
14. Ⓐ Ⓑ Ⓒ Ⓓ
15. Ⓐ Ⓑ Ⓒ Ⓓ
16. Ⓐ Ⓑ Ⓒ Ⓓ
17. Ⓐ Ⓑ Ⓒ Ⓓ
18. Ⓐ Ⓑ Ⓒ Ⓓ
19. Ⓐ Ⓑ Ⓒ Ⓓ
20. Ⓐ Ⓑ Ⓒ Ⓓ
21. Ⓐ Ⓑ Ⓒ Ⓓ
22. Ⓐ Ⓑ Ⓒ Ⓓ
23. Ⓐ Ⓑ Ⓒ Ⓓ
24. Ⓐ Ⓑ Ⓒ Ⓓ
25. Ⓐ Ⓑ Ⓒ Ⓓ
26. Ⓐ Ⓑ Ⓒ Ⓓ
27. Ⓐ Ⓑ Ⓒ Ⓓ
28. Ⓐ Ⓑ Ⓒ Ⓓ
29. Ⓐ Ⓑ Ⓒ Ⓓ
30. Ⓐ Ⓑ Ⓒ Ⓓ

31. Ⓐ Ⓑ Ⓒ Ⓓ
32. Ⓐ Ⓑ Ⓒ Ⓓ
33. Ⓐ Ⓑ Ⓒ Ⓓ
34. Ⓐ Ⓑ Ⓒ Ⓓ
35. Ⓐ Ⓑ Ⓒ Ⓓ
36. Ⓐ Ⓑ Ⓒ Ⓓ
37. Ⓐ Ⓑ Ⓒ Ⓓ
38. Ⓐ Ⓑ Ⓒ Ⓓ
39. Ⓐ Ⓑ Ⓒ Ⓓ
40. Ⓐ Ⓑ Ⓒ Ⓓ
41. Ⓐ Ⓑ Ⓒ Ⓓ
42. Ⓐ Ⓑ Ⓒ Ⓓ
43. Ⓐ Ⓑ Ⓒ Ⓓ
44. Ⓐ Ⓑ Ⓒ Ⓓ
45. Ⓐ Ⓑ Ⓒ Ⓓ
46. Ⓐ Ⓑ Ⓒ Ⓓ
47. Ⓐ Ⓑ Ⓒ Ⓓ
48. Ⓐ Ⓑ Ⓒ Ⓓ
49. Ⓐ Ⓑ Ⓒ Ⓓ
50. Ⓐ Ⓑ Ⓒ Ⓓ
51. Ⓐ Ⓑ Ⓒ Ⓓ
52. Ⓐ Ⓑ Ⓒ Ⓓ
53. Ⓐ Ⓑ Ⓒ Ⓓ
54. Ⓐ Ⓑ Ⓒ Ⓓ
55. Ⓐ Ⓑ Ⓒ Ⓓ
56. Ⓐ Ⓑ Ⓒ Ⓓ
57. Ⓐ Ⓑ Ⓒ Ⓓ
58. Ⓐ Ⓑ Ⓒ Ⓓ
59. Ⓐ Ⓑ Ⓒ Ⓓ
60. Ⓐ Ⓑ Ⓒ Ⓓ

61. Ⓐ Ⓑ Ⓒ Ⓓ
62. Ⓐ Ⓑ Ⓒ Ⓓ
63. Ⓐ Ⓑ Ⓒ Ⓓ
64. Ⓐ Ⓑ Ⓒ Ⓓ
65. Ⓐ Ⓑ Ⓒ Ⓓ
66. Ⓐ Ⓑ Ⓒ Ⓓ
67. Ⓐ Ⓑ Ⓒ Ⓓ
68. Ⓐ Ⓑ Ⓒ Ⓓ
69. Ⓐ Ⓑ Ⓒ Ⓓ
70. Ⓐ Ⓑ Ⓒ Ⓓ
71. Ⓐ Ⓑ Ⓒ Ⓓ
72. Ⓐ Ⓑ Ⓒ Ⓓ
73. Ⓐ Ⓑ Ⓒ Ⓓ
74. Ⓐ Ⓑ Ⓒ Ⓓ
75. Ⓐ Ⓑ Ⓒ Ⓓ
76. Ⓐ Ⓑ Ⓒ Ⓓ
77. Ⓐ Ⓑ Ⓒ Ⓓ
78. Ⓐ Ⓑ Ⓒ Ⓓ
79. Ⓐ Ⓑ Ⓒ Ⓓ
80. Ⓐ Ⓑ Ⓒ Ⓓ
81. Ⓐ Ⓑ Ⓒ Ⓓ
82. Ⓐ Ⓑ Ⓒ Ⓓ
83. Ⓐ Ⓑ Ⓒ Ⓓ
84. Ⓐ Ⓑ Ⓒ Ⓓ
85. Ⓐ Ⓑ Ⓒ Ⓓ
86. Ⓐ Ⓑ Ⓒ Ⓓ
87. Ⓐ Ⓑ Ⓒ Ⓓ
88. Ⓐ Ⓑ Ⓒ Ⓓ
89. Ⓐ Ⓑ Ⓒ Ⓓ
90. Ⓐ Ⓑ Ⓒ Ⓓ

Practice Test 1

Directions: You will have 1 hour and 50 minutes to complete the following 90 questions. For each question, select the choice that best answers the question, and mark that answer letter on your answer sheet. Remember, this test should be used to help you determine areas that require additional review. Each question represents a particular area of the PTCE blueprint, which can help you pinpoint areas of mastery or concepts that require additional studying. The official PTCE exam uses a scaled score to determine your grade. Only 80 out of 90 questions on the PTCE are scored, and unscored questions are not identified. You should be able to answer about 72 of the questions on this test correctly, averaging an overall percentage of 80% or more on your attempt at this test.

1. How many mL of 70% and 40% alcohol elixirs should be mixed to prepare 300 mL of 60% alcohol?

   (A) 200 mL of 70%, 100 mL of 40%
   (B) 100 mL of 70%, 200 mL of 40%
   (C) 75 mL of 70%, 25 mL of 40%
   (D) 50 mL of 70%, 250 mL of 40%

2. Which of the following vaccines should be kept in a freezer?

   (A) Varicella vaccine
   (B) MMR vaccine
   (C) Fluzone vaccine
   (D) Gardasil vaccine

3. Which of the following is an example of a Class II recall?

   (A) foreign objects that pose a physical hazard
   (B) a label mix-up on a life-saving drug
   (C) a medication container defect or malfunctioning drug delivery device
   (D) All of the above

4. The Roman numeral XXXVI is equal to
   _____.

   (A) 34
   (B) 36
   (C) 26
   (D) 24

5. Many terminally ill patients on pain medications require increasingly higher doses to obtain pain relief. This is known as _____.

   (A) tolerance
   (B) addiction
   (C) dependence
   (D) habituation

6. A Class III prescription balance requires recertification every _____.

   (A) year
   (B) 2 years
   (C) 4 years
   (D) 5 years

7. The physician orders cefaclor 450 mg TID. The drug is available as a 375 mg/5 mL suspension. How many mL should be given for each dose?

   (A) 2 mL
   (B) 6 mL
   (C) 12 mL
   (D) 18 mL

8. What is the appropriate form required for a pharmacy to order Schedule II medications from a distributor?

   (A) DEA form 222
   (B) DEA form 41
   (C) DEA form 106
   (D) None of the above

9. Hydrocortisone 0.5% cream in a 1-ounce tube contains _____.

   (A) hydrocortisone 141.75 mg in 28.35 g of cream
   (B) hydrocortisone 0.4175 g in 100 mg of cream
   (C) hydrocortisone 0.4175 g in 28.35 g of cream
   (D) hydrocortisone 28.35 mg in 141.75 g of cream

10. How many prednisone 5 mg tablets are needed to fill a prescription with the following directions?

    prednisone 5 mg tablets

    Take $\frac{1}{2}$ tab PO QID × 2 days

    $\frac{1}{2}$ tab PO TID × 2 days

    $\frac{1}{2}$ tab PO BID × 2 days

    $\frac{1}{2}$ tab PO QD × 2 days

    Then stop

    (A) 5
    (B) 10
    (C) 20
    (D) 30

11. How much gentamicin 40 mg/mL is needed for a 130 mg dose?

    (A) 2 mL
    (B) 2.25 mL
    (C) 3 mL
    (D) 3.25 mL

12. The four aspects of pharmacokinetics include _____.

    (A) absorption, distribution, mitosis, and excretion
    (B) absorption, distribution, migration, and excretion
    (C) absorption, distribution, metastasis, and excretion
    (D) absorption, distribution, metabolism, and excretion

13. Ibuprofen can be given to a child at a dose of 10 mg/kg. What is the dose for a 44 lb child?

    (A) 200 mg
    (B) 220 mg
    (C) 440 mg
    (D) 968 mg

14. Concentrated sodium chloride solution (23.4%) contains 4 mEq/mL. How much (in mL) is needed to provide 40 mEq of NaCl for a parenteral nutrition admixture?

    (A) 4 mL
    (B) 10 mL
    (C) 23.4 mL
    (D) 40 mL

15. When reading the volume of liquid in a graduated cylinder, you should _____.

    (A) read the top of the meniscus
    (B) read the middle of the meniscus
    (C) read the bottom of the meniscus
    (D) read the bubble that forms at the top of the meniscus

16. Which of the following is identified as an error-prone abbreviation by the ISMP?

    (A) cc
    (B) prn
    (C) IV
    (D) ac

17. A pharmacy can order Schedule III drugs _____.

    (A) using a DEA 222 form
    (B) using a standard invoice
    (C) through a reverse distributor
    (D) only one day a week

18. A failure to reconstitute a suspension is an example of an error that can occur during which of the following steps of the medication use process?

    (A) prescribing
    (B) transcribing
    (C) dispensing
    (D) administration

19. Look at the following sig.

    1 tab PO BID AC and HS

    What instructions should be typed on the customer label?

    (A) "Take one capsule by mouth twice a day before meals and at bedtime."
    (B) "Take one tablet by mouth twice a day before meals and at bedtime."
    (C) "Take one tablet by mouth twice a day after meals and at bedtime."
    (D) "Take one capsule by mouth twice a day after meals and at bedtime."

20. Which of the following liquid drug dosage forms contains concentrated sucrose solutions?

    (A) suspension
    (B) elixir
    (C) syrup
    (D) tincture

21. Pharmacy technicians check refrigerators that are used to hold medications daily and log temperature data. When checking the temperature of a refrigerator, an appropriate range is _____.

    (A) −4° to 14°F
    (B) 36° to 46°F
    (C) 46° to 59°F
    (D) 68° to 77°F

22. A compounded solid drug product should never have a BUD beyond _____.

    (A) 14 days
    (B) 3 months
    (C) 6 months
    (D) 1 year

23. How many teaspoons are in 1 ounce?

    (A) 1 teaspoon
    (B) 3 teaspoons
    (C) 6 teaspoons
    (D) 8 teaspoons

24. Which of the following medications is the brand name for omeprazole?

    (A) Prilosec
    (B) Protonix
    (C) AcipHex
    (D) Nexium

25. Which of the following supplements is commonly used as a sleep aid?

    (A) valerian root
    (B) ginseng
    (C) ginkgo biloba
    (D) resveratrol

26. Which DEA form is used to register with the DEA to dispense controlled substances?

    (A) Form 41
    (B) Form 106
    (C) Form 222
    (D) Form 224

27. Most prescriptions, with the exception of controlled substances, are valid for _____.

    (A) 6 months or 5 refills
    (B) a 3-month supply because of lower insurance copay
    (C) 12 months from the date written
    (D) 12 months from the date filled

28. A medication is to be taken "PC." It should be taken _____.

    (A) in the morning
    (B) in the evening
    (C) before meals
    (D) after meals

29. Oxycodone is a DEA Schedule II drug. This means that the drug has a _____ potential for abuse and _____ accepted medical uses in the United States.

    (A) high; no currently
    (B) low; no currently
    (C) high; currently
    (D) low; currently

30. The Combat Methamphetamine Epidemic Act (CMEA) restricts the sale of which of the following?

    (A) Robitussin
    (B) Delsym
    (C) Sudafed
    (D) Zyrtec

31. Which of the following is an example of a physical incompatibility that may result from the mixture of two or more substances?

    (A) increase in temperature
    (B) effervescence
    (C) precipitation
    (D) decomposition

32. What class of drugs is used to treat elevated blood pressure?

    (A) antihistamines
    (B) antihypertensives
    (C) anticoagulants
    (D) antihyperlipidemics

33. Pharmaceutical drugs are found in what hazardous drug list classification?

    (A) P-list
    (B) S-list
    (C) K-list
    (D) F-list

34. Look at the following look-alike/sound-alike (LASA) drug pairs. Which LASA pair contains an antihypertensive?

    (A) ALPRAZolam and LORazepam
    (B) methylPREDNISOLONE and medroxyPROGESTERone
    (C) hydrALAZINE and hydrOXYzine
    (D) vinBLASTine and vinCRISTine

35. What needle gauge size is used in the administration of insulin?

    (A) 18
    (B) 21
    (C) 26
    (D) 29

36. Xanax is listed as a Schedule IV drug in Ohio. Xanax expires after _____ and may have up to _____ refills.

    (A) 1 year; no
    (B) 6 months; no
    (C) 6 months; up to 5
    (D) 1 year; up to 5

37. Convert 86°F to degrees Celsius.

    (A) 20°C
    (B) 25°C
    (C) 30°C
    (D) 35°C

38. The Combat Methamphetamine Epidemic Act places _____ and _____ limits on the over-the-counter sale of products that contain pseudoephedrine.

    (A) daily, weekly
    (B) daily, monthly
    (C) weekly, monthly
    (D) monthly, yearly

39. How many mL are in 4 L of NS?

    (A) 40 mL
    (B) 400 mL
    (C) 4,000 mL
    (D) 40,000 mL

40. A patient weighs 50 kg. What is his weight in lbs?

    (A) 50 lbs
    (B) 100 lbs
    (C) 110 lbs
    (D) 200 lbs

41. A doctor has written a prescription for 10 mL of brand "X" antibiotic suspension to be taken twice daily. How many days will an 8-ounce bottle last?

    (A) 10 days
    (B) 12 days
    (C) 14 days
    (D) 16 days

42. Which of the following techniques is used to identify medications that are about to expire?

    (A) placing a colored sticker on the stock bottle
    (B) moving expired medication to the back of the shelf
    (C) organizing medications alphabetically by generic name
    (D) organizing medications by brand name

43. Mixing powders of unequal quantity is called _____.

    (A) geometric dilution
    (B) spatulation
    (C) levigation
    (D) emulsion

44. Which regulatory agency could initiate a Class II medication recall?

    (A) DEA
    (B) ASHP
    (C) TJC
    (D) FDA

45. What is the generic name for Cytomel?

    (A) levothyroxine
    (B) liothyronine
    (C) lamotrigine
    (D) levetiracetam

46. Which of the following is an autoimmune disease in which the thyroid is overactive and produces excessive amounts of thyroid hormones?

    (A) HIV/AIDS
    (B) hyperlipidemia
    (C) Graves disease
    (D) hypothyroidism

47. If two drugs are taken together and one of them intensifies the action of the other, what type of drug interaction has occurred?

    (A) additive
    (B) synergistic
    (C) potentiated
    (D) antagonistic

48. Which of the following herbal medications can be used to promote relaxation?

    (A) kava
    (B) ginseng
    (C) garlic
    (D) ephedra

49. Which of the following drugs has a narrow therapeutic index?

    (A) clindamycin
    (B) carbamazepine
    (C) labetalol
    (D) clopidogrel

50. The drug name Synthroid is also known as the _____ name.

    (A) chemical
    (B) generic
    (C) brand
    (D) supplier

51. Which of the following situations requires a pharmacist's intervention?

    (A) an automated refill request
    (B) a prior authorization request
    (C) an OTC recommendation
    (D) ordering non-controlled medications

52. The percent equivalent of a 1:80 ratio is _____%.

    (A) 1.5
    (B) 1.3
    (C) 1.25
    (D) 1

53. What method is used to prepare capsules?

    (A) punch method
    (B) flocculation
    (C) dry gum method
    (D) geometric dilution

54. Patients should be instructed to rinse well following corticosteroid use _____.

    (A) due to the potential for candidiasis
    (B) to help relieve headaches
    (C) to prevent future cavities
    (D) to freshen breath

55. What type of drug is metoprolol?

    (A) proton-pump inhibitor (PPI)
    (B) beta blocker
    (C) diuretic
    (D) antihistamine

56. A term that is used to describe the harmful and undesired effects produced by a medication when taken at normal doses is called _____.

    (A) potentiation
    (B) a contraindication
    (C) synergism
    (D) an adverse drug reaction

57. A patient's prescription reads: albuterol, 1–2 puffs q4–6 hours as needed for asthma. The patient approaches the pharmacy and indicates that she is using the inhaler every day, twice in the morning and twice in the evening, as a proactive approach for her asthma. What type of issue is this patient experiencing?

    (A) a drug interaction
    (B) an issue with adherence
    (C) therapeutic substitution
    (D) an adverse drug event

58. Where is a NuvaRing stored in the pharmacy?

    (A) at room temperature
    (B) in a refrigerator
    (C) in a freezer
    (D) in a refrigerator or a freezer

59. Mrs. Smith is picking up an order of drug "X" #50 tablets, which cost her $120. While you're ringing up her order, she asks, "How much does each tablet cost?" What is she being charged for each tablet?

    (A) $1.20
    (B) $1.80
    (C) $2.40
    (D) $2.80

60. What size needle has the largest diameter?

   (A) 24
   (B) 22
   (C) 18
   (D) 16

61. A drug patent lasts _____ years beginning on the _____ date.

   (A) 10; filing
   (B) 10; drug approval
   (C) 20; filing
   (D) 20; drug approval

62. What percentage strength of isopropyl alcohol is used to clean pharmacy counters and counting trays?

   (A) 50% isopropyl alcohol
   (B) 70% isopropyl alcohol
   (C) 95% isopropyl alcohol
   (D) 99% isopropyl alcohol

63. If the manufacturer's expiration date for a drug is 12/25, the drug is considered acceptable to dispense until which date?

   (A) 12/31/25
   (B) 12/01/25
   (C) 12/15/25
   (D) 12/07/25

64. What is the generic name for Advair?

   (A) tiotropium
   (B) salmeterol
   (C) salmeterol and fluticasone propionate
   (D) formoterol and budesonide

65. Nitroglycerin is provided as a sublingual tablet. This means that the tablet should be dissolved _____.

   (A) in a cup of water
   (B) under the tongue
   (C) in the eye
   (D) in normal saline

66. Which of the following NSAIDs is available OTC?

   (A) meloxicam
   (B) ibuprofen
   (C) ketorolac
   (D) celecoxib

67. The abbreviation "au" means _____.

   (A) right ear
   (B) both ears
   (C) left eye
   (D) both eyes

68. A script is presented for "Zocor 20 mg PO QHS." The pharmacy is currently out of Zocor 20 mg. Which of the following may the pharmacist substitute to fill the order?

   (A) atorvastatin
   (B) simvastatin
   (C) candesartan
   (D) losartan

69. A _____ protects a brand name drug from unauthorized use.

   (A) patent
   (B) copyright
   (C) trademark
   (D) symbol

70. Which clinical trial phase includes 20–100 individuals and tests for safety?

   (A) Phase I
   (B) Phase II
   (C) Phase III
   (D) Phase IV

71. What is the maximum number of refills allowed for a Schedule II medication?

   (A) 0 refills
   (B) 1 refill
   (C) 5 refills
   (D) 12 refills

72. Which of the following is a side effect that is associated with the ACE inhibitor lisinopril?

    (A) dry, hacking cough
    (B) leukopenia
    (C) muscle weakness
    (D) drowsiness

73. There are _____ ounces (oz) in a pound (lb).

    (A) 2
    (B) 8
    (C) 16
    (D) 24

74. What is the correct classification for furosemide?

    (A) loop diuretic
    (B) thiazide diuretic
    (C) potassium-sparing diuretic
    (D) beta blocker

75. Which of the following suffixes indicates a condition of enlargement?

    (A) -oma
    (B) -megaly
    (C) -osis
    (D) -itis

76. Pharmacies that handle hazardous medications must maintain which of the following documents?

    (A) package insert
    (B) medication guide
    (C) safety data sheet
    (D) compounding log

77. How would pharmacy personnel identify a medication in a drug recall situation?

    (A) check the medication name
    (B) check the lot number
    (C) check the medication instructions
    (D) look for opened medications

78. Medications and foods that should not be taken together would be identified in which of the following monitoring parameters?

    (A) drug-allergy interaction
    (B) drug-nutrient interaction
    (C) drug-drug interaction
    (D) drug-food interaction

79. A 70% HCl solution has a strength of 25 mEq/mL. How many mL are needed to prepare 60 mEq?

    (A) 1.2 mL
    (B) 1.7 mL
    (C) 2.1 mL
    (D) 2.4 mL

80. Which of the following medications for osteoporosis is taken once a month?

    (A) Fosamax
    (B) Boniva
    (C) Actonel
    (D) Reclast

81. Which of the following is an antibiotic that is indicated in the treatment of UTIs?

    (A) ketoconazole
    (B) miconazole
    (C) clotrimazole
    (D) metronidazole

82. Which of the following is NOT an example of a drug interaction?

    (A) drug-drug
    (B) drug-laboratory
    (C) therapeutic duplication
    (D) food-environment

83. Which of the following must appear on a written prescription for a controlled substance?

    (A) indication
    (B) patient's medication history
    (C) prescriber's DEA number
    (D) patient's social security number

84. What is the brand name for pravastatin?

(A) Pravachol
(B) Lipitor
(C) Zocor
(D) Crestor

85. What is the body surface area for a patient who weighs 22 kg and is 60 cm tall?

(A) 0.9 m^2
(B) 0.74 m^2
(C) 0.61 m^2
(D) 0.37 m^2

86. When calculating w/v%, the percentage refers to _____.

(A) mg/100 mL
(B) g/100 mL
(C) mg/100 L
(D) g/100 L

87. On average, how many drops are in 1 mL?

(A) 5 drops
(B) 10 drops
(C) 20 drops
(D) 30 drops

88. Lanoxin pediatric solution is available in 0.05 mg/mL. If a patient takes 0.25 mg of Lanoxin per day, what will be the dispensed quantity in mL for 30 days?

(A) 50 mL
(B) 100 mL
(C) 150 mL
(D) 200 mL

89. What is the name of the process that is used to grind tablets into a fine powder using a mortar and pestle?

(A) spatulation
(B) sifting
(C) trituration
(D) tumbling

90. Which of the following capsule sizes is the smallest?

(A) 00
(B) 0
(C) 1
(D) 5

ANSWER KEY
Practice Test 1

1. **A**	31. **C**	61. **C**
2. **A**	32. **B**	62. **B**
3. **A**	33. **A**	63. **A**
4. **B**	34. **C**	64. **C**
5. **A**	35. **D**	65. **B**
6. **A**	36. **C**	66. **B**
7. **B**	37. **C**	67. **B**
8. **A**	38. **B**	68. **B**
9. **A**	39. **C**	69. **A**
10. **B**	40. **C**	70. **A**
11. **D**	41. **B**	71. **A**
12. **D**	42. **A**	72. **A**
13. **A**	43. **A**	73. **C**
14. **B**	44. **D**	74. **A**
15. **C**	45. **B**	75. **B**
16. **A**	46. **C**	76. **C**
17. **B**	47. **C**	77. **B**
18. **C**	48. **A**	78. **D**
19. **B**	49. **B**	79. **D**
20. **C**	50. **C**	80. **B**
21. **B**	51. **C**	81. **D**
22. **C**	52. **C**	82. **D**
23. **C**	53. **A**	83. **C**
24. **A**	54. **A**	84. **A**
25. **A**	55. **B**	85. **C**
26. **D**	56. **D**	86. **B**
27. **C**	57. **B**	87. **C**
28. **D**	58. **B**	88. **C**
29. **C**	59. **C**	89. **C**
30. **C**	60. **D**	90. **D**

ANSWERS EXPLAINED

1. **(A)** You will need 200 mL of 70% solution and 100 mL of 40% solution. To answer this question, you need to follow five essential steps:

STEP 1 Set up your alligation problem using the sample setup below.

Strength of higher strength component (H)		P – L = relative amount of H needed to prepare P
	Desired strength of product (P)	
Strength of lower strength component (L)		H – P = relative amount of L needed to prepare P

70 (H)		P – L = 60 – 40 = 20 parts
	60 (P)	
40 (L)		H – P = 70 – 60 = 10 parts

STEP 2 Add the part values in the right-hand column together to get the total part value of the product.

$$10 + 20 = 30 \text{ parts}$$

STEP 3 Divide each part value by the total parts.

The amount of 70% alcohol is $\frac{20}{30}$ of the final product.

The amount of 40% alcohol is $\frac{10}{30}$ of the final product.

STEP 4 Solve for the volume of alcohol needed for each concentration.

To solve for the volume of 70% alcohol needed:

$$300 \text{ mL} \times \frac{20}{30} = 200 \text{ mL of 70\% alcohol needed}$$

To solve for the volume of 40% alcohol needed:

$$300 \text{ mL} \times \frac{10}{30} = 100 \text{ mL of 40\% alcohol needed}$$

STEP 5 Check your work to see if your answer makes sense.

When 200 mL of 70% alcohol are mixed with 100 mL of 40% alcohol, the resulting solution is 300 mL of 60% alcohol. Therefore, choice (A)—200 mL of 70%, 100 mL of 40%—is correct. Choice (B) is incorrect because it reverses the mL for 70% and 40%. Choice (C) cannot be the answer because the sum of the respective quantities does not equal the total amount of solution. Choice (D) incorrectly reflects a $\frac{1}{4}$ reduction in the total amount of 70% alcohol solution needed. The total amount of 40% alcohol solution is incorrect in choice (D) as well. (*Knowledge Domain 4.2*)

2. **(A)** The Varicella vaccine is one of a few vaccinations that should not be kept in a refrigerator. This preparation must be kept in a freezer until it is used. Choices (B), (C), and (D) are incorrect because the MMR, Fluzone, and Gardasil vaccines should be kept in a refrigerator, not in a freezer. (*Knowledge Domain 1.7*)

3. **(A)** Foreign objects that pose a physical hazard are an example of a Class II recall. This type of recall is defined by the FDA as "a situation in which use of, or exposure to, a violative product may cause temporary or medically reversible adverse health consequences or where the probability of serious adverse health consequences is remote." Choice (B) is an example of a Class I recall. This type of recall is defined as "a situation in which there is a reasonable probability that the use of, or exposure to, a violative product will cause serious adverse health consequences or death." Choice (C) is an example of a Class III recall, which is defined as a situation in which use of, or exposure to, a violative product is not likely to cause adverse health consequences." Since choices (B) and (C) are not examples of a Class II recall, choice (D) is incorrect as well. (*Knowledge Domain 2.5*)

4. **(B)** The Roman numeral XXXVI is equal to 36. Each X equals 10, each V equals 5, and each I equals 1. Therefore, 10 + 10 + 10 + 5 + 1 = 36. Choice (A) would be correct if the question asked for the equivalence of XXXIV. Since X equals 10 and IV equals 4, this Roman numeral equals 10 + 10 + 10 + 4 = 34. Choice (C) would be true if the question asked for the equivalence of XXVI. Since X equals 10, V equals 5, and I equals 1, this Roman numeral equals 10 + 10 + 5 + 1 = 26. Choice (D) would be right if the question asked for the equivalence of XXIV. Since X equals 10 and IV equals 4, this Roman numeral equals 10 + 10 + 4 = 24. (*Knowledge Domain 4.2*)

5. **(A)** Tolerance is defined as the need for larger or increased doses to achieve the desired response. Addiction, choice (B), is defined as a pattern of compulsive use, characterized by an overwhelming pattern of drug use and abuse. Dependence, choice (C), is defined as an altered state where continued administration of the drug is necessary to prevent physical and psychological withdrawal. Habituation, choice (D), is defined as becoming accustomed to a behavior or condition, including psychoactive drug use. (*Knowledge Domain 1.5*)

6. **(A)** A Class III prescription balance should be recertified every year. (*Knowledge Domain 4.1*)

7. **(B)** This problem can be solved by setting up a proportion.

$$\frac{375 \text{ mg}}{5 \text{ mL}} = \frac{450 \text{ mg}}{x \text{ mL}}$$

$$x = 6 \text{ mL}$$

6 mL is the volume that the patient will take per dose. (*Knowledge Domain 4.2*)

8. **(A)** DEA form 222 can be used to order both Schedule I and Schedule II drugs. DEA form 41, choice (B), is used to return or destroy drugs that are pending DEA approval. DEA form 106, choice (C), is used to report the theft or loss of controlled substances. (*Knowledge Domain 2.3*)

9. **(A)** A percentage weight in weight solution (w/w) is the number of grams of a constituent in 100 grams of mixture. So 0.5% cream is 0.5 grams in 100 grams of mixture. Perform the necessary calculations:

$$\frac{0.5 \text{ g}}{100 \text{ g}} = \frac{x}{28.35 \text{ g}}$$

$$(0.5 \text{ g})(28.35 \text{ g}) = x(100 \text{ g})$$

$$14.175 = 100x$$

$$x = 0.14175 \text{ g}$$

Since no answer contains this amount, convert grams to milligrams:

$$1,000 \text{ mg} = 1 \text{ g}$$

$$0.14175 \times 1,000 = 141.75 \text{ mg}$$

The correct amount is 141.75 mg in 28.35 g of cream, choice (A). (*Knowledge Domain 4.2*)

10. **(B)** To fill this prescription, 10 prednisone 5 mg tablets are needed. To answer this question, solve for how many tabs of QID, TID, BID, and QD are needed:

$$\frac{1}{2} \text{ tab PO QID} \times 2 \text{ days} = 2.5 \times 4 = 10 \text{ mg} \times 2 = 20 \text{ mg} = 4 \text{ tabs}$$

$$\frac{1}{2} \text{ tab PO TID} \times 2 \text{ days} = 2.5 \times 3 = 7.5 \text{ mg} \times 2 = 15 \text{ mg} = 3 \text{ tabs}$$

$$\frac{1}{2} \text{ tab PO BID} \times 2 \text{ days} = 2.5 \times 2 = 5 \text{ mg} \times 2 = 10 \text{ mg} = 2 \text{ tabs}$$

$$\frac{1}{2} \text{ tab PO QD} \times 2 \text{ days} = 2.5 \times 1 = 2.5 \text{ mg} \times 2 = 5 \text{ mg} = 1 \text{ tab}$$

$$4 \text{ tabs} + 3 \text{ tabs} + 2 \text{ tabs} + 1 \text{ tab} = 10 \text{ tablets}$$

The answer is 10 tablets. (*Knowledge Domain 4.2*)

11. **(D)**

$$\frac{40 \text{ mg}}{1 \text{ mL}} = \frac{130 \text{ mg}}{x}$$

$$40x = 130$$

$$x = 3.25 \text{ mL}$$

The answer is 3.25 mL, choice (D). (*Knowledge Domain 4.2*)

12. **(D)** The four aspects of pharmacokinetics include absorption, distribution, metabolism, and excretion. The acronym ADME can be used to remember this process. Choice (A) is wrong because mitosis is not a part of pharmacokinetics. Choices (B) and (C) mistakenly include "migration" and "metastasis," respectively, instead of "metabolism." (*Knowledge Domain 1.5*)

13. **(A)** The correct dose is 200 mg. Since 1 kg = 2.2 lbs:

$$\frac{1 \text{ kg}}{2.2 \text{ lbs}} = \frac{x}{44 \text{ lbs}}$$

$$2.2x = 44$$

$$x = 20 \text{ kg}$$

Therefore:

$$\frac{10\ \text{mg}}{1\ \cancel{\text{kg}}} \times 20\ \cancel{\text{kg}} = 200\ \text{mg dose}$$

Choice (B), 220 mg, reflects an error in the conversion calculation of lb to kg. When dividing 44 lb by 2.2 lb, 22 kg is mistakenly the answer, rather than 20 kg:

$$10\ \text{mg} \times 22\ \text{kg} = 220\ \text{mg dose}$$

Choice (C), 440 mg, reflects more than double the dose of ibuprofen that should be given to a 20 kg child. Choice (D), 968 mg, reflects more than quadruple the dose of ibuprofen that should be given to a 20 kg child. (*Knowledge Domain 4.2*)

14. **(B)** If NaCl = 4 mEq/mL, then:

$$\frac{4\ \text{mEq}}{1\ \text{mL}} = \frac{40\ \text{mEq}}{x}$$

Cross multiply and solve for *x*:

$$x = 10\ \text{mL}$$

The correct amount is 10 mL, choice (B). (*Knowledge Domain 4.2*)

15. **(C)** A graduated cylinder contains a concave meniscus that forms due to surface tension in the liquid. Therefore, the meniscus is read at eye level at the bottom of the curve. (*Knowledge Domain 4.1*)

16. **(A)** The Institute for Safe Medication Practices (ISMP) has compiled a list of abbreviations, symbols, and dose designations that have been reported to the ISMP MERP program as being frequently misinterpreted with the potential to be involved in harmful medication errors. According to the ISMP, the abbreviation "cc" is commonly mistaken for the abbreviation for "u" or units. Since 1 cc = 1 mL, it is suggested to use the abbreviation "mL" instead of "cc" to avoid a misinterpretation. The abbreviations described in choices (B), (C), and (D) are not identified as error-prone abbreviations by the ISMP. (*Knowledge Domain 3.2*)

17. **(B)** Schedule III–V medications are ordered using a standard invoice. Schedule II medications are ordered using a DEA 222 form. Reverse distributors remove expired medications from the pharmacy. (*Knowledge Domain 2.3*)

18. **(C)** A failure to reconstitute a suspension is an example of an error that can occur during the dispensing step of the medication use process. Other examples of dispensing errors include dispensing the wrong medication, dosage form, or dose. A failure to identify drug interactions or contraindications, or a dosage miscalculation, may also result in a dispensing error. Prescribing errors are those that occur during the prescription writing process. Transcribing errors occur due to data entry errors made by the human operator. Administration errors typically involve the patient, medication, time, dose, or route. (*Knowledge Domain 3.4*)

19. **(B)** The label should advise the customer to take one tablet by mouth twice a day before meals and at bedtime. Choice (A) is incorrect because "tab" refers to a tablet, not a capsule. Capsule is the incorrect dosage form. Choice (C) is incorrect because the sig "AC" refers to "before meals," not "after meals." Choice (D) contains the same errors as choices (A) and (C). (*Knowledge Domain 4.2*)

20. **(C)** Syrups are concentrated sucrose solutions where sugar is used to mask the taste of the medication. Suspensions, choice (A), are prepared when solid particles are dispersed but not completely dissolved in the solvent. Elixirs, choice (B), are sweetened liquids that contain concentrations of alcohol. Tinctures, choice (D), are alcoholic solutions of nonvolatile substances. (*Knowledge Domain 4.1*)

21. **(B)** *USP* <797> defines the temperature range of 36° to 46° F as "cold." When in this range, the temperature is maintained thermostatically. Choice (A) is the appropriate temperature range for a freezer. Choice (C) is a temperature range that the *USP* <797> defines as "cool." Choice (D) is an appropriate temperature range for working areas. (*Knowledge Domain 1.10*)

22. **(C)** *USP* <795> recommends that non-aqueous formulations have a beyond-use date of no later than the time remaining until the earliest expiration date of any active pharmaceutical ingredient (API) or 6 months, whichever comes first. (*Knowledge Domain 4.4*)

23. **(C)** One ounce is equal to 30 mL. One teaspoon is equal to 5 mL. Therefore, $\frac{30}{5}$ = 6 teaspoons, choice (C). (*Knowledge Domain 4.2*)

24. **(A)** Omeprazole is the generic name for the drug Prilosec. Pantoprazole is the generic name for Protonix. Rabeprazole is the generic name for AcipHex. Esomeprazole is the generic name for Nexium. (*Knowledge Domain 1.1*)

25. **(A)** Valerian root is a natural supplement that is used for sleep and anxiety. Ginseng is commonly used to increase energy levels. Ginkgo biloba is a supplement that is used to assist with dementia. Resveratrol is highly regarded as an antioxidant. (*Knowledge Domain 1.6*)

26. **(D)** DEA form 224 is used by an entity that is requesting permission to dispense controlled substances. DEA forms 41, 106, and 222 are used to destroy controlled substances, report a loss/theft of controlled substances, and order Schedule II substances, respectively. (*Knowledge Domain 2.3*)

27. **(C)** A majority of noncontrolled prescriptions are valid for 12 months from the date written. Choice (A) is wrong because although laws vary from state to state, some states may place limitations on Schedule III and IV controlled substances. Choice (B) is incorrect because insurance does not determine the validity of a prescription. Choice (D) is wrong because prescription filling laws are determined from the date the prescription is written, not the fill date. (*Knowledge Domain 2.2*)

28. **(D)** A medication that is "PC" should be taken after meals. In the morning, choice (A), is written as "AM." In the evening, choice (B), is written as "PM." Before meals, choice (C), is written as "AC." (*Knowledge Domain 4.2*)

29. **(C)** Oxycodone has a high potential for abuse and currently accepted medical uses in the United States. Choice (A) is the definition of a Schedule I drug. Choice (B) is not an appropriate definition of a scheduled drug. Choice (D) is the definition of a Schedule IV drug. (*Knowledge Domain 2.2*)

30. **(C)** Sudafed contains the active ingredient pseudoephedrine, which is restricted by the CMEA. None of the other drugs are restricted by the CMEA. (*Knowledge Domain 2.4*)

31. **(C)** Physical incompatibilities include insolubility, immiscibility, liquefaction, and precipitation. Chemical incompatibilities include temperature changes, effervescence, oxidation, and decomposition. (*Knowledge Domain 1.9*)

32. **(B)** Antihypertensives treat high blood pressure. Antihistamines, choice (A), treat allergies. Anticoagulants, choice (C), work to prevent the clotting of blood. Antihyperlipidemics, choice (D), lower lipid levels. (*Knowledge Domain 1.6*)

33. **(A)** Pharmaceutical agents are classified by the Resource Conservation and Recovery Act (RCRA) as P-list or U-list hazardous drugs. Classification is based on four characteristics: ignitability, corrosivity, toxicity, and reactivity. (*Knowledge Domain 2.1*)

34. **(C)** Hydralazine is a vasodilator that is used in the treatment of hypertension. Hydroxyzine is a first-generation H_1 antagonist that is used to treat allergies. Alprazolam and lorazepam are both benzodiazepines that are used in the treatment of anxiety. Methylprednisolone is a corticosteroid, and medroxyprogesterone is a steroidal progestin. Vinblastine and vincristine are both chemotherapeutic agents. (*Knowledge Domain 3.1*)

35. **(D)** Gauge size refers to the thickness of the needle. The higher the gauge size, the smaller the needle. Common gauge sizes for insulin needles are 28, 29, 30, and 31. (*Knowledge Domain 4.3*)

36. **(C)** Federal law states that Schedule III through Schedule V medications may be refilled up to 5 times in 6 months. (*Knowledge Domain 2.2*)

37. **(C)** $°C = (°F - 32) \times \dfrac{5}{9}$; $°C = (86 - 32) \times \dfrac{5}{9} = 54 \times \dfrac{5}{9} = 30°C$ (*Knowledge Domain 4.2*)

38. **(B)** The Combat Methamphetamine Epidemic Act (CMEA) places a maximum limit of 3.6 g/day and 9 g/month of base product. (*Knowledge Domain 2.4*)

39. **(C)** 1 L = 1,000 mL. Therefore, 4 L = 4,000 mL. (*Knowledge Domain 4.2*)

40. **(C)** 1 kg = 2.2 lbs. Therefore, 50 kg $\times$ 2.2 = 110 lbs. (*Knowledge Domain 4.2*)

41. **(B)** 1 oz = 30 mL and 8 oz = 240 mL. The patient is taking 20 mL a day. So the bottle will last $\dfrac{240}{20}$ = 12 days. (*Knowledge Domain 4.2*)

42. **(A)** Common techniques for identifying medications that are about to expire include placing colored stickers, or writing numbers to indicate the expiration month, on the stock bottle and moving stock that is going to expire to the front of the shelf. Alphabetizing medications by generic name is a common organizational tactic that is used in the pharmacy. Pharmacies do not typically organize medications by brand name because these names can vary. (*Knowledge Domain 4.5*)

43. **(A)** Geometric dilution is used when mixing powders of unequal quantity. Spatulation, choice (B), involves mixing powders with a spatula. Levigation, choice (C), is a technique that is used to reduce particle size by triturating with a solvent. A mixture of two drugs that are normally immiscible is an emulsion, choice (D). (*Knowledge Domain 4.1*)

44. **(D)** The FDA and/or the manufacturer may initiate recalls on medications. (*Knowledge Domain 2.5*)

45. **(B)** Liothyronine is the generic name for Cytomel. Levothyroxine is the generic name for Synthroid. Lamotrigine is the generic name for Lamictal. Levetiracetam is the generic name for Keppra. (*Knowledge Domain 1.1*)

46. **(C)** Graves disease results in the overproduction of thyroid hormones. HIV/AIDS, choice (A), is an infection caused by the human immunodeficiency virus. Choice (B) is incorrect because hyperlipidemia causes elevated lipid levels in the blood. Hypothyroidism, choice (D), causes an underactive thyroid, so this is incorrect. (*Knowledge Domain 1.6*)

47. **(C)** A potentiated interaction is an interaction that occurs when one drug intensifies the activity of another drug. An additive interaction, choice (A), is an interaction that results when two drugs given in combination have an effect equal to the sum of the individual effects. A synergistic interaction, choice (B), is an interaction where two drugs that are taken together produce greater effects than when they are taken separately. An antagonistic interaction, choice (D), happens when drugs given in combination cause a decreased, or diminished, effect in one or more drugs. (*Knowledge Domain 1.3*)

48. **(A)** Kava has properties that cause relaxation and may be taken to relieve anxiety. Ginseng, choice (B), is used for its stimulant effects. Garlic, choice (C), is rich in antioxidants and is used for its cardioprotective effects. Ephedra, choice (D), is a supplement that has been banned in the United States but has noted uses for nasal congestion, weight loss, and the ability to increase energy. (*Knowledge Domain 1.6*)

49. **(B)** Narrow therapeutic index drugs are drugs for which small differences in dose or blood concentration may lead to serious therapeutic failures and/or adverse drug reactions. Carbamazepine has been identified by the FDA as a NTI drug. Clindamycin, labetalol, and clopidogrel have not been identified by the FDA as NTI drugs. (*Knowledge Domain 1.8*)

50. **(C)** Synthroid is the brand name of this drug. Choice (A) is incorrect because it refers to the atomic structure of the drug. Choice (B) is incorrect because Synthroid is not the generic name of this drug. The generic name for Synthroid is levothyroxine. Choice (D) is incorrect because Synthroid does not refer to the name of the drug supplier. (*Knowledge Domain 1.1*)

51. **(C)** OTC recommendations, adverse drug events, misuse, adherence, post-immunization follow-up, therapeutic substitution, drug interactions, and allergies are all issues that require a pharmacist's intervention. The situations described in choices (A), (B), and (D) do not require a pharmacist's intervention. (*Knowledge Domain 3.3*)

52. **(C)** Percent is defined as parts per 100:

$$\frac{1}{80} = \frac{x}{100}$$

$$\frac{100}{80} = x$$

$$1.25 = x$$

The answer is 1.25, choice (C). (*Knowledge Domain 4.2*)

53. **(A)** The punch method is a method that is used to hand fill capsules. Flocculation is a process by which small particles clump together or floc. The dry gum method is used to mix immiscible oils. Geometric dilution is a process that is used to mix a small amount of

a drug with an appropriate amount of diluent to ensure equal distribution. (*Knowledge Domain 4.1*)

54. **(A)** Inhaled corticosteroids can depress your immune system. This can lead to an increased chance for thrush to form and accumulate in the oral cavity. (*Knowledge Domain 1.4*)

55. **(B)** Metoprolol is a beta blocker that is used in the treatment of hypertension. Examples of proton-pump inhibitors (PPIs), choice (A), are omeprazole and esomeprazole. PPIs are used in the treatment of GERD and excess stomach acid. Diuretics, choice (C), include triamterene and furosemide. They are used in the treatment of hypertension. Antihistamines, choice (D), may include loratadine and diphenhydramine, which are used in the treatment of allergies. (*Knowledge Domain 1.1*)

56. **(D)** An adverse drug reaction is a term that is used to describe an unintended side effect. A reaction that occurs when one drug intensifies the activity of another drug is called potentiation, choice (A). A contraindication, choice (B), is the possibility of unwanted side effects. A contraindication is a reason why a patient should not take a particular medication. In a synergism reaction, choice (C), two drugs that are taken together produce greater effects than when either drug is taken separately. (*Knowledge Domain 4.4*)

57. **(B)** This patient should be counseled by the pharmacist on proper medication adherence. She is not taking the medication as prescribed, and this could contribute to an exacerbation of her asthma and issues with refilling her medication in the future. The issues described in choices (A), (C), and (D) do not pertain to this particular patient and situation. (*Knowledge Domain 3.3*)

58. **(B)** Prior to dispensing, NuvaRing (etonogestrel/ethinyl estradiol vaginal ring) is stored in a pharmacy refrigerator. Once dispensed, NuvaRing may be stored at room temperature for up to 4 months. (*Knowledge Domain 1.10*)

59. **(C)** To figure out the cost per tablet, you need to take the total cost and divide it by the number of tablets. In this case, $\frac{120 \text{ dollars}}{50 \text{ tablets}} = \$2.40$. (*Knowledge Domain 4.2*)

60. **(D)** The smaller the size of the needle, the larger the diameter. (*Knowledge Domain 4.3*)

61. **(C)** A drug patent is valid for 20 years beginning on the date the application was originally filed. (*Knowledge Domain 1.1*)

62. **(B)** The United States Pharmacopeia found that 70% isopropyl alcohol is the best concentration to use for disinfection. (*Knowledge Domain 3.6*)

63. **(A)** The drug is considered valid until the last day of that month. (*Knowledge Domain 4.4*)

64. **(C)** Advair is a combination of two medications: salmeterol (a bronchodilator) and fluticasone propionate (a corticosteroid). Tiotropium is the generic name for Spiriva. Serevent is the brand name for the inhaler that only contains salmeterol. Formoterol and budesonide are active ingredients in the drug Symbicort. (*Knowledge Domain 1.2*)

65. **(B)** The term *sublingual* means to dissolve "under the tongue." (*Knowledge Domain 4.2*)

66. **(B)** Ibuprofen is available OTC as a 200 mg tablet, liquid, or capsule. Meloxicam (Mobic), ketorolac (Toradol), and celecoxib (Celebrex) are available by prescription. (*Knowledge Domain 1.4*)

67. **(B)** The abbreviation "au" refers to both ears. The abbreviation "ad" is used to indicate the right ear. The abbreviation "os" is used to indicate the left eye. The abbreviation "ou" refers to both eyes. (*Knowledge Domain 4.2*)

68. **(B)** Simvastatin is the generic therapeutic equivalent for the brand name drug Zocor. Atorvastatin, choice (A), is the generic therapeutic equivalent for the brand name drug Lipitor. Candesartan, choice (C), is the generic therapeutic equivalent for the brand name drug Atacand. Losartan, choice (D), is the generic therapeutic equivalent for the brand name drug Cozaar. (*Knowledge Domain 1.2*)

69. **(A)** A patent is a right granted to an entity and prohibits others from copying or selling that product for a set period of time. A copyright, choice (B), gives an entity the right to copy, print, and use material. A trademark, choice (C), is a proprietary term that represents a company or an organization. Choice (D) does not answer the question. (*Knowledge Domain 1.1*)

70. **(A)** Phase I clinical trials include 20–100 individuals, may take several months, and are the phase when testing safety begins. Phase II clinical trials include 100–500 participants, may take months to years, and are the phase when an emphasis is made on efficacy while still testing for safety. Phase III clinical trials include several thousand participants, may take several years, and are the phase when testing focuses on dosing while still looking at safety and efficacy. Phase IV clinical trials are performed after the product is on the market and focus on long-term side effects. (*Knowledge Domain 1.1*)

71. **(A)** Schedule II medications are not refillable. The patient must present a new hard copy of a prescription to receive more of the medication. (*Knowledge Domain 2.2*)

72. **(A)** A dry, hacking cough, a rash, and angioedema are all potential side effects that may occur while using ACE inhibitors. These are important counseling points that should be emphasized by the pharmacist. Leukopenia, muscle weakness, and drowsiness are not side effects that are associated with ACE inhibitor use. (*Knowledge Domain 1.5*)

73. **(C)** There are 16 ounces in 1 pound. (*Knowledge Domain 4.2*)

74. **(A)** Furosemide (Lasix) is classified as a loop diuretic. Chlorothiazide (Diuril) and hydrochlorothiazide (Microzide) are examples of thiazide diuretics. Potassium-sparing diuretics include spironolactone (Aldactone) and triamterene (Dyrenium). Beta blockers are not diuretics, but they can be used as adjuvant therapy in the treatment of hypertension. (*Knowledge Domain 1.1*)

75. **(B)** The suffix -megaly indicates a condition of enlargement. -oma is used to identify a tumor. -osis refers to an abnormal condition, process, or state. -itis means inflammation. (*Knowledge Domain 4.2*)

76. **(C)** Safety data sheets are required for all hazardous substances. They provide information on receiving, handling, preparing, dispensing, and disposing of these substances. (*Knowledge Domain 2.1*)

77. **(B)** In a recall situation, the pharmacy would be provided with the specific lot number(s) affected. (*Knowledge Domain 2.5*)

78. **(D)** Drug-food interactions identify medication and food combinations that are contraindicated. Drug-allergy monitoring parameters identify potentially harmful reactions that may occur when a prescribed medication could interact with a potential allergen

listed in the patient's profile. Drug-nutrient monitoring parameters detect interactions between medications and vitamins and minerals. Drug-drug monitoring parameters would identify medications that should not be taken together. (*Knowledge Domain 1.3*)

79. **(D)** In order to solve this problem, set up a proportion, and solve for *x*.

$$\frac{25 \text{ mEq}}{1 \text{ mL}} = \frac{60 \text{ mEq}}{x}$$
$$x = 2.4 \text{ mL}$$

The answer is 2.4 mL, choice (D). (*Knowledge Domain 4.2*)

80. **(B)** Boniva is an oral medication that is taken monthly for the treatment of osteoporosis. Fosamax and Actonel can be taken daily or weekly. Reclast is taken once a year. (*Knowledge Domain 1.4*)

81. **(D)** Metronidazole is an antibiotic that is indicated in the treatment of UTIs. Ketoconazole, miconazole, and clotrimazole have antifungal indications. (*Knowledge Domain 1.6*)

82. **(D)** A food-environment allergy occurs when the safety and quality of food is affected by the environment. Drug interactions can affect the activity of another drug (drug-drug). Medication administration can affect a laboratory result (drug-laboratory). Drug interactions also can occur when one drug reacts with another that has a similar indication (therapeutic duplication). (*Knowledge Domain 1.3*)

83. **(C)** The prescriber's DEA number is required to be present on all controlled substances. (*Knowledge Domain 2.2*)

84. **(A)** Pravachol is the brand name for pravastatin. Lipitor is the brand name for atorvastatin. Zocor is the brand name for simvastatin. Crestor is the brand name for rosuvastatin. (*Knowledge Domain 1.1*)

85. **(C)** Body surface area (BSA) can be solved using the following equation:

$$\text{BSA m}^2 = \sqrt{\frac{(\text{height in cm}) \times (\text{weight in kg})}{3,600}}$$
$$\text{BSA m}^2 = \sqrt{\frac{(60 \text{ cm}) \times (22 \text{ kg})}{3,600}}$$
$$\text{BSA m}^2 = 0.61 \text{ m}^2$$

The answer is 0.61 m². (*Knowledge Domain 4.2*)

86. **(B)** w/v% refers to g/100 mL. (*Knowledge Domain 4.2*)

87. **(C)** On average, 20 drops are equivalent to 1 mL. (*Knowledge Domain 4.2*)

88. **(C)** Set up a proportion.

$$\frac{0.05 \text{ mg}}{1 \text{ mL}} = \frac{0.25 \text{ mg}}{x \text{ mL}}$$
$$x = 5 \text{ mL}$$

Then, determine how much is needed for a 30 day supply.

$$\frac{5 \text{ mL}}{1 \text{ day}} = \frac{x \text{ mL}}{30 \text{ days}}$$
$$x = 150 \text{ mL}$$

The answer is 150 mL. (*Knowledge Domain 4.2*)

89. **(C)** Trituration is the process of grinding a tablet into a fine powder. Spatulation is the process of mixing compounds by moving a spatula on a sheet of parchment paper or a tile. Sifting is a process that is used to mix substances by passing them through a sieve. Tumbling is the process of mixing powders in a large container using an electronic mixer. (*Knowledge Domain 4.1*)

90. **(D)** Capsule sizes are inversely proportional. 00 is the largest capsule size of these answer choices, whereas 5 is the smallest capsule size. (*Knowledge Domain 4.1*)

ANSWER SHEET
Practice Test 2

1. Ⓐ Ⓑ Ⓒ Ⓓ
2. Ⓐ Ⓑ Ⓒ Ⓓ
3. Ⓐ Ⓑ Ⓒ Ⓓ
4. Ⓐ Ⓑ Ⓒ Ⓓ
5. Ⓐ Ⓑ Ⓒ Ⓓ
6. Ⓐ Ⓑ Ⓒ Ⓓ
7. Ⓐ Ⓑ Ⓒ Ⓓ
8. Ⓐ Ⓑ Ⓒ Ⓓ
9. Ⓐ Ⓑ Ⓒ Ⓓ
10. Ⓐ Ⓑ Ⓒ Ⓓ
11. Ⓐ Ⓑ Ⓒ Ⓓ
12. Ⓐ Ⓑ Ⓒ Ⓓ
13. Ⓐ Ⓑ Ⓒ Ⓓ
14. Ⓐ Ⓑ Ⓒ Ⓓ
15. Ⓐ Ⓑ Ⓒ Ⓓ
16. Ⓐ Ⓑ Ⓒ Ⓓ
17. Ⓐ Ⓑ Ⓒ Ⓓ
18. Ⓐ Ⓑ Ⓒ Ⓓ
19. Ⓐ Ⓑ Ⓒ Ⓓ
20. Ⓐ Ⓑ Ⓒ Ⓓ
21. Ⓐ Ⓑ Ⓒ Ⓓ
22. Ⓐ Ⓑ Ⓒ Ⓓ
23. Ⓐ Ⓑ Ⓒ Ⓓ
24. Ⓐ Ⓑ Ⓒ Ⓓ
25. Ⓐ Ⓑ Ⓒ Ⓓ
26. Ⓐ Ⓑ Ⓒ Ⓓ
27. Ⓐ Ⓑ Ⓒ Ⓓ
28. Ⓐ Ⓑ Ⓒ Ⓓ
29. Ⓐ Ⓑ Ⓒ Ⓓ
30. Ⓐ Ⓑ Ⓒ Ⓓ

31. Ⓐ Ⓑ Ⓒ Ⓓ
32. Ⓐ Ⓑ Ⓒ Ⓓ
33. Ⓐ Ⓑ Ⓒ Ⓓ
34. Ⓐ Ⓑ Ⓒ Ⓓ
35. Ⓐ Ⓑ Ⓒ Ⓓ
36. Ⓐ Ⓑ Ⓒ Ⓓ
37. Ⓐ Ⓑ Ⓒ Ⓓ
38. Ⓐ Ⓑ Ⓒ Ⓓ
39. Ⓐ Ⓑ Ⓒ Ⓓ
40. Ⓐ Ⓑ Ⓒ Ⓓ
41. Ⓐ Ⓑ Ⓒ Ⓓ
42. Ⓐ Ⓑ Ⓒ Ⓓ
43. Ⓐ Ⓑ Ⓒ Ⓓ
44. Ⓐ Ⓑ Ⓒ Ⓓ
45. Ⓐ Ⓑ Ⓒ Ⓓ
46. Ⓐ Ⓑ Ⓒ Ⓓ
47. Ⓐ Ⓑ Ⓒ Ⓓ
48. Ⓐ Ⓑ Ⓒ Ⓓ
49. Ⓐ Ⓑ Ⓒ Ⓓ
50. Ⓐ Ⓑ Ⓒ Ⓓ
51. Ⓐ Ⓑ Ⓒ Ⓓ
52. Ⓐ Ⓑ Ⓒ Ⓓ
53. Ⓐ Ⓑ Ⓒ Ⓓ
54. Ⓐ Ⓑ Ⓒ Ⓓ
55. Ⓐ Ⓑ Ⓒ Ⓓ
56. Ⓐ Ⓑ Ⓒ Ⓓ
57. Ⓐ Ⓑ Ⓒ Ⓓ
58. Ⓐ Ⓑ Ⓒ Ⓓ
59. Ⓐ Ⓑ Ⓒ Ⓓ
60. Ⓐ Ⓑ Ⓒ Ⓓ

61. Ⓐ Ⓑ Ⓒ Ⓓ
62. Ⓐ Ⓑ Ⓒ Ⓓ
63. Ⓐ Ⓑ Ⓒ Ⓓ
64. Ⓐ Ⓑ Ⓒ Ⓓ
65. Ⓐ Ⓑ Ⓒ Ⓓ
66. Ⓐ Ⓑ Ⓒ Ⓓ
67. Ⓐ Ⓑ Ⓒ Ⓓ
68. Ⓐ Ⓑ Ⓒ Ⓓ
69. Ⓐ Ⓑ Ⓒ Ⓓ
70. Ⓐ Ⓑ Ⓒ Ⓓ
71. Ⓐ Ⓑ Ⓒ Ⓓ
72. Ⓐ Ⓑ Ⓒ Ⓓ
73. Ⓐ Ⓑ Ⓒ Ⓓ
74. Ⓐ Ⓑ Ⓒ Ⓓ
75. Ⓐ Ⓑ Ⓒ Ⓓ
76. Ⓐ Ⓑ Ⓒ Ⓓ
77. Ⓐ Ⓑ Ⓒ Ⓓ
78. Ⓐ Ⓑ Ⓒ Ⓓ
79. Ⓐ Ⓑ Ⓒ Ⓓ
80. Ⓐ Ⓑ Ⓒ Ⓓ
81. Ⓐ Ⓑ Ⓒ Ⓓ
82. Ⓐ Ⓑ Ⓒ Ⓓ
83. Ⓐ Ⓑ Ⓒ Ⓓ
84. Ⓐ Ⓑ Ⓒ Ⓓ
85. Ⓐ Ⓑ Ⓒ Ⓓ
86. Ⓐ Ⓑ Ⓒ Ⓓ
87. Ⓐ Ⓑ Ⓒ Ⓓ
88. Ⓐ Ⓑ Ⓒ Ⓓ
89. Ⓐ Ⓑ Ⓒ Ⓓ
90. Ⓐ Ⓑ Ⓒ Ⓓ

Practice Test 2

Directions: You will have 1 hour and 50 minutes to complete the following 90 questions. For each question, select the choice that best answers the question, and mark that answer letter on your answer sheet. Remember, this test should be used to help you determine areas that require additional review. Each question represents a particular area of the PTCE blueprint, which can help you pinpoint areas of mastery or concepts that require additional studying. The official PTCE exam uses a scaled score to determine your grade. Only 80 out of 90 questions on the PTCE are scored, and unscored questions are not identified. You should be able to answer about 72 of the questions on this test correctly, averaging an overall percentage of 80% or more on your attempt at this test.

1. Which of the following is a true statement?

   (A) Syrups contain sugar, usually to mask the taste of the medication.
   (B) Elixirs contain oil and water and should be shaken well before use.
   (C) Suspensions are liquid preparations that contain one or more active ingredients dissolved in a liquid vehicle.
   (D) Capsules are made of hard, compressed medication in round, oval, or square shapes.

2. Which of the following is true regarding storage of the MMRV vaccine?

   (A) The vaccine should be stored at room temperature.
   (B) The vaccine should be stored in a refrigerator.
   (C) The vaccine should be stored in a freezer.
   (D) The vaccine may be stored at room temperature or placed in a refrigerator.

3. Zetia is indicated for the treatment of

   _____.

   (A) hypertension
   (B) gout
   (C) rheumatoid arthritis
   (D) hyperlipidemia

4. Cranberry is a supplement that is commonly used for the prevention of what condition?

   (A) diabetes mellitus
   (B) urinary tract infections (UTIs)
   (C) gout
   (D) hyperlipidemia

5. Which of the following dosage forms bypasses the digestive system?

   (A) elixir
   (B) suspension
   (C) sublingual tablet
   (D) ointment

6. Which of the following capsule sizes is the largest?

   (A) 000
   (B) 0
   (C) 1
   (D) 5

7. According to the Controlled Substances Act, which of the following drugs is classified as a controlled substance?

   (A) warfarin (Coumadin)
   (B) tramadol (Ultram)
   (C) minocycline (Minocin, Solodyn)
   (D) mometasone (Nasonex)

8. A prescription for a controlled substance must include which of the following statements on the label?

   (A) "Caution: State law prohibits the sale of this drug to any person"
   (B) "Caution: Federal law prohibits the transfer of this drug to any person other than the patient for whom it was prescribed"
   (C) "Caution: State law prohibits the sale of this drug to any person other than the patient for whom it was prescribed"
   (D) "Caution: State law prohibits the sale of this drug"

9. Which of the following nasal corticosteroids is available over-the-counter?

   (A) Omnaris
   (B) Dymista
   (C) Flonase
   (D) Rhinocort

10. Which auxiliary label should be placed onto a prescription vial containing metronidazole (Flagyl)?

    (A) "Refrigerate"
    (B) "Shake before use"
    (C) "Do not drink alcohol"
    (D) "Take with food"

11. Which of the following prescription medications should NOT be handled by a pharmacy technician who is pregnant?

    (A) famotidine
    (B) furosemide
    (C) fexofenadine
    (D) finasteride

12. How many mg of magnesium sulfate are in 3 mL of a 50% solution?

    (A) 1,000 mg
    (B) 1,500 mg
    (C) 1,750 mg
    (D) 2,000 mg

13. How many mL of a 2% (w/v) solution are needed to make 8 oz of a 1:200 solution?

    (A) 15 mL
    (B) 30 mL
    (C) 60 mL
    (D) 80 mL

14. What is the antibiotic classification of the drug azithromycin (Zithromax)?

    (A) tetracycline
    (B) penicillin
    (C) macrolide
    (D) cephalosporin

15. Which of the following look-alike/sound-alike drug pairs contains an H_1 antagonist?

    (A) buPROPion and busPIRone
    (B) dimenhyDRINATE and diphenhydrAMINE
    (C) predniSONE and prednisoLONE
    (D) rOPINIRole and risperiDONE

16. The acronym NDC is used when identifying a drug product. It also relays information pertaining to the manufacturer and the medication package size. What does the acronym NDC stand for?

    (A) Nationwide Drug Carrier
    (B) National District Code
    (C) Nationwide District Code
    (D) National Drug Code

17. A root-cause analysis is a method that is used to _____.

    (A) prevent an error from reoccurring
    (B) assess the appropriateness of drug therapy
    (C) identify an adverse drug reaction
    (D) promote MTM services

18. Which of the following forms is issued by a reverse distributor who is picking up expired CII medications from a pharmacy?

    (A) DEA form 222
    (B) pharmacy invoice
    (C) purchase order
    (D) DEA form 41

19. In the NDC number 0084-6571-10, what does the number 0084 indicate?

    (A) package size
    (B) product strength
    (C) manufacturer
    (D) dosage form

20. How many 250 mg capsules are needed to prepare 75 mL of a 1% solution?

    (A) 1 capsule
    (B) 2 capsules
    (C) 3 capsules
    (D) 4 capsules

21. Which of the following patient service principles should NOT be used by pharmacy personnel when dealing with a patient's complaint?

    (A) Avoid passing judgment on the patient.
    (B) Provide accurate information to the patient.
    (C) Maintain a positive attitude toward the patient.
    (D) Provide a follow-up survey to gauge the patient's feedback.

22. Which government agency enforces the Controlled Substances Act?

    (A) DEA
    (B) OSHA
    (C) FDA
    (D) CDC

23. CCXI is equal to _____.

    (A) 209
    (B) 210
    (C) 211
    (D) 212

24. What is the minimum sensitivity reading on a Class III prescription balance?

    (A) 2 mg
    (B) 6 mg
    (C) 8 mg
    (D) 10 mg

25. A pharmacy technician is filling out a controlled medication order on a DEA 222 form. Which copy of the paper form is kept by the pharmacy?

    (A) top copy
    (B) middle copy
    (C) bottom copy
    (D) top and bottom copies

26. What is the brand name of the drug rabeprazole?

    (A) Aciphex
    (B) Nexium
    (C) Prilosec
    (D) Protonix

27. Nitrostat 0.4 mg is exempt from the child-resistant cap requirement according to which pharmacy-specific law?

    (A) Poison Prevention Packaging Act of 1970
    (B) Isotretinoin Safety and Risk Management Act of 2004
    (C) Combat Methamphetamine Epidemic Act of 2005
    (D) Health Insurance Portability and Accountability Act of 1996

28. How many tablets should be dispensed, given the following order?

prednisone 5 mg sig:
ii tabs PO TID × 2 days
ii tabs PO BID × 2 days
i tab PO TID × 2 days
ii tabs PO QD × 2 days
i tab PO QD × 2 days
Then stop

(A) 22 tablets
(B) 30 tablets
(C) 32 tablets
(D) 38 tablets

29. A patient is to receive 8 doses of azithromycin 500 mg. If the pharmacy only has 1-gram vials available, how many vials are needed to prepare this prescription?

(A) 2
(B) 3
(C) 4
(D) 5

30. The convex or concave curve located at the top of a volume of liquid in a graduated cylinder is known as a(n) _____.

(A) levigation
(B) meniscus
(C) ointment
(D) troches

31. Which of the following abbreviations is on ISMP's list of error-prone abbreviations?

(A) cap
(B) prn
(C) qhs
(D) inj

32. Which of the following is NOT a solid dosage form?

(A) powder
(B) capsule
(C) suspension
(D) suppository

33. A patient receives a prescription for an otic preparation. Where is an otic product instilled?

(A) in the eye
(B) in the nose
(C) in the rectum
(D) in the ear

34. A medication is to be kept at room temperature. What is the appropriate temperature range for this medication?

(A) –4°F to 14°F
(B) 36°F to 46°F
(C) 68°F to 77°F
(D) 90°F to 110°F

35. What is the maximum number of refills permitted for a Class III prescription according to federal law?

(A) 0 refills
(B) 1 refill
(C) 5 refills in 6 months
(D) 11 refills in 12 months

36. All of the following are classified as high-alert medications by the Institute for Safe Medication Practices (ISMP) EXCEPT

_____.

(A) metformin
(B) warfarin
(C) midazolam
(D) ampicillin

37. What is the name of the mandatory distribution program for products that contain isotretinoin?

(A) VAERS
(B) iPLEDGE
(C) ETASU
(D) MedGUIDE

38. Non-aqueous solutions, such as a capsule without water, have a maximum beyond-use date (BUD) of no later than _____.

(A) 14 days
(B) 30 days
(C) 6 months
(D) 1 year

39. Convert 1.22 mg to micrograms.

(A) 12.2 mcg
(B) 122 mcg
(C) 1,220 mcg
(D) 12,220 mcg

40. A patient is requesting that her Class IV prescription be transferred to a pharmacy that does not share the same online database. What is the maximum number of times a Class IV prescription can be transferred to this pharmacy?

(A) 1 time
(B) 2 times
(C) 5 times
(D) unlimited times

41. Biennial inventory is inventory of all controlled substances on hand that is to be conducted _____.

(A) twice a year
(B) once a year
(C) every 2 years
(D) every 5 years

42. Which of the following is NOT a strategy used to decrease the potential for expired drugs to be on pharmacy shelves?

(A) using colored stickers to indicate the month of expiration
(B) placing medications with similar drug names away from each other
(C) writing the month of expiration on the stock bottle
(D) placing new products behind old products on the shelves

43. Which of the following forms is required to order methylphenidate (Ritalin)?

(A) DEA 224 form
(B) DEA 222 form
(C) DEA 106 form
(D) DEA 41 form

44. A bothersome or unwanted effect that results from the use of a drug and is unrelated to the intended effect of the drug is called a(an) _____.

(A) side effect
(B) contraindication
(C) allergy
(D) drug interaction

45. Which of the following error prevention strategies is used to avoid variation or complexity?

(A) the use of electronic processing software
(B) the integration of a computer with the pharmacy register
(C) the use of a scanner to match the NDC of the selected drug to the profiled medication
(D) the use of preprinted prescription blanks that contain frequently prescribed medications

46. When a prescription is filled with the wrong quantity of a medication as a result of illegible handwriting, this should be classified as a(an) _____.

(A) unauthorized drug error
(B) prescribing error
(C) wrong drug preparation error
(D) administration error

47. What is the therapeutic equivalent for Claritin?

(A) diphenhydramine
(B) cetirizine
(C) loratadine
(D) fexofenadine

48. Counting trays should be _____.

   (A) tossed, and new trays should be purchased, every 6 months

   (B) labeled when used with hazardous medications

   (C) made of glass

   (D) kept in the compounding area

49. What type of prescriptions may NOT be prescribed over the phone?

   (A) Class II prescriptions

   (B) Class III prescriptions

   (C) Class IV prescriptions

   (D) noncontrolled prescriptions

50. In which controlled substance schedule does morphine belong?

   (A) Schedule I

   (B) Schedule II

   (C) Schedule III

   (D) Schedule IV

51. How many 5 mL doses can be packaged from a pint of medication (round to the nearest whole number)?

   (A) 37

   (B) 78

   (C) 95

   (D) 112

52. Which instrument is used to grind tablets into fine powders?

   (A) spatula and ointment slab

   (B) electronic balance and spatula

   (C) stir rod and beaker

   (D) mortar and pestle

53. According to federal law, how long should Schedule II prescriptions be kept in the pharmacy?

   (A) 1 year

   (B) 2 years

   (C) 5 years

   (D) 7 years

54. Which of the following prefixes means "bladder"?

   (A) chol-

   (B) cardi-

   (C) costo-

   (D) cyst-

55. Which of the following vitamins is fat-soluble?

   (A) vitamin A

   (B) vitamin B12

   (C) vitamin B6

   (D) vitamin C

56. What is the minimum weighable quantity for a Class III prescription balance?

   (A) 6 mg

   (B) 120 mg

   (C) 6 mL

   (D) 120 mL

57. Which measuring device would be the most appropriate for dispensing liquid for an infant?

   (A) oral syringe

   (B) medication cup

   (C) oral dropper

   (D) teaspoon

58. Which of the following is a long-acting insulin?

   (A) insulin glulisine

   (B) insulin aspart

   (C) insulin glargine

   (D) insulin lispro

59. A sig states that a medication should be taken QID. The medication should be taken _____ a day.

   (A) once

   (B) twice

   (C) three times

   (D) four times

60. Which of the following dosage forms is taken orally and is designed to be quickly absorbed into the bloodstream?

(A) chewable tablet
(B) syrup
(C) sublingual tablet
(D) elixir

61. Which of the following drugs is a calcium channel blocker?

(A) atenolol
(B) furosemide
(C) lidocaine
(D) verapamil

62. How many gallons are in 240 pints?

(A) 10 gallons
(B) 20 gallons
(C) 30 gallons
(D) 40 gallons

63. According to federal law, who may perform the final check for all prescriptions processed and filled in the pharmacy?

(A) pharmacy technician
(B) pharmacist
(C) physician
(D) pharmacy intern

64. How many grams of drug are in 300 mL of a 50% solution?

(A) 90 g
(B) 130 g
(C) 150 g
(D) 220 g

65. How much dextrose is in 1,000 mL of D10W?

(A) 100 g
(B) 1,000 g
(C) 100 mg
(D) 1,000 mg

66. Which of the following is an acceptable temperature to store insulin at in the pharmacy's refrigerator?

(A) 1°C
(B) 5°C
(C) 12°C
(D) 15°C

67. Which organ(s) is mainly affected by hepatotoxicity?

(A) kidneys
(B) stomach
(C) liver
(D) lungs

68. Why should medication stock be rotated in a pharmacy?

(A) to ensure that short-dated medications are used first
(B) to ensure that long-dated medications are used first
(C) to ensure that the pharmacy supply is maximized
(D) to ensure that the stock is facing properly

69. Which of the following best describes information that should be included on unit dose packaged medications?

(A) the medication name, the strength, the manufacturer's name, the NDC, the lot number, and the expiration date
(B) the medication name, the strength, the manufacturer's name, the NDC, the lot number, and the instructions for patient use
(C) the medication name, the strength, and the instructions for patient use
(D) the medication name, the strength, and the manufacturer's name

70. Glucovance is a combination product that contains which of the following medications?

(A) metformin and glipizide
(B) rosiglitazone and glimepiride
(C) rosiglitazone and metformin
(D) metformin and glyburide

71. Which of the following could increase the likelihood of a medication error?

(A) using leading zeros
(B) using trailing zeros
(C) avoiding confusing abbreviations
(D) using barcoding systems

72. A physician orders an IV drip rate of a medication to be infused at 15 mL/hr for a total of 36 hours. What is the total volume of medication to be administered?

(A) 240 mL
(B) 480 mL
(C) 540 mL
(D) 615 mL

73. Which FDA recall classification is the least severe?

(A) Class I
(B) Class II
(C) Class III
(D) Class IV

74. The doctor has prescribed antihistamine drops to treat seasonal allergy symptoms. The directions state 1–2 gtts os TID. What should be typed on the prescription label?

(A) Instill 1–2 drops in each eye three times a day.
(B) Instill 1–2 drops in the right eye three times a day.
(C) Instill 1–2 drops in the left eye three times a day.
(D) Instill 1–2 drops in the left ear three times a day.

75. The pharmacy should complete which of the following steps after receiving an alert from the FDA about a drug recall from a specific manufacturer?

(A) pull the offending drug from pharmacy shelves and, if deemed appropriate, call patients who are taking this medication to inform them of the significant medication problem
(B) pull the offending drug from pharmacy shelves but do not contact patients who are taking this medication until it is time for the next medication refill
(C) continue to use the offending drug until stock runs out but do not order more for future fills
(D) continue to use the offending drug but post an alert in the pharmacy for patients to see information about the significant medication problem

76. Which of the following is an angiotensin II receptor blocker (ARB)?

(A) metoprolol
(B) lisinopril
(C) lovastatin
(D) candesartan

77. The expiration date of a bottle reads 9/28. What is the last day this medication may be used?

(A) 09/01/2028
(B) 09/30/2028
(C) 10/01/2028
(D) 08/31/2028

78. The Combat Methamphetamine Epidemic Act of 2005 was enacted to regulate over-the-counter sales of which of the following substances?

(A) dextromethorphan
(B) pseudoephedrine
(C) guaifenesin
(D) phenylephrine

79. The pharmacy receives a prescription for 500 mL of 15% solution "X." The pharmacy carries 30% and 5% stock solutions. How much of the 30% and 5% solutions, respectively, should be used to mix this order?

(A) 100 mL of 30% solution, 400 mL of 5% solution

(B) 200 mL of 30% solution, 300 mL of 5% solution

(C) 300 mL of 30% solution, 200 mL of 5% solution

(D) 400 mL of 30% solution, 100 mL of 5% solution

80. What volume of a 125 mg/mL injectable should be drawn up for a 275 mg dose?

(A) 1.4 mL

(B) 2.2 mL

(C) 2.8 mL

(D) 3.1 mL

81. Which of the following eye drops is kept in a refrigerator prior to opening?

(A) latanoprost

(B) timolol

(C) ofloxacin

(D) olopatadine

82. Which organization oversees the Medication Error Reporting Program (MERP)?

(A) FDA

(B) CDC

(C) DEA

(D) ISMP

83. What is the color of the "C" stamped on controlled substance prescriptions and manufacturer bottles?

(A) green

(B) blue

(C) red

(D) black

84. A patient receives her medication at 1800 military hours. At what standard time did she receive her medication?

(A) 9:00 P.M.

(B) 6:00 P.M.

(C) 9:00 A.M.

(D) 6:00 A.M.

85. What should a pharmacy technician do if he or she receives an incomplete prescription order?

(A) Call the prescriber to inquire about the missing information.

(B) Ask the patient, and fill in the missing information.

(C) Refuse to fill the prescription.

(D) Fill the prescription using information from a previous fill.

86. According to *USP* <795>, what type of water should be used when compounding non-sterile drug preparations?

(A) tap water

(B) alkaline water

(C) purified water

(D) hypertonic water

87. Capsules and tablets are counted in multiples of what number?

(A) 2

(B) 3

(C) 5

(D) 10

88. What is the technical name for the stem of a needle?

(A) shaft

(B) bevel

(C) hub

(D) lumen

89. Which of the following is NOT an advantage of barcoding technology?

(A) It ensures that the patient receives the correct drug.
(B) It ensures that the correct dose is given to the patient.
(C) It ensures that the patient receives the medication at the best cost.
(D) It ensures that the correct patient receives the dose.

90. What is the term for "solid particles dispersed in a liquid medium"?

(A) suspension
(B) emulsion
(C) elixir
(D) solution

ANSWER KEY
Practice Test 2

1. **A**	31. **C**	61. **D**
2. **C**	32. **C**	62. **C**
3. **D**	33. **D**	63. **B**
4. **B**	34. **C**	64. **C**
5. **C**	35. **C**	65. **A**
6. **A**	36. **D**	66. **B**
7. **B**	37. **B**	67. **C**
8. **B**	38. **C**	68. **A**
9. **C**	39. **C**	69. **A**
10. **C**	40. **A**	70. **D**
11. **D**	41. **C**	71. **B**
12. **B**	42. **B**	72. **C**
13. **C**	43. **B**	73. **C**
14. **C**	44. **A**	74. **C**
15. **B**	45. **D**	75. **A**
16. **D**	46. **B**	76. **D**
17. **A**	47. **C**	77. **B**
18. **A**	48. **B**	78. **B**
19. **C**	49. **A**	79. **B**
20. **C**	50. **B**	80. **B**
21. **D**	51. **C**	81. **A**
22. **A**	52. **D**	82. **D**
23. **C**	53. **B**	83. **C**
24. **B**	54. **D**	84. **B**
25. **C**	55. **A**	85. **C**
26. **A**	56. **B**	86. **C**
27. **A**	57. **A**	87. **C**
28. **C**	58. **C**	88. **A**
29. **C**	59. **D**	89. **C**
30. **B**	60. **C**	90. **A**

ANSWERS EXPLAINED

1. **(A)** Syrups are concentrated aqueous solutions of sugar. Flavoring constituents can be added to mask the bitter or unpleasant tastes of medications. Elixirs are typically flavored, clear liquid preparations that contain concentrated amounts of ethanol. Suspensions contain one or more insoluble active ingredients suspended in a liquid vehicle. Capsules are medications that are contained in a gelatin container. (*Knowledge Domain 4.1*)

2. **(C)** The MMRV vaccine is a vaccine that must be frozen in order to maintain the integrity of the medication. The MMR vaccine, on the other hand, may be refrigerated or frozen prior to reconstitution. (*Knowledge Domain 1.10*)

3. **(D)** Zetia is a medication that is used to treat hyperlipidemia by inhibiting intestinal absorption of cholesterol. (*Knowledge Domain 1.6*)

4. **(B)** Cranberry is often used to prevent UTIs. (*Knowledge Domain 1.6*)

5. **(C)** Sublingual tablets bypass the digestive system because they diffuse into the bloodstream. Elixirs and suspensions are ingested and follow the gastrointestinal tract before entering the bloodstream. Ointments are used topically for local administration and therefore are not systemically absorbed. (*Knowledge Domain 1.4*)

6. **(A)** Capsule sizes are inversely proportional. The smallest number indicates the largest capsule size. The largest number is indicative of the smallest capsule size.

7. **(B)** Tramadol (Ultram) is classified as a Schedule IV controlled substance under the Controlled Substances Act. Warfarin (Coumadin), minocycline (Minocin, Solodyn), and mometasone (Nasonex) are not classified as controlled substances under the Controlled Substances Act. (*Knowledge Domain 2.2*)

8. **(B)** Controlled prescriptions must include the following statement on the prescription label "Caution: Federal law prohibits the transfer of this drug to any person other than the patient for whom it was prescribed." Choices (A), (C), and (D) are all incorrect because this statement is a federal law, not a state law. In addition, the correct statement should not reference the "sale" but, rather, the "transfer" of the drug. (*Knowledge Domain 2.2*)

9. **(C)** Flonase is approved as an over-the-counter treatment for hay fever. Omnaris, Dymista, and Rhinocort are prescription nasal sprays that are indicated for the treatment of allergic rhinitis. (*Knowledge Domain 1.1*)

10. **(C)** Metronidazole (Flagyl) is an antibiotic that is used to treat anaerobic bacterial infections. The concomitant consumption of alcohol while taking metronidazole can produce a disulfiram-like reaction, resulting in tachycardia, flushing, and hypotension. (*Knowledge Domain 1.4*)

11. **(D)** Finasteride (Proscar, Propecia) is a pregnancy category X drug, indicating that, in clinical studies, this drug has been shown to cause abnormal effects and risks to the human fetus. Famotidine (Pepcid), furosemide (Lasix), and fexofenadine (Allegra) are not categorized as pregnancy category X drugs and may be handled by a pharmacy technician during her pregnancy. (*Knowledge Domain 1.4*)

12. **(B)** A proportion can be used to solve this problem:

$$\frac{50 \text{ g}}{100 \text{ mL}} = \frac{x}{3 \text{ mL}}$$

$$100x = 150$$

$$x = 1.5 \text{ g}$$

Since none of the answer choices are in grams (g), we must convert this answer to milligrams (mg):

$$\frac{1,000 \text{ mg}}{1 \text{ g}} = \frac{x}{1.5 \text{ g}}$$

$$x = 1,500 \text{ mg}$$

The answer is 1,500 mg. (*Knowledge Domain 4.2*)

13. **(C)** This problem can be solved using the following equation: (IS)(IV) = (FS)(FV). The initial strength (IS) is 2%. You must solve for the initial volume (IV). The final strength (FS) is 1:200. The strength is presented as a ratio in this problem and should be converted to a percentage. To convert to a percentage, you must first realize that 1:200 is a ratio written as $\frac{1}{200}$. Multiply $\frac{1}{200}$ by 100 to get 0.5%. The final volume (FV) is 8 oz, which is the same as 240 mL $\left(\frac{1 \text{ oz}}{30 \text{ mL}} = \frac{8 \text{ oz}}{x}\right)$. Now plug the numbers into the equation, and solve for x:

$$(2\%)(x \text{ mL}) = (0.5\%)(240 \text{ mL})$$

$$2x \text{ mL} = 120 \text{ mL}$$

$$x = 60 \text{ mL}$$

The answer is 60 mL. (*Knowledge Domain 4.2*)

14. **(C)** Azithromycin (Zithromax) is classified as a macrolide antibiotic. (*Knowledge Domain 1.1*)

15. **(B)** Diphenhydramine is an H_1 antagonist. Dimenhydrinate is an antiemetic that has antihistamine properties. Bupropion is classified as an antidepressant and smoking cessation aid. Buspirone is an anxiolytic. Prednisone and prednisolone are both corticosteroids. Ropinirole is used to treat Parkinson's disease. Risperidone is used in the treatment of schizophrenia and bipolar disorder. (*Knowledge Domain 3.1*)

16. **(D)** The acronym NDC stands for National Drug Code. (*Knowledge Domain 4.4*)

17. **(A)** A root-cause analysis is a method that is used to identify the root cause of a problem, with the end of goal of finding a way to prevent that error from reoccurring in the future. (*Knowledge Domain 3.4*)

18. **(A)** A reverse distributor will provide DEA form 222 for any CII medications. (*Knowledge Domain 2.3*)

19. **(C)** The first set of numbers in a National Drug Code (NDC) identifies the labeler, defined as the manufacturer or the distributor of the drug. The second set of numbers identifies the product, and the third set identifies the package size. (*Knowledge Domain 4.4*)

20. **(C)** First, set up a proportion to find the number of milligrams required:

$$\frac{1\ g}{100\ mL} = \frac{x}{75\ mL}$$

$$100x = 75$$

$$x = 0.75\ g = 750\ mg$$

Then, set up another proportion to find the number of capsules needed:

$$\frac{250\ mg}{1\ capsule} = \frac{750\ mg}{x}$$

$$250x = 750$$

$$x = 3$$

The answer is 3 capsules. (*Knowledge Domain 4.2*)

21. **(D)** A follow-up survey may be provided by the pharmacy to collect data regarding patient satisfaction, but it is *not* an example of a patient service principle that may be used when speaking with a patient. When dealing with a patient's complaint, pharmacy personnel should avoid passing judgment, provide accurate information to the patient, and maintain a positive attitude toward the patient. (*Knowledge Domain 3.3*)

22. **(A)** The Drug Enforcement Administration (DEA) enforces the Controlled Substances Act. Choice (B) is incorrect because the Occupational Safety and Health Administration (OSHA), is a federal agency that regulates workplace safety and health. Choice (C) is incorrect because the Food and Drug Administration (FDA) assures the safety and efficacy of drugs, foods, medical devices, and other biological products. Choice (D) is incorrect because the Centers for Disease Control and Research (CDC) supports health promotion, awareness, and preparedness. (*Knowledge Domain 2.2*)

23. **(C)** C equals 100, X equals 10, and I equals 1. Therefore, CCXI = 100 + 100 + 10 + 1 = 211. (*Knowledge Domain 4.2*)

24. **(B)** The minimum sensitivity reading required to move the pointer on the scale is 6 mg. (*Knowledge Domain 4.1*)

25. **(C)** The bottom copy is kept by the pharmacy and will be used to notate receipt of the medications ordered. The top copy, choice (A), is forwarded to the supplier. The middle copy, choice (B), is forwarded to the special agent in charge of the Drug Enforcement Administration in the local area of the supplier. The top and bottom copies, choice (D), are not both kept by the pharmacy. (*Knowledge Domain 2.3*)

26. **(A)** Aciphex is the brand name for rabeprazole. Nexium, choice (B), is the brand name for esomeprazole. Prilosec, choice (C), is the brand name for omeprazole. Protonix, choice (D), is the brand name for pantoprazole. (*Knowledge Domain 1.1*)

27. **(A)** The Poison Prevention Packaging Act of 1970 has some exemptions to the child-resistant packaging requirement. These exemptions including effervescent aspirin, oral contraceptives, sublingual nitroglycerin, and hormone replacement therapy. The Isotretinoin Safety and Risk Management Act of 2004, choice (B), was enacted to restrict the use of isotretinoin (Accutane). The Combat Methamphetamine Epidemic Act of 2005, choice (C), places restrictions on products that contain pseudoephedrine, ephedrine,

and/or phenylpropanolamine. The Health Insurance Portability and Accountability Act of 1996, choice (D), places safeguards on all protected health information (PHI). (*Knowledge Domain 1.4*)

28. **(C)**

$$\text{ii tabs PO TID} \times 2 \text{ days: } 2 \times 3 = 6 \times 2 = 12 \text{ tablets}$$
$$\text{ii tabs PO BID} \times 2 \text{ days: } 2 \times 2 = 4 \times 2 = 8 \text{ tablets}$$
$$\text{i tab PO TID} \times 2 \text{ days: } 1 \times 3 = 3 \times 2 = 6 \text{ tablets}$$
$$\text{ii tabs PO QD} \times 2 \text{ days: } 2 \times 1 = 2 \times 2 = 4 \text{ tablets}$$
$$\text{i tab PO QD} \times 2 \text{ days: } 1 \times 1 = 1 \times 2 = 2 \text{ tablets}$$
$$12 + 8 + 6 + 4 + 2 = 32 \text{ tablets}$$

The answer is 32 tablets, choice (C). (*Knowledge Domain 4.2*)

29. **(C)** This problem can be solved in three steps:

STEP 1 Convert mg to g.

$$\frac{1 \text{ g}}{1,000 \text{ mg}} = \frac{x \text{ g}}{500 \text{ mg}}$$
$$x = 0.5 \text{ g}$$

STEP 2 Determine the total number of grams for 8 doses.
$$0.5 \text{ g} \times 8 \text{ doses} = 4 \text{ g}$$

STEP 3 Determine the total number of vials needed to fill this prescription.

$$\frac{1 \text{ g}}{1 \text{ vial}} = \frac{4 \text{ g}}{x \text{ vials}}$$
$$x = 4 \text{ vials}$$

The answer is 4 vials. (*Knowledge Domain 4.2*)

30. **(B)** A meniscus is the curved surface that appears at the top of a volume of liquid in a graduated cylinder. Levigation, choice (A), is the process of grinding a powder through the incorporation of a liquid. Ointment, choice (C), is a water in oil (w/o) emulsion. Troches, choice (D), are tablets designed to be dissolved in the mouth. (*Knowledge Domain 4.1*)

31. **(C)** "qhs" is designated on ISMP's list of error-prone abbreviations, symbols, and dose designations. (*Knowledge Domain 3.2*)

32. **(C)** A suspension is an example of a liquid dosage form where the active ingredient is dispersed in the liquid vehicle. Powders, capsules, and suppositories are all examples of solid dosage forms. (*Knowledge Domain 1.4*)

33. **(D)** Otic = ear; ophthalmic = eye; nasal = nose; and rectal = rectum. (*Knowledge Domain 4.2*)

34. **(C)** Medications kept at room temperature should be maintained at temperatures of 68°F to 77°F. Medications that need to be frozen are maintained at temperatures of −4°F to 14°F. Refrigerated medications are maintained at temperatures of 36°F to 46°F. Medications should not be kept at temperatures exceeding those of room temperature. (*Knowledge Domain 1.10*)

35. **(C)** Class III, IV, and V prescriptions may be refilled up to 5 times in 6 months. (*Knowledge Domain 2.2*)

36. **(D)** Ampicillin is not classified as a high-alert medication as indicated by the Institute for Safe Medication Practices (ISMP). Oral hypoglycemics (e.g., metformin), anticoagulants (e.g., warfarin), and intravenous sedative agents (e.g., midazolam) are all classified by the ISMP for their potential to cause patient harm when used in error. (*Knowledge Domain 3.1*)

37. **(B)** Risk Evaluation and Mitigation Strategies (REMS) vary, but for isotretinoin, the REMS program is a web-based system called iPLEDGE. (*Knowledge Domain 2.4*)

38. **(C)** Non-aqueous solutions have a beyond-use date of no later than 6 months. Oral solutions that contain water have a beyond-use date of no later than 14 days. Topical solutions that contain water have a beyond-use date of no later than 30 days. (*Knowledge Domain 4.4*)

39. **(C)** Set up a proportion:

$$\frac{1 \text{ g}}{1,000 \text{ mg}} = \frac{1.22 \text{ mg}}{x \text{ mcg}}$$

$$x = 1,220 \text{ mcg}$$

The answer is 1,220 mcg. (*Knowledge Domain 4.2*)

40. **(A)** Class III and Class IV prescriptions may be transferred only 1 time when a transfer to a pharmacy that does not share a real-time online database is requested. If the pharmacy does share an online database, the prescription may be transferred as many times as needed or until the prescription expires or the refills are out. (*Knowledge Domain 2.2*)

41. **(C)** The term "biennial" means every other year. (*Knowledge Domain 2.3*)

42. **(B)** It is true that medications with similar drug names (e.g., look-alike/sound-alike drugs) should not be placed next to each other on a pharmacy shelf. This, however, is an example of an error prevention strategy, not a strategy used to prevent finding expired drugs on pharmacy shelves. Using colored stickers that indicate the month of expiration, writing the month of expiration on pharmacy stock bottles, and placing new stock bottles behind old stock bottles (e.g., rotating stock) are all common strategies used to prevent expired products from being found on pharmacy shelves. (*Knowledge Domain 4.5*)

43. **(B)** The purchasing and returning of Class II medications such as Ritalin are made using a DEA 222 form. A DEA 224 form is used by a pharmacy that is looking to dispense controlled substances. A DEA 106 form is used to report lost or stolen substances. A DEA 41 form is used to document the destruction of controlled substances. (*Knowledge Domain 2.3*)

44. **(A)** An undesirable effect of a drug is known as a side effect. A contraindication is a condition or factor that would make prescribing a certain drug unwise or unsafe. An allergy is an immune system's abnormal reaction to a drug. A drug interaction occurs when a substance affects the activity or response of a drug when both the substance and the drug are administered simultaneously. (*Knowledge Domain 1.5*)

45. **(D)** The use of preprinted prescription blanks with commonly used protocols or frequently prescribed medications is an example of a standardization technique that is used to avoid variation or complexity. Electronic processing software is an example of automa-

tion and computerization. Fail-safe and constraints, such as the integration of pharmacy computers with the pharmacy register, may be implemented as an error prevention strategy. Pharmacies may also use forcing functions to provide a stop in the system, requiring verification before proceeding to fill the prescription. An example of this would be the use of a scanner to match the selected medication to the profiled medication. (*Knowledge Domain 3.2*)

46. **(B)** An illegible prescription that results in filling a prescription with the wrong quantity is categorized as a prescribing error. An unauthorized drug error results in the administration of a drug that is not authorized for the patient. A wrong drug preparation error is a result of incorrectly formulating or manipulating a drug before administration. Administration errors vary but can include wrong time or rate of administration. (*Knowledge Domain 3.5*)

47. **(C)** Loratadine is the therapeutic equivalent for Claritin. Diphenhydramine is the therapeutic equivalent for Benadryl. Cetirizine is the therapeutic equivalent for Zyrtec. Fexofenadine is the therapeutic equivalent for Allegra. (*Knowledge Domain 1.2*)

48. **(B)** Counting trays that are used to count antibiotics or hazardous medications should be labeled and should only be used for counting those specific medications. General counting trays can be used to count all other medications. Counting trays are not made of glass. They are typically made of plastic or metal to avoid accidental breakage. Counting trays should be kept in an accessible area, typically the pharmacy filling area. They should not be kept in the compounding area of the pharmacy. (*Knowledge Domain 3.6*)

49. **(A)** Class II prescriptions must be presented in person or sent in electronically (check with your state laws) and therefore may not be prescribed over the phone. Class III, Class IV, and noncontrolled prescriptions may all be called into the pharmacy by the prescriber. (*Knowledge Domain 2.2*)

50. **(B)** Morphine is a Schedule II controlled substance. (*Knowledge Domain 2.2*)

51. **(C)** Set up a proportion to solve for how many 5 mL doses are in 1 pint. Note that 1 pint = 473 mL.

$$\frac{5 \text{ mL}}{1 \text{ dose}} = \frac{473 \text{ mL}}{x \text{ doses}}$$

$$x = 94.6 \text{ doses} \approx 95 \text{ doses}$$

The answer is 95 doses. (*Knowledge Domain 4.2*)

52. **(D)** A mortar and pestle are used to grind tablets or granules into a fine powder. A spatula may be used in conjunction with an ointment slab to mix ointments. A spatula may be used on an electronic balance to transfer a compound to be weighed. A stir rod is used in a beaker to mix an aqueous solution. (*Knowledge Domain 4.1*)

53. **(B)** Federal law mandates that Schedule II prescriptions must be maintained in the pharmacy for at least 2 years. (*Knowledge Domain 2.3*)

54. **(D)** The prefix "cyst-" means "bladder." The prefix "chol-" means "bile." The prefix "cardi-" means "heart." The prefix "costo-" means "ribs." (*Knowledge Domain 4.2*)

55. **(A)** Fat-soluble vitamins can be remembered using the acronym "ADEK," referring to vitamins A, D, E, and K. (*Knowledge Domain 1.6*)

56. **(B)** The minimum weighable quantity for a Class III prescription balance is 120 mg. The prescription balance is used to measure mass, not volume, and has a minimum sensitivity reading of 6 mg. (*Knowledge Domain 4.1*)

57. **(A)** The oral syringe is most appropriate when dispensing liquid for an infant because the caregiver can draw up the correct amount of medication into the syringe. A medication cup would not be appropriate because an infant is not able to drink from a cup. An oral dropper is difficult to use, and the caregiver may not accurately count the number of drops given to the child. A teaspoon is a household unit of measure that should not be used when dosing a patient. (*Knowledge Domain 4.3*)

58. **(C)** Insulin glargine (Lantus, Toujeo) is classified as a long-acting insulin. Insulin glulisine (Apidra), insulin aspart (NovoLog), and insulin lispro (Humalog) are all classified as rapid-acting insulin. (*Knowledge Domain 1.7*)

59. **(D)** QID is an acronym that means "four times a day." QD means once a day, BID means twice a day, and TID means three times a day. (*Knowledge Domain 4.2*)

60. **(C)** Sublingual administration refers to the route of administration by which substances diffuse into the bloodstream by absorption through tissues. Chewable tablets, syrups, and elixirs must enter the gastrointestinal system before being diffused into the bloodstream. (*Knowledge Domain 1.4*)

61. **(D)** Verapamil is classified as a calcium channel blocker. Atenolol is classified as a beta blocker. Furosemide is a loop diuretic. Lidocaine is an amide local anesthetic. (*Knowledge Domain 1.1*)

62. **(C)** This problem can be solved by setting up a proportion:

$$\frac{1 \text{ gallon}}{8 \text{ pints}} = \frac{x \text{ gallons}}{240 \text{ pints}}$$

$$8x = 240$$

$$x = 30$$

The answer is 30 gallons. (*Knowledge Domain 4.2*)

63. **(B)** The final check, which includes a comprehensive drug utilization review, must be performed only by a licensed pharmacist. (*Knowledge Domain 3.3*)

64. **(C)** A 50% solution means that there are 50 g of drug in 100 mL of solution. Calculate how many grams of drug are in 300 mL of solution by setting up a proportion.

$$\frac{50 \text{ g}}{100 \text{ mL}} = \frac{x \text{ g}}{300 \text{ mL}}$$

$$x = 150 \text{ g}$$

The answer is 150 g. (*Knowledge Domain 4.2*)

65. **(A)** This problem may be solved by setting up a proportion. Recall that D10W is a solution that contains 10% dextrose in water:

$$\frac{10\text{ g}}{100\text{ mL}} = \frac{x}{1{,}000\text{ mL}}$$

$$100x = 10{,}000$$

$$x = 100$$

The answer is 100 g. (*Knowledge Domain 4.2*)

66. **(B)** The pharmacy's refrigerator should be between 2°C and 8°C (36°F and 46°F). (*Knowledge Domain 1.10*)

67. **(C)** The prefix "hepato-" refers to the liver. The prefix "nephr-" would indicate the kidneys. The prefix "gastro-"" would indicate the stomach. The prefix "pneumo-" would indicate the lungs. (*Knowledge Domain 4.2*)

68. **(A)** Medication stock is rotated in order to minimize stock loss by placing short-dated medications near the front of the shelf and long-dated medications at the back of the shelf. (*Knowledge Domain 4.5*)

69. **(A)** Unit dose packaged medications should include the medication name, the strength, the manufacturer's name, the NDC, the lot number, and the expiration date. They may also include barcoding technology to identify the medication. They do not include instructions for patient use. (*Knowledge Domain 4.3*)

70. **(D)** Glucovance is a medication that is indicated for the treatment of type 2 diabetes and contains metformin and glyburide. Metaglip is a combination drug that contains metformin and glipizide. Avandaryl contains rosiglitazone and glimepiride. Avandamet contains rosiglitazone and metformin. (*Knowledge Domain 1.1*)

71. **(B)** Using trailing zeros can result in a 10-fold error. *Not* using leading zeros, *using* confusing abbreviations, and *not* using barcoding systems could also result in a medication error. (*Knowledge Domain 3.2*)

72. **(C)** This problem can be solved by setting up a proportion:

$$\frac{15\text{ mL}}{1\text{ hr}} = \frac{x\text{ mL}}{36\text{ hr}}$$

$$x = 540$$

The answer is 540 mL. (*Knowledge Domain 4.2*)

73. **(C)** The FDA classifies recalls according to severity. Class III recalls are not likely to cause adverse health consequences. Class I recalls are initiated when the likelihood of causing an adverse health consequence, or even death, is possible. Class II recalls are initiated when the use of a product may cause temporary health problems and the probability of a serious adverse health consequence is minimal. The FDA currently classifies recalls based on one of three categories and does not recognize a Class IV recall. (*Knowledge Domain 2.5*)

74. **(C)** The sig "1–2 gtts os TID" can be translated to mean "Instill 1–2 drops in the left eye three times a day." "os" refers to the "left eye," "ou" refers to "both eyes," "od" refers to the "right eye," and "as" refers to the "left ear." (*Knowledge Domain 4.2*)

75. **(A)** Upon receipt of a drug recall, pharmacy staff should pull the offending drug from pharmacy shelves immediately and contact patients who are taking this medication. The offending drug should not be left on pharmacy shelves nor should it be used to fill additional prescriptions. In addition, an attempt to order additional quantities of the offending drug should be avoided. (*Knowledge Domain 2.5*)

76. **(D)** Angiotensin II receptor blockers (ARBs) are used to treat hypertension by causing vasodilation. These agents, also known as angiotensin antagonists, can be recognized by the suffix "-sartan" and are often referred to as "sartans." An example of an ARB is candesartan. Metoprolol is a beta receptor agonist that is used in the treatment of hypertension. Beta receptor blockers, also knows as beta blockers, are often recognized by the suffix "-olol." Lisinopril is an ACE inhibitor that is used to treat hypertension. ACE inhibitors can be recognized by the suffix "-pril." Lovastatin is an HMG-CoA reductase inhibitor that is used in the treatment of hyperlipidemia. HMG-CoA reductase inhibitors are often recognized by the suffix "-statin" and are often referred to as "statins." (*Knowledge Domain 1.6*)

77. **(B)** Medication bottles are assumed to expire at the end of the month unless otherwise stated. (*Knowledge Domain 4.4*)

78. **(B)** The Combat Methamphetamine Epidemic Act of 2005 was enacted to regulate the sale of products that contain pseudoephedrine, ephedrine, and phenylpropanolamine. (*Knowledge Domain 2.4*)

79. **(B)** This problem can be solved by using an alligation. Set up a tic-tac-toe grid as follows:

30 (H)		10 (P – L)
	15 (P)	
5 (L)		15 (H – P)

(STEP 1) Set up an alligation by placing 30 in the top left corner and 5 in the bottom left corner. The final preparation concentration is placed in the middle.

(STEP 2) Determine the number of parts by subtracting as indicated above.

(STEP 3) Add the number of parts together to determine the total number of parts:

$$10 + 15 = 25 \text{ total parts}$$

(STEP 4) Set up a proportion to determine the quantity needed for each solution:

$$30\%: \frac{10}{25} = \frac{x}{500 \text{ mL}}$$

$$25x = 5,000$$

$$x = 200 \text{ mL}$$

$$5\%: \frac{15}{25} = \frac{x}{500 \text{ mL}}$$

$$25x = 7,500$$

$$x = 300 \text{ mL}$$

The answer is 200 mL of 30% solution and 300 mL of 5% solution. (*Knowledge Domain 4.2*)

80. **(B)** This problem can be solved by setting up a proportion:

$$\frac{125 \text{ mg}}{1 \text{ mL}} = \frac{275 \text{ mg}}{x}$$

$$125x = 275$$

$$x = 2.2$$

The answer is 2.2 mL. (*Knowledge Domain 4.2*)

81. **(A)** Latanoprost (Xalatan) is kept in a refrigerator prior to opening the bottle. Timolol, ofloxacin, and olopatadine do not need to be refrigerated. (*Knowledge Domain 1.10*)

82. **(D)** The ISMP oversees the Medication Error Reporting Program. The FDA oversees the MedWatch medication error reporting system. The CDC aims to improve public health by supporting health promotion, preparation, and preparedness. The DEA oversees the Controlled Substances Act. (*Knowledge Domain 3.4*)

83. **(C)** The "C" stamped or printed on controlled substance prescriptions and manufacturer bottles is red in color. (*Knowledge Domain 2.3*)

84. **(B)** Military time can be converted to standard time by subtracting 1200 for military times 1300 and larger (e.g., 1800 − 1200 = 6:00 P.M.). Military times less than 1300 can similarly be converted by adding 1200 to the military time. (*Knowledge Domain 4.2*)

85. **(C)** Pharmacy technicians should refuse to fill incomplete prescriptions and bring the prescription to the attention of the pharmacist. Pharmacy technicians should never contact the prescriber directly to verify a prescription. Pharmacy technicians should never fill the script based on the patient's recollection or past trends. (*Knowledge Domain 3.3*)

86. **(C)** *USP* <795> suggests that only purified water should be used in the compounding of non-sterile drug preparations. (*Knowledge Domain 4.1*)

87. **(C)** Capsules and tablets are typically counted in multiples of 5 when using a counting tray. (*Knowledge Domain 4.1*)

88. **(A)** The shaft is the stem of the needle that provides the overall length. The bevel is the angled surface at the top of the needle. The hub is the portion of the needle that attaches to the syringe. The lumen is the hollow center of the needle. (*Knowledge Domain 4.3*)

89. **(C)** Barcoding technology is not used to identify cost-saving strategies at this time. Verification of the correct drug, correct dose, and correct patient are all ways that barcoding technology is implemented to improve patient outcome and enhance patient safety. (*Knowledge Domain 3.2*)

90. **(A)** A suspension is a liquid dosage form where the active ingredient, most commonly a solid particle, is dispersed in a liquid medium. An emulsion is a mixture of two or more liquids that are immiscible. An elixir is a hydroalcoholic solution that contains water and alcohol. A solution is a liquid dosage form where the active ingredient is dissolved in the liquid medium. (*Knowledge Domain 1.4*)

Appendixes

For any recent updates to the information contained in the following appendixes, visit *http://bit.ly/Barrons-PTCE* to access an online version of all of these appendixes.

*Be sure to have your copy of *PTCE: Pharmacy Technician Certification Exam, Second Edition* on hand to complete the registration process.

Appendix A:
Top 200 Drugs
by Brand Name

Brand Name	Generic Name	Classification and Use
Abilify	aripiprazole	Antipsychotic
Aciphex	rabeprazole	Gastric antisecretory and GERD
Actonel	risedronate	Bisphosphonate
Actos	pioglitazone	Antidiabetic
Adderall XR	amphetamine and dextroamphetamine	Stimulant
Advair Diskus	fluticasone and salmeterol	Topical corticosteroid and bronchodilator combination
Aleve	naproxen	Nonsteroidal anti-inflammatory
Allegra	fexofenadine	Antihistamine
Allegra-D	fexofenadine and pseudoephedrine	Antihistamine and decongestant combination
Altace	ramipril	Antihypertensive
Amaryl	glimepiride	Antidiabetic
Ambien	zolpidem	Anxiolytics and sedatives and hypnotics
Amoxil	amoxicillin	Antibiotic
Ancef	cefazolin	Antibiotic
Aricept	donepezil	Neurodegenerative agent
Ativan	lorazepam	Anxiolytics and sedatives and hypnotics
Atropen	atropine	Antimuscarinic
Atrovent	ipratropium bromide	Bronchodilator
Augmentin	amoxicillin and clavulanate	Antibiotic
Avodart	dutasteride	Anti-testosterone
Bactrim	trimethoprim and sulfamethoxazole	Antibiotic
Bactroban	mupirocin	Topical antibiotic
Bayer	aspirin	Nonsteroidal anti-inflammatory and antiplatelet
Benadryl	diphenhydramine	Antihistamine
Benicar	olmesartan	Antihypertensive

Brand Name	Generic Name	Classification and Use
Biaxin	clarithromycin	Antibiotic
Bystolic	nebivolol	Antihypertensive
Caduet	amlodipine and atorvastatin	Antihypertensive and hypolipidemic
Calan	verapamil	Antihypertensive and antiarrhythmic
Calciferol	ergocalciferol	Vitamin derivative
Catapres	clonidine	Antihypertensive
Celebrex	celecoxib	Nonsteroidal anti-inflammatory
Celexa	citalopram	Antidepressant
Cialis	tadalafil	Vasodilator
Cipro	ciprofloxacin	Antibiotic
Claforan	cefotaxime	Antibiotic
Claritin	loratadine	Antihistamine
Claritin-D 24-Hour	loratadine and pseudoephedrine	Antihistamine and decongestant combination
Colace	docusate sodium	Laxative
Combivent Respimat	ipratropium bromide and albuterol	Bronchodilator combination
Compazine	prochlorperazine	Antiemetic
Concerta	methylphenidate ER	Stimulant
Cordarone	amiodarone	Antiarrhythmic
Coreg	carvedilol	Antihypertensive
Cortizone 10	hydrocortisone	Topical corticosteroid
Coumadin	warfarin	Anticoagulant
Cozaar	losartan	Antihypertensive
Crestor	rosuvastatin	Hypolipidemic
Cymbalta	duloxetine	Antidepressant
Decadron	dexamethasone	Systemic adrenal corticosteroid
Delsym	dextromethorphan	Antitussive
Deltasone	prednisone	Systemic adrenal corticosteroid
Desyrel	trazodone	Antidepressant
Detrol LA	tolterodine	Non-vascular smooth muscle relaxant
Diflucan	fluconazole	Antifungal
Diovan	valsartan	Antihypertensive
Diovan HCT	valsartan and hydrochlorothiazide	Antihypertensive and diuretic combination
Diprivan	propofol	General anesthetic and sedative and hypnotic
Dobutrex	dobutamine	Inotrope
Dopastat	dopamine	Inotrope and pressor
Duragesic	fentanyl	Opioid analgesic
Effexor	venlafaxine	Antidepressant
Elavil	amitriptyline	Antidepressant
Eliquis	apixaban	Anticoagulant

Brand Name	Generic Name	Classification and Use
Epogen	epoetin alfa	Growth factor
Flexeril	cyclobenzaprine	Skeletal muscle relaxant
Flomax	tamsulosin	Alpha blocker
Flonase	fluticasone	Topical corticosteroid
Flovent HFA	fluticasone	Inhaled corticosteroid
FluMist	influenza vaccine live	Vaccine
Fluzone	inactivated influenza vaccine	Vaccine
Focalin XR	dexmethylphenidate	Stimulant
Fosamax	alendronate	Bisphosphonate
Glucophage	metformin	Antidiabetic
Humalog	insulin lispro	Antidiabetic
Humulin N	insulin NPH (human)	Antidiabetic
Humulin R	insulin regular (human)	Antidiabetic
Hydrodiuril	hydrochlorothiazide	Diuretic
Imitrex	sumatriptan	Antimigraine and central vasoconstrictor
Inderal	propranolol	Antihypertensive
Ismo	isosorbide mononitrate	Antianginal
Isordil	isosorbide dinitrate	Antianginal
Januvia	sitagliptin	Antidiabetic
Keflex	cephalexin	Antibiotic
Klonopin	clonazepam	Anxiolytics and sedatives and hypnotics
Lamisil	terbinafine	Topical antifungal
Lanoxin	digoxin	Inotrope
Lantus	insulin glargine	Antidiabetic
Lasix	furosemide	Diuretic
Levaquin	levofloxacin	Antibiotic
Levemir	insulin detemir	Antidiabetic
Lexapro	escitalopram	SSRI antidepressant
Lipitor	atorvastatin	Hypolipidemic
Loestrin	ethinyl estradiol and norethindrone	Contraceptive
Lotensin	benazepril	Antihypertensive
Lotrel	amlodipine and benazepril	Antihypertensive
Lovaza	omega-3-acid ethyl esters	Hypolipidemic
Lovenox	enoxaparin	Anticoagulant
Lunesta	eszopiclone	Anxiolytics and sedatives and hypnotics
Lyrica	pregabalin	Anticonvulsant
Maxzide	triamterene and hydrochlorothiazide	Diuretic
Medrol	methylprednisolone	Systemic adrenal corticosteroid

Brand Name	Generic Name	Classification and Use
Micro-K	potassium chloride	Electrolyte
Micronase	glyburide	Antidiabetic
MiraLAX	polyethylene glycol 3350	Laxative
Mobic	meloxicam	Nonsteroidal anti-inflammatory
Motrin	ibuprofen	Nonsteroidal anti-inflammatory
MS Contin	morphine	Opioid analgesic
Namenda	memantine	Neurodegenerative agent
Narcan	naloxone	Opioid antagonist
Nasonex	mometasone furoate	Topical corticosteroid
Neosporin	neomycin and polymyxin B and bacitracin	Topical antibiotic
Neurontin	gabapentin	Anticonvulsant
Nexium	esomeprazole	Gastric antisecretory and GERD
Nitrostat	nitroglycerin	Antianginal
Norvasc	amlodipine	Antihypertensive
NuvaRing	etonogestrel and ethinyl estradiol	Contraceptive
Os-Cal	calcium carbonate	Vitamin derivative
Oxycontin	oxycodone	Opioid analgesic
Paxil	paroxetine	Antidepressant
Pepcid AC	famotidine	Gastric antisecretory and GERD
Pepto Bismol	bismuth subsalicylate	Gastric antisecretory and GERD
Percocet	oxycodone and acetaminophen	Opioid analgesic and non-opioid analgesic combination
Phenergan	promethazine	Antihistamine
Phenergan with Codeine	promethazine and codeine	Antitussive combination
Plavix	clopidogrel	Anticoagulant
Pradaxa	dabigatran etexilate	Anticoagulant
Pravachol	pravastatin	Hypolipidemic
Premarin	conjugated estrogens	Female sex hormone
Prevacid 24-Hour	lansoprazole	Gastric antisecretory and GERD
Prilosec	omeprazole	Gastric antisecretory and GERD
Prinzide	lisinopril and hydrochlorothiazide	Antihypertensive and diuretic combination
Pristiq	desvenlafaxine	Antidepressant
Protonix	pantoprazole	Gastric antisecretory and GERD
Prozac	fluoxetine	Antidepressant
Qvar	beclomethasone	Topical corticosteroid
Restoril	temazepam	Anxiolytics and sedatives and hypnotics
Rhinocort	budesonide	Topical corticosteroid

Brand Name	Generic Name	Classification and Use
Robitussin	guaifenesin	Expectorant
Rocaltrol	calcitriol	Vitamin derivative
Rocephin	ceftriaxone	Antibiotic
Senokot	senna	Laxative
Seroquel	quetiapine	Antipsychotic
Singulair	montelukast	Immune modulator
Solu-Cortef	hydrocortisone	Systemic adrenal corticosteroid
Soma	carisoprodol	Skeletal muscle relaxant
Spiriva HandiHaler	tiotropium bromide	Bronchodilator
Sublimaze	fentanyl	Opioid analgesic
Suboxone	buprenorphine and naloxone	Opioid analgesic and opioid antagonist combination
Sudafed	pseudoephedrine	Decongestant
Sudafed PE	phenylephrine	Pressor and vasoconstrictor
Symbicort	budesonide and formoterol	Topical corticosteroid and bronchodilator combination
Synthroid	levothyroxine	Thyroid agent
Tamiflu	oseltamivir	Antiviral
Tenormin	atenolol	Antihypertensive
Toprol XL	metoprolol succinate	Antihypertensive
Toradol	ketorolac	Nonsteroidal anti-inflammatory
Tricor	fenofibrate	Hypolipidemic
Tylenol	acetaminophen	Analgesic and antipyretic
Tylenol with Codeine	acetaminophen and codeine	Opioid analgesic and non-opioid analgesic combination
Ultram	tramadol	Opioid analgesic
Valium	diazepam	Anxiolytics and sedatives and hypnotics
Valtrex	valacyclovir	Antiviral
Vancocin	vancomycin	Antibiotic
Ventolin	albuterol	Bronchodilator
Versed	midazolam	Anxiolytics and sedatives and hypnotics
VESIcare	solifenacin	Non-vascular smooth muscle relaxant
Viagra	sildenafil	Vasodilator
Vicodin	hydrocodone and acetaminophen	Opioid analgesic and non-opioid analgesic combination
Vytorin	ezetimibe and simvastatin	Hypolipidemic
Vyvanse	lisdexamfetamine	Stimulant
Wellbutrin	bupropion	Antidepressant
Xalatan	latanoprost	Topical prostaglandin analog
Xanax	alprazolam	Anxiolytics and sedatives and hypnotics

Brand Name	Generic Name	Classification and Use
Xarelto	rivaroxaban	Anticoagulant
Xopenex	levalbuterol	Bronchodilator
Xylocaine	lidocaine	Local anesthetic
Yaz	ethinyl estradiol and drospirenone	Contraceptive
Zantac	ranitidine	Gastric antisecretory
Zestril	lisinopril	Antihypertensive
Zetia	ezetimibe	Hypolipidemic
Zithromax	azithromycin	Antibiotic
Zocor	simvastatin	Hypolipidemic
Zofran	ondansetron	Antiemetic
Zoloft	sertraline	Antidepressant
Zosyn	piperacillin and tazobactam	Antibiotic
Zovirax	acyclovir	Antiviral
Zyloprim	allopurinol	Gout
Zyprexa	olanzapine	Antipsychotic
Zyrtec	cetirizine	Antihistamine
	echinacea*	Immune stimulator
	ferrous sulfate*	Iron preparation
	*Ginkgo biloba**	Stimulant
	green tea*	Anti-inflammatory and antioxidant
	heparin*	Anticoagulant
	magnesium sulfate*	Electrolyte
	penicillin*	Antibiotic
	potassium chloride*	Electrolyte
	triamcinolone*	Topical corticosteroid
	vitamin D3*	Vitamin derivative

*No brand name formulation is currently available.

**Note that the Pharmacy Technician Certification Board does not endorse any one list of the top 200 brand name drugs because this information is constantly being updated. However, this list should provide you with a general idea of some of the most common brand name drugs that you should be familiar with.

Appendix B:
Top 200 Drugs by Classification and Use

Classification and Use	Brand Name	Generic Name
Alpha blocker	Flomax	tamsulosin
Analgesic and antipyretic	Tylenol	acetaminophen
Antianginal	Ismo	isosorbide mononitrate
Antianginal	Isordil	isosorbide dinitrate
Antianginal	Nitrostat	nitroglycerin
Antiarrhythmic	Cordarone	amiodarone
Antibiotic	Amoxil	amoxicillin
Antibiotic	Ancef	cefazolin
Antibiotic	Augmentin	amoxicillin and clavulanate
Antibiotic	Bactrim	trimethoprim and sulfamethoxazole
Antibiotic	Biaxin	clarithromycin
Antibiotic	Cipro	ciprofloxacin
Antibiotic	Claforan	cefotaxime
Antibiotic	Keflex	cephalexin
Antibiotic	Levaquin	levofloxacin
Antibiotic	Rocephin	ceftriaxone
Antibiotic	Vancocin	vancomycin
Antibiotic	Zithromax	azithromycin
Antibiotic	Zosyn	piperacillin and tazobactam
Antibiotic		penicillin*
Anticoagulant	Coumadin	warfarin
Anticoagulant	Eliquis	apixaban
Anticoagulant	Lovenox	enoxaparin
Anticoagulant	Plavix	clopidogrel
Anticoagulant	Pradaxa	dabigatran etexilate
Anticoagulant	Xarelto	rivaroxaban
Anticoagulant		heparin*
Anticonvulsant	Lyrica	pregabalin
Anticonvulsant	Neurontin	gabapentin
Antidepressant	Celexa	citalopram
Antidepressant	Cymbalta	duloxetine
Antidepressant	Desyrel	trazodone
Antidepressant	Effexor	venlafaxine

Classification and Use	Brand Name	Generic Name
Antidepressant	Elavil	amitriptyline
Antidepressant	Paxil	paroxetine
Antidepressant	Pristiq	desvenlafaxine
Antidepressant	Prozac	fluoxetine
Antidepressant	Wellbutrin	bupropion
Antidepressant	Zoloft	sertraline
Antidiabetic	Actos	pioglitazone
Antidiabetic	Amaryl	glimepiride
Antidiabetic	Glucophage	metformin
Antidiabetic	Humalog	insulin lispro
Antidiabetic	Humulin N	insulin NPH (human)
Antidiabetic	Humulin R	insulin regular (human)
Antidiabetic	Januvia	sitagliptin
Antidiabetic	Lantus	insulin glargine
Antidiabetic	Levemir	insulin detemir
Antidiabetic	Micronase	glyburide
Antiemetic	Compazine	prochlorperazine
Antiemetic	Zofran	ondansetron
Antifungal	Diflucan	fluconazole
Antihistamine	Allegra	fexofenadine
Antihistamine	Benadryl	diphenhydramine
Antihistamine	Claritin	loratadine
Antihistamine	Phenergan	promethazine
Antihistamine	Zyrtec	cetirizine
Antihistamine and decongestant combination	Allegra-D	fexofenadine and pseudoephedrine
Antihistamine and decongestant combination	Claritin-D 24-Hour	loratadine and pseudoephedrine
Antihypertensive	Altace	ramipril
Antihypertensive	Benicar	olmesartan
Antihypertensive	Bystolic	nebivolol
Antihypertensive	Catapres	clonidine
Antihypertensive	Coreg	carvedilol
Antihypertensive	Cozaar	losartan
Antihypertensive	Diovan	valsartan
Antihypertensive	Inderal	propranolol
Antihypertensive	Lotensin	benazepril
Antihypertensive	Lotrel	amlodipine and benazepril
Antihypertensive	Norvasc	amlodipine
Antihypertensive	Tenormin	atenolol
Antihypertensive	Toprol XL	metoprolol succinate
Antihypertensive	Zestril	lisinopril

Classification and Use	Brand Name	Generic Name
Antihypertensive and antiarrhythmic	Calan	verapamil
Antihypertensive and diuretic combination	Diovan HCT	valsartan and hydrochlorothiazide
Antihypertensive and diuretic combination	Prinzide	lisinopril and hydrochlorothiazide
Antihypertensive and hypolipidemic	Caduet	amlodipine and atorvastatin
Anti-inflammatory and antioxidant		green tea*
Antimigraine and central vasoconstrictor	Imitrex	sumatriptan
Antimuscarinic	Atropen	atropine
Antipsychotic	Abilify	aripiprazole
Antipsychotic	Seroquel	quetiapine
Antipsychotic	Zyprexa	olanzapine
Anti-testosterone	Avodart	dutasteride
Antitussive	Delsym	dextromethorphan
Antitussive combination	Phenergan with Codeine	promethazine and codeine
Antiviral	Tamiflu	oseltamivir
Antiviral	Valtrex	valacyclovir
Antiviral	Zovirax	acyclovir
Anxiolytics and sedatives and hypnotics	Ambien	zolpidem
Anxiolytics and sedatives and hypnotics	Ativan	lorazepam
Anxiolytics and sedatives and hypnotics	Klonopin	clonazepam
Anxiolytics and sedatives and hypnotics	Lunesta	eszopiclone
Anxiolytics and sedatives and hypnotics	Restoril	temazepam
Anxiolytics and sedatives and hypnotics	Valium	diazepam
Anxiolytics and sedatives and hypnotics	Versed	midazolam
Anxiolytics and sedatives and hypnotics	Xanax	alprazolam
Bisphosphonate	Actonel	risedronate
Bisphosphonate	Fosamax	alendronate
Bronchodilator	Atrovent	ipratropium bromide
Bronchodilator	Spiriva HandiHaler	tiotropium bromide
Bronchodilator	Ventolin	albuterol
Bronchodilator	Xopenex	levalbuterol
Bronchodilator combination	Combivent Respimat	ipratropium bromide and albuterol

Classification and Use	Brand Name	Generic Name
Contraceptive	Loestrin	ethinyl estradiol and norethindrone
Contraceptive	NuvaRing	etonogestrel and ethinyl estradiol
Contraceptive	Yaz	ethinyl estradiol and drospirenone
Decongestant	Sudafed	pseudoephedrine
Diuretic	Hydrodiuril	hydrochlorothiazide
Diuretic	Lasix	furosemide
Diuretic	Maxzide	triamterene and hydrochlorothiazide
Electrolyte	Micro-K	potassium chloride
Electrolyte		magnesium sulfate*
Electrolyte		potassium chloride*
Expectorant	Robitussin	guaifenesin
Female sex hormone	Premarin	conjugated estrogens
Gastric antisecretory	Pepcid AC	famotidine
Gastric antisecretory	Pepto Bismol	bismuth subsalicylate
Gastric antisecretory	Zantac	ranitidine
Gastric antisecretory and GERD	Aciphex	rabeprazole
Gastric antisecretory and GERD	Nexium	esomeprazole
Gastric antisecretory and GERD	Prevacid 24-Hour	lansoprazole
Gastric antisecretory and GERD	Prilosec	omeprazole
Gastric antisecretory and GERD	Protonix	pantoprazole
General anesthetic and sedative and hypnotic	Diprivan	propofol
Gout	Zyloprim	allopurinol
Growth factor	Epogen	epoetin alfa
Hypolipidemic	Crestor	rosuvastatin
Hypolipidemic	Lipitor	atorvastatin
Hypolipidemic	Lovaza	omega-3-acid ethyl esters
Hypolipidemic	Pravachol	pravastatin
Hypolipidemic	Tricor	fenofibrate
Hypolipidemic	Vytorin	ezetimibe and simvastatin
Hypolipidemic	Zetia	ezetimibe
Hypolipidemic	Zocor	simvastatin
Immune modulator	Singulair	montelukast
Immune stimulator		echinacea*
Inhaled corticosteroid	Flovent HFA	fluticasone
Inotrope	Dobutrex	dobutamine
Inotrope	Lanoxin	digoxin
Inotrope and pressor	Dopastat	dopamine

Classification and Use	Brand Name	Generic Name
Iron preparation		ferrous sulfate*
Laxative	Colace	docusate sodium
Laxative	MiraLAX	polyethylene glycol 3350
Laxative	Senokot	senna
Local anesthetic	Xylocaine	lidocaine
Neurodegenerative agent	Aricept	donepezil
Neurodegenerative agent	Namenda	memantine
Nonsteroidal anti-inflammatory	Aleve	naproxen
Nonsteroidal anti-inflammatory	Celebrex	celecoxib
Nonsteroidal anti-inflammatory	Mobic	meloxicam
Nonsteroidal anti-inflammatory	Motrin	ibuprofen
Nonsteroidal anti-inflammatory	Toradol	ketorolac
Nonsteroidal anti-inflammatory and antiplatelet	Bayer	aspirin
Non-vascular smooth muscle relaxant	Detrol LA	tolterodine
Non-vascular smooth muscle relaxant	VESIcare	solifenacin
Opioid analgesic	Duragesic	fentanyl
Opioid analgesic	MS Contin	morphine
Opioid analgesic	Oxycontin	oxycodone
Opioid analgesic	Sublimaze	fentanyl
Opioid analgesic	Ultram	tramadol
Opioid analgesic and non-opioid analgesic combination	Percocet	oxycodone and acetaminophen
Opioid analgesic and non-opioid analgesic combination	Tylenol with Codeine	acetaminophen and codeine
Opioid analgesic and non-opioid analgesic combination	Vicodin	hydrocodone and acetaminophen
Opioid analgesic and opioid antagonist combination	Suboxone	buprenorphine and naloxone
Opioid antagonist	Narcan	naloxone
Pressor and vasoconstrictor	Sudafed PE	phenylephrine
Skeletal muscle relaxant	Flexeril	cyclobenzaprine
Skeletal muscle relaxant	Soma	carisoprodol
SSRI antidepressant	Lexapro	escitalopram
Stimulant	Adderall XR	amphetamine and dextroamphetamine
Stimulant	Concerta	methylphenidate ER
Stimulant	Focalin XR	dexmethylphenidate
Stimulant	Vyvanse	lisdexamfetamine
Stimulant		*Ginkgo biloba**
Systemic adrenal corticosteroid	Decadron	dexamethasone
Systemic adrenal corticosteroid	Deltasone	prednisone
Systemic adrenal corticosteroid	Medrol	methylprednisolone

Classification and Use	Brand Name	Generic Name
Systemic adrenal corticosteroid	Solu-Cortef	hydrocortisone
Thyroid agent	Synthroid	levothyroxine
Topical antibiotic	Bactroban	mupirocin
Topical antibiotic	Neosporin	neomycin and polymyxin B and bacitracin
Topical antifungal	Lamisil	terbinafine
Topical corticosteroid	Cortizone 10	hydrocortisone
Topical corticosteroid	Flonase	fluticasone
Topical corticosteroid	Nasonex	mometasone furoate
Topical corticosteroid	Qvar	beclomethasone
Topical corticosteroid	Rhinocort	budesonide
Topical corticosteroid		triamcinolone*
Topical corticosteroid and bronchodilator combination	Advair Diskus	fluticasone and salmeterol
Topical corticosteroid and bronchodilator combination	Symbicort	budesonide and formoterol
Topical prostaglandin analog	Xalatan	latanoprost
Vaccine	FluMist	influenza vaccine live
Vaccine	Fluzone	inactivated influenza vaccine
Vasodilator	Cialis	tadalafil
Vasodilator	Viagra	sildenafil
Vitamin derivative	Calciferol	ergocalciferol
Vitamin derivative	Os-Cal	calcium carbonate
Vitamin derivative	Rocaltrol	calcitriol
Vitamin derivative		vitamin D3*

*No brand name formulation is currently available.

**Note that the Pharmacy Technician Certification Board does not endorse any one list of the top 200 brand name drugs because this information is constantly being updated. However, this list should provide you with a general idea of some of the most common brand name drugs that you should be familiar with.

Appendix C: Commonly Refrigerated Prescription Medications

Brand Name	Generic Name
Amoxil*	amoxicillin
Apidra	insulin glulisine
Augmentin*	amoxicillin and clavulanic acid
Avonex	interferon beta-1a
Benzamycin gel	erythromycin and benzoyl peroxide
Byetta	exenatide
Ceclor*	cefaclor
Ceftin*	cefuroxime axetil
Cipro	ciprofloxacin
CombiPatch	estradiol and norethindrone
DDAVP	desmopressin
Duac	clindamycin and benzoyl peroxide
Duricef*	cefadroxil
Enbrel	etanercept
Epogen	epoetin alfa
Foradil	formoterol
Forteo	teriparatide
Humalog	insulin lispro
Humira	adalimumab
Humulin N	NPH insulin
Humulin R	regular insulin
Iletin	insulin
Infergen	interferon alfacon-1
Kaletra	lopinavir and ritonavir
Keflex*	cephalexin
Kineret	anakinra
Lantus	insulin glargine
Levemir	insulin detemir
Miacalcin	calcitonin
Neulasta	pegfilgrastim
Neupogen	filgrastim
Novolin N	NPH insulin
Novolin R	regular insulin

Brand Name	Generic Name
NovoLog	insulin aspart
NuvaRing	etonogestrel and ethinyl estradiol vaginal ring
Phenergan suppository	promethazine
Procrit	epoetin alfa
Rebetron	interferon alfa-2b and ribavirin
Suprax	cefixime
Tamiflu*	oseltamivir
V-Cillin K*	penicillin V potassium
Veetids*	penicillin V
Vibramycin	doxycycline
Victoza	liraglutide
Viroptic	trifluridine
Xalatan	latanoprost
Zithromax*	azithromycin

*Indicates anti-infective therapy that may require refrigeration after reconstitution

Appendix D: Vaccines

Vaccine Name	Uses	Storage
DTaP	Diphtheria, tetanus, and acellular pertussis	Refrigerator
Hep A: Havrix, VAQTA	Hepatitis A	Refrigerator
Hep B: Engerix-B	Hepatitis B	Refrigerator
Hib	Haemophilus influenzae type B	Refrigerator
HPV 2: Cervarix	Human papillomavirus types 16 and 18	Refrigerator
HPV 4: Gardasil 9	Human papillomavirus types 16, 18, 31, 33, 45, 52, and 58	Refrigerator
IPV: IPOL	Poliovirus	Refrigerator
LAIV: FluMist	Influenza virus vaccine, quad, intranasal use	Refrigerator
Menactra and Menveo	Meningococcal conjugate	Refrigerator
MMR	Measles, mumps, and rubella	Refrigerator
MPSV4	Meningitis	Refrigerator
PCV13: Prevnar 13	Pneumococcal conjugate	Refrigerator
Quadrivalent IIV: Fluzone	Influenza virus vaccine, quad, intradermal use	Refrigerator
RV1: Rotarix or RV5: RotaTeq	Rotavirus	Refrigerator
Td: Tenivac and Tdap: Adacel and Boostrix	Tetanus and diphtheria toxoids	Refrigerator
MMRV: ProQuad	Measles, mumps, rubella, and varicella (chickenpox)	Freezer
VAR: VARIVAX	Varicella (chickenpox)	Freezer
Zostavax	Herpes zoster, shingles	Freezer

Appendix E: Vitamins

Common Name	Alternate Name	Function in the Body
Vitamin A	Retinol	Essential for vision, bone growth, and skin; antioxidant
Vitamin B complex	Comprised of B1, B2, B3, B5, B6, B7, and B12	Helps convert food into energy
Vitamin B1	Thiamine	Helps convert food into energy; coenzyme is used in the production of ATP
Vitamin B2	Riboflavin	Helps convert food into energy
Vitamin B3	Niacin	Helps convert food into energy; aids in the conversion of carbohydrates into energy; increases good cholesterol
Vitamin B5	Pantothenic acid	Helps convert food into energy; aids in the synthesis of fatty acids and cholesterol
Vitamin B6	Pyridoxine	May reduce the risk of heart disease; aids in the production of RBCs; plays a role in the production of key indicators that are essential to sleep, mood, and appetite
Vitamin B7	Biotin	Helps bone and hair growth; helps to synthesize glucose and convert food into energy
Vitamin B9	Folate	Synthetic folic acid is taken during pregnancy to prevent spinal cord and brain defects
Vitamin B12	Cobalamin	May reduce the risk of heart disease; aids in the production of new cells while also encouraging the normal growth of cells; protects nerve cells; aids in the production of RBCs
Vitamin C	Ascorbic acid	Helps to produce collagen, serotonin, and norepinephrine; antioxidant
Vitamin D	Calciferol	Helps maintain normal levels of calcium and phosphorus; essential for teeth and bones
Vitamin E	Alpha-tocopherol	Antioxidant; essential for nerve function
Vitamin K	Phylloquinone	Essential in the blood clotting cascade

Appendix F: Common Over-the-Counter Products

Brand Name	Generic Name	Classification
Abreva	docosanol	Cold sores
Afrin	oxymetazoline	Nasal decongestant
Aleve	naproxen	Anti-inflammatory
Allegra	fexofenadine	Antihistamine
Alli	orlistat	Weight loss
Benadryl	diphenhydramine	Antihistamine, sleep aid
Benefiber	wheat dextrin	Constipation
Bonine	meclizine	Nausea, motion sickness
Caladryl	calamine lotion	Topical anti-itch
Chlor-Trimeton	chlorpheniramine	Antihistamine
Citrucel	methylcellulose	Bulk laxative
Claritin	loratadine	Antihistamine
Clearasil	benzoyl peroxide	Acne
Colace	docusate	Stool softener
Cortizone	hydrocortisone	Topical corticosteroid
Debrox	carbamide peroxide	Earwax removal
Delsym	dextromethorphan	Antitussive
Dramamine	dimenhydrinate	Nausea, motion sickness
Dulcolax	bisacodyl	Stimulant laxative
Ecotrin	aspirin (enteric coated)	Anti-inflammatory
Emetrol	dextrose, levulose, phosphoric acid	Antiemetic
Excedrin	acetaminophen and aspirin and caffeine	Analgesic, anti-inflammatory, diuretic
Fibercon	polycarbophil	Laxative
Fleet suppositories	glycerin	Laxative
Flonase	fluticasone nasal	Corticosteroid used in allergic rhinitis
Gas-X, Phazyme	simethicone	Antiflatulent
Gyne-Lotrimin-3, Gyne-Lotrimin-7	clotrimazole	Vaginal antifungal
Imodium A-D	loperamide	Antidiarrheal

Brand Name	Generic Name	Classification
Ivy-Dry	benzyl alcohol	Urushiol-induced contact dermatitis
Kaopectate	bismuth subsalicylate	Antidiarrheal
Lactaid	lactase	Lactose intolerance
Lamisil AT	terbinafine	Topical antifungal
Lotrimin AF	clotrimazole	Topical antifungal
Maalox	magnesium and aluminum and simethicone	Heartburn, antacid
Melatonin	melatonin	Sleep aid
Metamucil	psyllium fiber	Fiber laxative
MiraLAX	polyethylene glycol 3350	Osmotic laxative
Monistat-3, Monistat-7	miconazole	Vaginal antifungal
Motrin, Advil	ibuprofen	Anti-inflammatory
Murine, Artificial Tears	artificial tears	Ocular lubricant
Mylanta	magnesium and aluminum and simethicone	Heartburn, antacid
Naphcon-A	naphazoline and pheniramine	Ocular antihistamine and decongestant
Nasacort	triamcinolone	Corticosteroid used in allergic rhinitis
NasalCrom	cromolyn sodium	Nasal antihistamine
Neosporin	neomycin and bacitracin and polymyxin	Topical antibiotic
Nexium	esomeprazole	GERD
Nix	permethrin	Topical scabicide
NoDoz	caffeine	Stimulant
Ocean	normal saline	Nasal moisturizer
Orajel	benzocaine	Topical anesthetic
Oxy Clean	salicylic acid	Acne
Pepcid	famotidine	Antiulcer
Pepto Bismol	bismuth subsalicylate	Indigestion, antidiarrheal
Peroxyl Oral Cleanser	hydrogen peroxide	Oral antiseptic
Phillips Milk of Magnesia	magnesium hydroxide	Constipation
Plan B	levonogestrel	Emergency contraceptive
Polysporin	bacitracin and polymyxin	Topical antibiotic
Prevacid OTC	lansoprazole	GERD
Prilosec OTC	omeprazole	GERD
RID	piperonyl and pyrethrins	Pediculicide
Robitussin, Mucinex	guaifenesin	Expectorant
Rogaine	minoxidil	Hair growth
Rolaids	calcium and magnesium	Antacid
Senokot	senna	Laxative
Sudafed	pseudoephedrine	Decongestant

Brand Name	Generic Name	Classification
Sudafed PE	phenylephrine	Decongestant
Tagamet	cimetidine	Antacid
Tinactin	tolnaftate	Topical antifungal
Tums	calcium carbonate	Antacid
Tylenol	acetaminophen	Analgesic
Vagistat-1, Vagistat-3	miconazole	Vaginal antifungal
Visine-A	naphazoline and pheniramine	Ocular antihistamine
Zanfel	polyethylene granules	Urushiol-induced contact dermatitis
Zantac 75	ranitidine	Antiulcer
Zostrix	capsaicin	Topical neuralgia
Zyrtec	cetirizine	Antihistamine

Appendix G:
Natural Supplements

Supplement	Indication
Black Cohosh	For symptoms of menopause
Chondroitin Sulfate	For joint inflammation
Coenzyme Q10	Increases energy; antioxidant
Cranberry	For UTIs; antioxidant
Echinacea	For immune support
Elderberry	For immune support
Fish Oil	Lowers triglycerides
Ginger	For nausea and motion sickness
Ginkgo Biloba	For dementia, fatigue
Ginseng	For an immune stimulant; for fatigue and inflammation
Glucosamine	For inflammation and joint pain
Kava	Helps with relaxation and anxiety
Melatonin	Regulates the sleep-wake cycle
Milk Thistle	For liver conditions; lowers cholesterol
Resveratrol	Antioxidant
Saw Palmetto	For BPH
St. John's Wort	For depression
Valerian	For insomnia

Appendix H:
Commonly Used
Pharmacy Abbreviations

Pharmacy technicians must be able to identify pharmacy abbreviations. Check your knowledge using this list of common pharmacy abbreviations. The use of these abbreviations, as well as the placement of periods and capitalization, varies. Refer to ISMP's list of error-prone abbreviations located in Appendix J.

Each of the following tables list common abbreviations in the left column and the definitions of those abbreviations in the right column. Test your knowledge by covering the definitions. Do you remember what the abbreviations mean?

Table H-1. Frequency

Abbreviation	Definition
AC	Before meals
PC	After meals
AM	Morning
PM	Evening
HS	At nighttime
Q	Every
Q __ H	Every __ hour(s)
QD	Every day
BID	Twice a day
TID	Three times a day
QID	Four times a day
PRN	As needed

Table H-2. Formulation

Abbreviation	Definition
amp	Ampule
cap	Capsule
elix	Elixir
inj	Injection
IUD	Intrauterine device
lot	Lotion
loz	Lozenge
MDI	Metered-dose inhaler
supp	Suppository
susp	Suspension
syr	Syrup
tab	Tablet
tbsp	Tablespoon
tinct	Tincture
TPN	Total parenteral nutrition
tsp	Teaspoon
ung, oint	Ointment

Table H-3. Route of Administration

Abbreviation	Definition
ad	Right ear
as	Left ear
au	Both ears
IM	Intramuscular
IV	Intravenous
IVP	Intravenous push
IVPB	Intravenous piggyback
od	Right eye
os	Left eye
ou	Both eyes
PO	By mouth
PR	Rectal
PV	Vaginal
subq, SC	Subcutaneous
top	Topical

Table H-4. Units

Abbreviation	Definition
cc	Cubic centimeter
fl oz	Fluid ounce
g or G	Gram
gal	Gallon
gr	Grain
kg	Kilogram
L	Liter
lb	Pound
mcg	Microgram
mg	Milligram
mL	Milliliter
oz	Ounce
pt	Pint
qt	Quart

Table H-5. Other

Abbreviation	Definition
aa	Of each
c or $\overline{c}$	With
disp	Dispense
div	Divide
non rep	Do not repeat
NR	No refills
Rx	Prescription
s or $\overline{s}$	Without
sig	Label, write
ss	One half
ud	As directed

Appendix I:
Medical Terminology

Table I-1. Prefixes

Prefix	Meaning
a-, an-	without
ab-	away
ad-	toward, near
ana-	up, again
ante-	before
anti-	against
apo-	upon
bi-	two
brady-	slow
cata-	down
con-	together
contra-	against
de-	from, down from
dia-	thorough, complete
dis-	to undo, free from
ect-	outer, outside
end-	within, inner
epi-	on, upon, over
eso-	inward
eu-	normal, good
extra-	outside of, beyond
hemi-	half
hyp-, hypo-	under, deficient
hyper-	above, beyond, excessive

Prefix	Meaning
in-	in, into
infra-	beneath, below
inter-	between
intra-	within
mal-	bad
meso-	middle
meta-	after, beyond
micro-	small
multi-	many
neo-	new
nulli-	none
pan-	all, total
para-	beside, beyond
per-	through
peri-	around
poly-	many, excessive
post-	after
pre-	before, in front of
pro-	before
re-	back
retro-	back, behind
semi-	half
sub-	under
super-	over, above
supra-	above
sym-, syn-	together, joined
tachy-	fast, rapid
tetra-	four
trans-	through, across
tri-	three
ultra-	beyond, excess
uni-	one

Table I-2. Suffixes

Suffix	Meaning
-agra	excessive pain
-algia	pain
-apheresis	removal
-ase	enzyme
-asthenia	weakness
-atresia	absence of a normal body opening
-capnia	carbon dioxide
-cele	hernia, protrusion
-centesis	surgical puncture to remove fluid
-cidal	killing
-clasis, -clast	break
-coccus	berry-shaped
-crine	Secrete
-crit	Separate
-cyte	Cell
-desis	surgical fixation, fusion
-drome	run, running
-ectasis	stretching out, dilation
-ectomy	cut out, excision
-ectopia	displacement
-emesis	Vomiting
-emia	blood condition
-esis, -iasis, -osis	state or condition
-en	substance or agent that produces or causes
-genesis	origin, cause
-genic	producing, originating, causing
-gram, -graphy	recording, written
-ia	disease or pathological condition
-iatry	physician, treatment
-ician	one who
-ictal	a blow, strike, stroke, or thrust
-ism	state of

Suffix	Meaning
-ites, -itis	Inflammation
-lepsy	Seizure
-lysis	loosening, separating, breaking down
-lytic	Destroy
-malacia	softening
-mania	madness, insanity
-megaly	enlargement
-meter	instrument used to measure
-metry	measure
-morph	form, shape
-odia	smell
-odynia	pain
-oid	resembling
-ologist	specialist, one who studies
-ology	study of
-oma	tumor
-oorhagia	rapid flow of blood
-oorhaphy	suturing, repairing
-opia	vision
-opsy	to view
-orrhea	flow
-orrhexis	rupture
-osis	abnormal condition
-ostomy	creation of an artificial opening
-oxia	oxygen
-paresis	slight paralysis
-pathy	Disease
-penia	deficiency, lack of
-pepsia	digestion
-pexy	surgical fixation
-phagia	eating
-phil, -philia	Love
-phobia	abnormal fear or aversion
-phonia	sound or voice

Suffix	Meaning
-phoria	feeling
-physis	growth
-plasia	formation, growth
-plasm	growth, substance
-plasty	surgical shaping
-pnea	breathing
-poiesis	formation
-porosis	passage
-prandial	meal
-praxia	in front of, before
-ptosis	dropping, sagging
-ptysis	spitting
-rrhaphy	suture
-rrhea	flow or discharge
-salpinx	fallopian tube
-sarcoma	malignant tumor
-schisis	split, fissure
-sclerosis	hardening
-scope, -scopic, -scopy	instrument used for visual examination; to examine
-sepsis	infection
-sis	state of
-spasm	sudden involuntary muscle contraction
-stalsis	contraction
-stasis	control, stop
-stenosis	constriction, narrowing
-stomy	surgical opening
-thorax	chest
-tocia	birth, labor
-tome	instrument used to cut
-tomy	cutting, incision
-tripsy	surgical crushing
-trophy	nourishment
-ule	little
-uria	urine, urination

Table I-3. Root Words

Root Word	Meaning
abdomen	abdomen
Acanth	thorny, spiny
acetabul	acetabulum
acou	Hearing
acr	extremities
actin	ray, radius
aden	gland
adenoid	adenoids
adren, adrenal	adrenal gland
aer	air, gas
albumin	albumin
algesi	pain
alveol	alveolus
ambly	dull, dim
amni	amnion
amyl	starch
andr	male
angi	vessel
anis	unequal
ankyl	crooked, bent
aort	aorta
appendic	appendix
arche	first, beginning
arteri	artery
arteriol	arteriole
arthr	joint
articul	joint
atel	imperfect, incomplete
ather	yellowish, fatty plaque
atri	atrium
aur	ear
aut	self

Root Word	Meaning
axill	armpit
azot	urea, nitrogen
bacteri	bacteria
bil	bile
bio	life
blast	developing cell
blephar	eyelid
brachi	arm
bronch	bronchus
bronchiol	bronchiole
bucc	cheek
burs	bursa
calc	calcium
carcin	cancer
cardi	heart
carp	carpals
caud	tail, toward the lower part of the body
cec	cecum
celi	abdomen
cephal	head
cerebell	cerebellum
cerebr	cerebrum
cerumen	earwax
cervic	cervix
cheil	lip
chir	hand
chol	gall, bile
cholangi	bile duct
choledoch	common bile duct
chondr	cartilage
chori	chorion
chrom	color
clavic, clavicul	clavicle

Root Word	Meaning
col	colon
colp	vagina
coni	dust
conjunctiv	conjunctiva
cor, core	pupil
corne	cornea
coron	heart
cortic	cortex
cost	rib
crani	cranium
cry	cold
crypt	hidden
cutane	skin
cyan	blue
cyes	pregnancy
cyt	cell
dacry	tear, tear duct
dactyl	fingers or toes
dent	tooth
derm, dermat	skin
dextr	right
diaphor	sweat
diaphragmat	diaphragm
dipl	two, double
dips	thirst
disk	intervertebral disk
diverticul	diverticulum
dors	back of the body
duoden	duodenum
dur	hard, dura mater
dynam	power or strength
ech	sound
ectop	located away from a usual place

Root Word	Meaning
electr	electricity
embry	embryo
emmetr	a normal measure
encephal	brain
endocrin	endocrine
enter	intestines
epididym	epididymis
epiglott	epiglottis
episi	vulva
epitheli	epithelium
erythr	red
esophag	esophagus
esthesi	sensation
eti	cause
faci	face
femor	femur
fet	fetus
fibr	fibrous tissue
fibul	fibula
gangli	ganglion
gastr	stomach
ger, geront	old age
gingiv	gum
glomerul	glomerulus
gloss	tongue
gluc	sweetness, sugar
glyc, glycos	sugar
gnath	jaw
gnos	knowledge
gon	seed
gravid	pregnancy
gyn, gynec	woman
hem, hemat	blood

Root Word	Meaning
hepat	liver
herni	hernia
heter	other
hidr	sweat
hist	tissue
home	unchanging
hor	boundary
humer	humerus
hydr	water
hymen	membrane
hypn	sleep
hyster	uterus
iatr	medicine, physician
ichthy	fish
ile	ileum
ili	ilium
immun	immune
ir, irid	iris
is	equal, same
isch	deficiency, blockage
ischi	ischium
jejun	jejunum
kal	potassium
kary	nucleus
kerat	cornea, hard tissue
kin	movement
kinesi	movement, motion
kyph	hump
labi	lip
labyrinth	maze, inner ear
lacrim	tear duct, tear
lact	milk
lamin	lamina

Root Word	Meaning
lapar	abdomen
laryng	larynx
later	side
lei	smooth
leuk	white
lingu	tongue
lip	fat
lith	stone, calculus
lob	lobe
lord	curve, bent forward
lymph	water
macro	abnormal largeness
mamm	breast
mandibul	mandible
mast	breast
mastoid	shaped like a nipple or breast
maxill	maxilla
meat	meatus
melan	black
men	menstruation
mening	meninges
menisc	meniscus
ment	mind
metr	uterus
mon	one
morph	form, shape
muc	mucus
my	muscle
myc	fungus
myel, myelon	bone marrow
myos	muscle
myring	eardrum
narc	stupor

Root Word	Meaning
nas	nose
nat	birth
necr	death
nephr	kidney
neur	nerve
noct	night
nyct, nyctal	night
ocul	eye
olig	scanty, few
onc	tumor
onych	nail
oo	egg, ovum
oophor	ovary
ophthalm	eye
opt	vision
or	mouth
orch, orchi, orchid	testis, testicle
organ	organ
orth	straight
oste	bone
ot	ear
ov	egg
ox	oxygen
pachy	thick
palat	palate
pancreat	pancreas
papill	nipple
para	bear, give birth to
parathyroid	parathyroid gland
part	bear, give birth to
patell	patella
path	disease
pector	chest

Root Word	Meaning
ped	child, foot
pelv	pelvis
perine	perineum
peritone	peritoneum
petr	stone
phac	lens of the eye
phag	eat, swallow
phak	lens of the eye
phalang	phalange (finger or toe joint)
phas	speech
phleb	vein
phot	light
phren	mind
physic	nature
plasm	plasma
pleur	pleura
pneum, pneumat, pneumon	lung, air
pod	foot
poikil	varied, irregular
poli	gray matter
polyp	small growth
poster	back of body
prim	first
proct	rectum
prostat	prostate gland
pseud	fake, false
psych	mind
pub	pubis
pulmon	lung
pupill	pupil
py	pus
pyel	renal pelvis
pylor	pylorus

Root Word	Meaning
pyr	fever, heat
quadr	four
rachi	vertebra
radi	radius
radicul	nerve root
rect	rectum
ren	kidney
retin	retina
rhabd	rod-shaped
rhin	nose
rhiz	nerve root
rhytid	wrinkle
salping	fallopian tube
sarc	flesh, connective tissue
scapul	scapula
scler	sclera
scoli	crooked, curved
seb	sebum
sept	septum
sial	saliva
sigmoid	sigmoid colon
sin	sinus
somat	body
somn	sleep
son	sound
sperm, spermat	spermatozoa, sperm cells
sphygm	pulse
spir	breathe, breathing
splen	spleen
spondyl	vertebra
staped	stapes
staphyl	grape-like clusters
stern	sternum

Root Word	Meaning
steth	chest
stomat	mouth
strept	twisted chains
synovi	synovia
tars	tarsal, tarsus
tendin	tendon
test	testis, testicle
therm	heat
thorac	thorax
thromb	clot
thym	thymus gland
thyr	thyroid gland
tibi	tibia
tom	cut, section
ton	tension, pressure
tonsil	tonsils
top	place
toxic	poison
trache	neck, neck-like, trachea
trich	hair
tympan	eardrum, middle ear
uln	ulna
ungu	nail
ur, urin	urine, urinary tract
urethr	urethra
uter	uterus
uvul	uvula
vagin	vagina
valv, valvul	valve
vas	vessel, duct
ven	vein
ventricul	ventricle
vertebr	vertebra

Root Word	Meaning
vesic	bladder
vesicul	seminal vesicles
viscer	internal organs
vulv	vulva
xanth	yellow
xer	dry

Appendix J: Institute for Safe Medication Practices's (ISMP's) List of Error-Prone Abbreviations, Symbols, and Dose Designations

The use of pharmacy abbreviations, acronyms, and symbols may be misinterpreted due to ambiguities, which could result in significant patient safety concerns. These errors are often reported to the Institute for Safe Medication Practices National Medication Errors Reporting Program (ISMP MERP). The ISMP maintains this voluntary practitioner error-reporting program to learn more about these errors and share information learned with the health care community. Examples of these errors include those made when prescribing, transcribing, dispensing, and administering medications/vaccines. The ISMP has argued that these abbreviations, acronyms, and symbols should be avoided in all medical communications, including written communications, telephone/verbal communications, computer-generated labels and storage bin labels, computer order entry screens, and medication administration records. Examples of these dose designations, medication abbreviations, and symbols can be found in the following table.

ISMP's List of *Error-Prone Abbreviations, Symbols,* and *Dose Designations*

The abbreviations, symbols, and dose designations found in this table have been reported to ISMP through the ISMP National Medication Errors Reporting Program (ISMP MERP) as being frequently misinterpreted and involved in harmful medication errors. They should **NEVER** be used when communicating medical information. This includes internal communications, telephone/verbal prescriptions, computer-generated labels, labels for drug storage bins, medication administration records, as well as pharmacy and prescriber computer order entry screens.

Abbreviations	Intended Meaning	Misinterpretation	Correction
µg	Microgram	Mistaken as "mg"	Use "mcg"
AD, AS, AU	Right ear, left ear, each ear	Mistaken as OD, OS, OU (right eye, left eye, each eye)	Use "right ear," "left ear," or "each ear"
OD, OS, OU	Right eye, left eye, each eye	Mistaken as AD, AS, AU (right ear, left ear, each ear)	Use "right eye," "left eye," or "each eye"
BT	Bedtime	Mistaken as "BID" (twice daily)	Use "bedtime"
cc	Cubic centimeters	Mistaken as "u" (units)	Use "mL"
D/C	Discharge or discontinue	Premature discontinuation of medications if D/C (intended to mean "discharge") has been misinterpreted as "discontinued" when followed by a list of discharge medications	Use "discharge" and "discontinue"
IJ	Injection	Mistaken as "IV" or "intrajugular"	Use "injection"
IN	Intranasal	Mistaken as "IM" or "IV"	Use "intranasal" or "NAS"
HS	Half-strength	Mistaken as bedtime	Use "half-strength" or "bedtime"
hs	At bedtime, hours of sleep	Mistaken as half-strength	
IU**	International unit	Mistaken as IV (intravenous) or 10 (ten)	Use "units"
o.d. or OD	Once daily	Mistaken as "right eye" (OD-oculus dexter), leading to oral liquid medications administered in the eye	Use "daily"
OJ	Orange juice	Mistaken as OD or OS (right or left eye); drugs meant to be diluted in orange juice may be given in the eye	Use "orange juice"
Per os	By mouth, orally	The "os" can be mistaken as "left eye" (OS-oculus sinister)	Use "PO," "by mouth," or "orally"
q.d. or QD**	Every day	Mistaken as q.i.d., especially if the period after the "q" or the tail of the "q" is misunderstood as an "i"	Use "daily"
qhs	Nightly at bedtime	Mistaken as "qhr" or every hour	Use "nightly"
qn	Nightly or at bedtime	Mistaken as "qh" (every hour)	Use "nightly" or "at bedtime"
q.o.d. or QOD**	Every other day	Mistaken as "q.d." (daily) or "q.i.d. (four times daily) if the "o" is poorly written	Use "every other day"
q1d	Daily	Mistaken as q.i.d. (four times daily)	Use "daily"
q6PM, etc.	Every evening at 6 PM	Mistaken as every 6 hours	Use "daily at 6 PM" or "6 PM daily"
SC, SQ, sub q	Subcutaneous	SC mistaken as SL (sublingual); SQ mistaken as "5 every;" the "q" in "sub q" has been mistaken as "every" (e.g., a heparin dose ordered "sub q 2 hours before surgery" misunderstood as every 2 hours before surgery)	Use "subcut" or "subcutaneously"
ss	Sliding scale (insulin) or ½ (apothecary)	Mistaken as "55"	Spell out "sliding scale;" use "one-half" or "½"
SSRI	Sliding scale regular insulin	Mistaken as selective-serotonin reuptake inhibitor	Spell out "sliding scale (insulin)"
SSI	Sliding scale insulin	Mistaken as Strong Solution of Iodine (Lugol's)	
i/d	One daily	Mistaken as "tid"	Use "1 daily"
TIW or tiw	3 times a week	Mistaken as "3 times a day" or "twice in a week"	Use "3 times weekly"
U or u**	Unit	Mistaken as the number 0 or 4, causing a 10-fold overdose or greater (e.g., 4U seen as "40" or 4u seen as "44"); mistaken as "cc" so dose given in volume instead of units (e.g., 4u seen as 4cc)	Use "unit"
UD	As directed ("ut dictum")	Mistaken as unit dose (e.g., diltiazem 125 mg IV infusion "UD" misinterpreted as meaning to give the entire infusion as a unit [bolus] dose)	Use "as directed"
Dose Designations and Other Information	**Intended Meaning**	**Misinterpretation**	**Correction**
Trailing zero after decimal point (e.g., 1.0 mg)**	1 mg	Mistaken as 10 mg if the decimal point is not seen	Do not use trailing zeros for doses expressed in whole numbers
"Naked" decimal point (e.g., .5 mg)**	0.5 mg	Mistaken as 5 mg if the decimal point is not seen	Use zero before a decimal point when the dose is less than a whole unit
Abbreviations such as mg. or mL. with a period following the abbreviation	mg mL	The period is unnecessary and could be mistaken as the number 1 if written poorly	Use mg, mL, etc. without a terminal period

ISMP's List of *Error-Prone Abbreviations, Symbols,* and *Dose Designations* (continued)

Dose Designations and Other Information	Intended Meaning	Misinterpretation	Correction
Drug name and dose run together (especially problematic for drug names that end in "l" such as Inderal40 mg; Tegretol300 mg)	Inderal 40 mg Tegretol 300 mg	Mistaken as Inderal 140 mg Mistaken as Tegretol 1300 mg	Place adequate space between the drug name, dose, and unit of measure
Numerical dose and unit of measure run together (e.g., 10mg, 100mL)	10 mg 100 mL	The "m" is sometimes mistaken as a zero or two zeros, risking a 10- to 100-fold overdose	Place adequate space between the dose and unit of measure
Large doses without properly placed commas (e.g., 100000 units; 1000000 units)	100,000 units 1,000,000 units	100000 has been mistaken as 10,000 or 1,000,000; 1000000 has been mistaken as 100,000	Use commas for dosing units at or above 1,000, or use words such as 100 "thousand" or 1 "million" to improve readability

Drug Name Abbreviations	Intended Meaning	Misinterpretation	Correction
To avoid confusion, do not abbreviate drug names when communicating medical information. Examples of drug name abbreviations involved in medication errors include:			
APAP	acetaminophen	Not recognized as acetaminophen	Use complete drug name
ARA A	vidarabine	Mistaken as cytarabine (ARA C)	Use complete drug name
AZT	zidovudine (Retrovir)	Mistaken as azathioprine or aztreonam	Use complete drug name
CPZ	Compazine (prochlorperazine)	Mistaken as chlorpromazine	Use complete drug name
DPT	Demerol-Phenergan-Thorazine	Mistaken as diphtheria-pertussis-tetanus (vaccine)	Use complete drug name
DTO	Diluted tincture of opium, or deodorized tincture of opium (Paregoric)	Mistaken as tincture of opium	Use complete drug name
HCl	hydrochloric acid or hydrochloride	Mistaken as potassium chloride (The "H" is misinterpreted as "K")	Use complete drug name unless expressed as a salt of a drug
HCT	hydrocortisone	Mistaken as hydrochlorothiazide	Use complete drug name
HCTZ	hydrochlorothiazide	Mistaken as hydrocortisone (seen as HCT250 mg)	Use complete drug name
MgSO4**	magnesium sulfate	Mistaken as morphine sulfate	Use complete drug name
MS, MSO4**	morphine sulfate	Mistaken as magnesium sulfate	Use complete drug name
MTX	methotrexate	Mistaken as mitoxantrone	Use complete drug name
NoAC	novel/new oral anticoagulant	No anticoagulant	Use complete drug name
PCA	procainamide	Mistaken as patient controlled analgesia	Use complete drug name
PTU	propylthiouracil	Mistaken as mercaptopurine	Use complete drug name
T3	Tylenol with codeine No. 3	Mistaken as liothyronine	Use complete drug name
TAC	triamcinolone	Mistaken as tetracaine, Adrenalin, cocaine	Use complete drug name
TNK	TNKase	Mistaken as "TPA"	Use complete drug name
TPA or tPA	tissue plasminogen activator, Activase (alteplase)	Mistaken as TNKase (tenecteplase), or less often as another tissue plasminogen activator, Retavase (retaplase)	Use complete drug names
ZnSO4	zinc sulfate	Mistaken as morphine sulfate	Use complete drug name

Stemmed Drug Names	Intended Meaning	Misinterpretation	Correction
"Nitro" drip	nitroglycerin infusion	Mistaken as sodium nitroprusside infusion	Use complete drug name
"Norflox"	norfloxacin	Mistaken as Norflex	Use complete drug name
"IV Vanc"	intravenous vancomycin	Mistaken as Invanz	Use complete drug name

Symbols	Intended Meaning	Misinterpretation	Correction
℥	Dram	Symbol for dram mistaken as "3"	Use the metric system
♏	Minim	Symbol for minim mistaken as "mL"	
x3d	For three days	Mistaken as "3 doses"	Use "for three days"
> and <	More than and less than	Mistaken as opposite of intended; mistakenly use incorrect symbol; "< 10" mistaken as "40"	Use "more than" or "less than"
/ (slash mark)	Separates two doses or indicates "per"	Mistaken as the number 1 (e.g., "25 units/10 units" misread as "25 units and 110" units)	Use "per" rather than a slash mark to separate doses
@	At	Mistaken as "2"	Use "at"
&	And	Mistaken as "2"	Use "and"
+	Plus or and	Mistaken as "4"	Use "and"
°	Hour	Mistaken as a zero (e.g., q2° seen as q 20)	Use "hr," "h," or "hour"
Φ or ⊘	zero, null sign	Mistaken as numerals 4, 6, 8, and 9	Use 0 or zero, or describe intent using whole words

**These abbreviations are included on The Joint Commission's "minimum list" of dangerous abbreviations, acronyms, and symbols that must be included on an organization's "Do Not Use" list, effective January 1, 2004. Visit www.jointcommission.org for more information about this Joint Commission requirement.

© ISMP 2015. Permission is granted to reproduce material with proper attribution for internal use within healthcare organizations. Other reproduction is prohibited without written permission from ISMP. Report actual and potential medication errors to the ISMP National Medication Errors Reporting Program (ISMP MERP) via the Web at www.ismp.org or by calling 1-800-FAIL-SAF(E).

ISMP
INSTITUTE FOR SAFE MEDICATION PRACTICES
www.ismp.org

Appendix K: Important Math Conversions to Remember

Avoirdupois Measurement	• 1 grain (gr) = 64.8 mg (permissible to round to 65 mg)
Apothecary Measurements	• 1 pint = 473 mL • 1 fluid ounce = 29.6 mL (permissible to round to 30 mL)
Common or Household Measurements	• 1 gallon (gal) = 4 quarts • 1 quart (qt) = 2 pints • 1 pint (pt) = 2 cups • 1 cup = 8 fluid ounces • 1 fluid ounces (fl oz) = 2 tablespoonfuls = 30 mL • 1 tablespoonful (T or tbsp) = 3 teaspoonfuls • 1 teaspoonful (tsp) = 5 mL • 1 pound (lb) = 16 ounces (oz)
Metric System Measurements	• 1 inch (in) = 2.54 centimeters (cm) • 1 liter (L) = 1,000 milliliters (mL) • 1 kilogram (kg) = 1,000 grams (g) • 1 milligram (mg) = 1,000 micrograms (mcg)
Other Measurements	• 1 cubic centimeter (cc) is synonymous with 1 milliliter (mL) (1 cc = 1 mL) • 1 kg = 2.2 lbs • 1 lb = 454 g • 1 oz = 28.35 g • Insulin U-100 = 100 IU per mL (100 international units per mL) • Ophthalmic and otic drops are assumed to be 20 gtts per mL unless stated otherwise • $°F = (°C \times \frac{9}{5}) + 32$ • $°C = (°F - 32) \times \frac{5}{9}$ • I or i = 1 • V or v = 5 • X or x = 10 • L or l = 50 • C or c = 100 • D or d = 500 • M or m = 1,000

Appendix L:
References

Academy of Managed Care Pharmacy. "Drug Utilization Review," last modified in November 2009. http://www.amcp.org/WorkArea/DownloadAsset.aspx?id=9296

American Journal of Health-System Pharmacy. "Introduction to the New Prescription Drug Labeling by the Food and Drug Administration," 2007; 64(23):2488–2494.

American Society of Health-System Pharmacists. "ASHP Technical Assistance Bulletin on Compounding Nonsterile Products in Pharmacies," *American Journal of Health-System Pharmacy*, 1994; 51:1441–1448.

Chaffee, Bruce, and Josephine Bonasso. "Strategies for Pharmacy Integration and Pharmacy Information System Interfaces, Part 1: History and Pharmacy Integration Options," *American Journal of Health-System Pharmacy*, 2004; 61(5): 502–506.

Chaffee, Bruce, and Josephine Bonasso. "Strategies for Pharmacy Integration and Pharmacy Information System Interfaces, Part 2: Scope of Work and Technical Aspects of Interfaces," *American Journal of Health-System Pharmacy*, 2004; 61(5): 506–514.

Institute for Safe Medication Practices. "ISMP's List of High-Alert Medications in Acute Care Settings," last modified in 2014.

Institute for Safe Medication Practices. "ISMP's List of High-Alert Medications in Community/Ambulatory Health Care," last modified in 2011.

National Council for Presciption Drug Programs. "EPrescribing Fact Sheet," last retrieved March 7, 2019. https://www.ncpdp.org/NCPDP/media/pdf/EprescribingFactSheet.pdf

National Council for Prescription Drug Programs. "Standards Information," last retrieved March 7, 2019. https://www.ncpdp.org/Standards/Standards-Info

Pharmacy Technician Certification Board. "Pharmacy Technician Certification Examination (PTCE) Content Outline." November 2018. https://www.ptcb.org/docs/default-source/about-ptcb/ptce-content-outline-effective-january-1-2020.pdf?

Riffkin, Rebecca. "Americans Rate Nurses Highest on Honesty, Ethical Standards," Gallup, last modified December 18, 2014. http://www.gallup.com/poll/180260/americans-rate-nurses-highest-honesty-ethical-standards.aspx

Shrewsbury, Robert P. "Excipients Used in Pharmaceutical Compounding," The Pharmaceutics and Compounding Laboratory. http://pharmlabs.unc.edu/appendix_resources.htm.

"Technician Tutorial, Keep it Cool: Storing Meds in the Fridge or Freezer." *Pharmacist's Letter/Pharmacy Technician's Letter.* September 2016.

U.S. Consumer Product Safety Commission. "Poison Prevention Packaging: A Guide for Health Care Professionals," last modified in 2005. http://www.cpsc.gov/s3fs-public/384.pdf

U.S. Department of Health and Human Services – Substance Abuse and Mental Health Services Administration Center for Behavioral Health Statistics and Quality. "Drug Abuse Warning Network, 2011: National Estimates of Drug-Related Emergency Department Visits," last modified in 2013. https://www.samhsa.gov/data/sites/default/files/DAWN2k11ED/ DAWN2k11ED/DAWN2k11ED.pdf

U.S. Food and Drug Administration. "Are You Taking Medication as Prescribed?" last modified in 2018. https://www.fda.gov/ForConsumers/ConsumerUpdates/ucm164616.htm

U.S. Department of Health and Human Services – Substance Abuse and Mental Health Services Administration Center for Behavioral Health Statistics and Quality. "Drug Abuse Warning Network, 2011: National Estimates of Drug-Related Emergency Department Visits," last modified in 2013. https://www.samhsa.gov/data/sites/default/files/DAWN2k11ED/ DAWN2k11ED/DAWN2k11ED.pdf

U.S. Drug Enforcement Administration. "Drug Scheduling," last retrieved March 7, 2019. www.dea.gov/druginfo/ds.shtml

U.S. Food and Drug Administration. "Background and Definitions," last modified in 2009.

U.S. Food and Drug Administration. "Disposal of Unused Medicines: What You Should Know," last modified in 2019. https://www.fda.gov/drugs/resourcesforyou/consumers/ buyingusingmedicinesafely/ensuringsafeuseofmedicine/safedisposalofmedicines/ ucm186187.htm#Medicines_recommended

U.S. Food and Drug Administration. "FY2015 Regulatory Science Research Report: Narrow Therapeutic Index Drugs," last modified in 2017. https://www.fda.gov/ForIndustry/UserFees/ GenericDrugUserFees/ucm500577.htm

U.S. Food and Drug Administration. "Product-Specific Guidances for Generic Drug Development," last modified in 2019. http://www.fda.gov/Drugs/GuidanceCompliance RegulatoryInformation/Guidances/ucm075207.htm

U.S. Food and Drug Administration. "Sulfanilamide Disaster," last modified in 2018. www.FDA.gov/History/ProductRegulation/ucm2007257.htm

U.S. Government Publishing Office. "General Administrative Requirements. 45 C.F.R. § 160.103 (2000)," last modified in 2013. http://www.ecfr.gov/cgi-bin/text-idx?SID=128171e8 10d2f66d37c119fe90729f95&mc=true&node=se45.1.160_1103&rgn=div8

U.S. Pharmacopeial Convention. "Pharmaceutical compounding—Nonsterile preparations (revision bulletin chapter 795).

Van Dusen, Virgil, PharmacyTimes.com. "A Review of Federal Legislation Affecting Pharmacy Practice," last modified December, 2006. http://www.pharmacytimes.com/publications/ issue/2006/2006-12/2006-12-6154#sthash.2NH7ru0F.dpuf

http://www.medscape.com/pharmacists

https://www.ashp.org/-/media/assets/policy-guidelines/docs/guidelines/handling-hazardous-drugs.ashx

https://www.jointcommission.org/assets/1/6/CAMH_2012_Update2_24_SE.pdf

https://www.nccmerp.org/consumer-information

Index

non-sterile, 38
oral solutions, 38
semisolid formulations, 38
topical solutions, 38
Bipolar disorder, medications for, 92
Birth control, and isotretinoin, 108
Blending, 138
Blood clot formation, miscellaneous agents, 63
Body surface area, calculations based on, 161
Body weight, calculations based on, 161
Brand name, 34, 219–224
Bronchodilation, 85

C

Calcium channel blockers (CCB), 59–61
Calculations
alligations, 158
cash register, 154
copays, 154
days supply, 148–151
dispensing fees, 154
infusion rates/drip rates, 160
math conversions, 267
strengths, 155
Caplet, dosage forms, 34
Capsule
calculating days supply, 148
in compounding, 140
dosage forms, 34
Capsule machine method, 140
Carbapenems, 52
Cardiovascular agents, 59–63
Cash register calculations, 154
C-C motif chemoreceptor 5 (CCR5), 56, 58
Center for Drug Evaluation and Research (CDER), 37
Cephalosporins, 49
Characteristic waste, 110
Chemical compatibility, 38, 42–43
Chemical name, 34
Childproof containers, 107
Claravis, 108
Class III prescription balance, directions for using, 136–137
Cleaning standards, 129–130
Clinical trials, 37

Comminution, 138
Compounding
a capsule, 140
equipment and supplies, 136–138
extemporaneous, 134
non-sterile, 134–135
solution, 140–141
sterile, 134
techniques for preparing, 138
See also Non-sterile compounding
Comprehensive Drug Abuse Prevention and Control Act of 1970. *See* Controlled Substances Act
Computerization, of prescription filling, 120
Continuous quality improvement (CQI), 119–120
Contraceptives
common, 83–84
emergency, 84
Controlled Substances Act
DEA 222 form, 103
DEA number, 104–105
documenting requirements under, 103–104
inventory, 104
National Provider Identifier (NPI), 105
opioid-based medications, 76–77
registration for, 103
requirements for, 102
scheduled listed chemical products, 108
schedules for, 102–103
transfer restrictions, 105
See also Prescription
Copays, 154
Corticosteroids, 85
Cost, selection of an agent, 47
Cough medications, with codeine, 84
Creams
calculating days supply, 151
determining supply, 64
dosage forms, 34
strengths, 155
Cyclic lipopeptide, information charts for, 53

D

DEA 41 form, 106
DEA 106 form, 106

Intradermal pellet, dosage forms, 35
Inventory
 under Controlled Substances Act, 104
 product, 135
Investigational New Drug (IND)
  application, 37
iPLEDGE program, 64, 108
Isotretinoin, 108

K
Ketolide, 51

L
Labels
 adulterated, 100
 auxiliary, 38–39
 over-the-counter, 101–102
 prescription, 101
 requirements, 101
Leukotriene inhibitors, 85
Levigation, 138
Light, medication storage concerns for, 43
Lincosamide, information charts for, 53
Liquids, strengths, 155
Look-alike/sound-alike (LASA)
  medications, 124
Loop diuretics, 59
Lot number, 146
Lotion, dosage forms, 35
Lozenge, dosage forms, 35

M
Macrolides, 50
Medical terminology, 147, 247–262
Medication errors
 abuse and misuse, 122–123
 causes of, 116
 error prevention strategies, 116–117
 reporting, 115–116
Medication Errors Reporting Program
  (MERP), 129
Medications
 adherence, 123
 Alzheimer's disease, 90–91
 attention-deficit hyperactivity disorder
  (ADHD), 91
 bipolar disorder, 92

codeine-related cough, 84
gastroesophageal reflux, 73
gout, 93
guides, 109
high-alert, 124, 125–126
look alike/sound alike (LASA), 124
migraines, 93
misuse, 122
opioid-based, 76–77
Parkinson's disease, 90–91
schizophrenia, 92
smoking cessation, 94
storage of, 42–43
See also Stems
Medication-specific numbers, 146–147
MedWatch, 129
Micropump, dosage forms, 35
Migraines, medications for, 93
Miscellaneous agents, 62–63
Misuse, drug, 122–123
Monobactams, 52
Muscular medications, 76–81
Myorisan, 108

N
Narrow therapeutic index (NTI), 41–42
National Coordinating Council for
  Medication Error Reporting and
  Prevention (NCCMERP), 115–116
National Drug Code (NDC), 146
National Provider Identifier (NPI), 105
Near miss errors, 129
New Drug Application, 37
Nitrofuran antibacterial, 53
Nonaqueous solutions, beyond-use date, 38
Non-hazardous substances, handling and
  disposal of, 110–111
Non-nucleoside reverse transcriptase
  inhibitors (NNRTIs), 56–57
Non-sterile, beyond-use date, 38
Non-sterile compounding
 commonly used active ingredients for,
  139
 overview of, 134–135
 preparations, 139
 procedures, 140
 See also Compounding

Prevention strategies
    continuous quality improvement, 119–120
    error, 116–119
Product expiration date, 146
Product inventory, 135
Professional Compounding Centers of America (PCCA), 135
Protease inhibitors (PIs), 56, 58
Pseudoephedrine-containing products, 108
Pulverization, 138
Punch filling method, 140
Pure Food and Drug Act of 1906, 100

Q

Quality control, in prescription filing, 120
Quality-related events (QRE), 120–121
Quinolones, 51

R

Rapid insulin secretors, 70
Recalls, classification of, 109
Receiving, under Controlled Substances Act, 103–104
Recertification, 7–8
Recordkeeping
    under Controlled Substances Act, 103–104
    pseudoephedrine-containing products, 108
Regulations, prescription return, destruction, and theft regulations, 106, 115–116
Reinstatement, 8
Reproductive agents, 81–83
Rescue inhalers, 85
Resource Conservation and Recovery Act, 110–111
Respiratory agents, 84–88
Restrictions, prescription, 104–105
Risk Evaluation and Mitigation Strategies (REMS), 64, 107
Root-cause analysis (RCA), 128–129

S

Safety concerns, medication storage concerns for, 43

Safety data sheets (SDS), 110–111
Scheduled listed chemical products, 108
Schizophrenia, medications for, 92
Sedative agent stems, 44–46
Selective sodium-glucose transporter-2 (SGLT2) inhibitors, 70
Semisolid formulations, beyond-use date, 38
Senses' agents, stems for, 66
Sensitivity, medication storage concerns for, 43
Sentinel event, 124
Side effects
    gastrointestinal agents, 73
    general, 36
    skeletal, muscular, and osteoporosis medications, 77
    smoking cessation, 94
Sifting, 138
Skeletal medications, 76–81
Smoking cessation, 94
Solution
    in compounding, 140–141
    diluting stock, 157
    dosage forms, 35
    strengths, 155
Spacers, 146
Spatulation, 138
Spectrum of prescription drug abuse, 122
Spirit, dosage forms, 35
Spray, aerosol, 34
Stability, definition of, 38
Standardization, of prescription filling, 120
State Board of Pharmacy, 3
Statins, 60
Stems
    ACE inhibitor, 59
    anti-anxiety, 44
    antidepressant, 44
    antiepileptic, 44
    antifungal, 60
    anti-infective agents, 47
    antiretroviral, 56
    beta blockers, 59
    cardiovascular, 59
    definition of, 34